XYROFIN   1994

Ice Cream

Fourth Edition

ICE CREAM

Fourth Edition

W. S. ARBUCKLE

Emeritus Professor of Dairy Science
University of Maryland
College Park, Maryland

An **avi** Book
Published by Van Nostrand Reinhold
New York

Library of Congress Catalog Card Number 85-28651
ISBN 0-87055-479-4

Van Nostrand Reinhold
115 Fifth Avenue
New York, New York 10003

Chapman and Hall
2-6 Boundary Row
London SE1 8HN, England

Thomas Nelson Australia
102 Dodds Street
South Melbourne 3205
Victoria, Australia

Nelson Canada
1120 Birchmount Road
Scarborough, Ontario M1K 5G4, Canada

16   15   14   13   12   11   10   9   8   7   6   5   4

Library of Congress Cataloging-in-Publication Data

Arbuckle, W. S. (Wendell Sherwood), 1911–
    Ice cream.

    Bibliography: p.
    Includes index.
    1. Ice cream industry.   I. Title.
TX795.A69 1986   637'.4   85-28651
ISBN 0-87055-479-4

Contents

4

Composition and Properties

5

Ice Cream Ingredients

6

Stabilizers and Emulsifiers

7

Flavoring and Coloring Materials

8

Calculation of Ice Cream Mixes

9

Restandardizing and Calculating Some Unusual Mixes

10

Calculating Cost and Percentage of Overrun

11

Mix Processing

12

The Freezing Process

13

Packaging, Hardening, and Shipping

14

Soft-Frozen Dairy Products and Special Formulas

15

Sherbets and Ices

16

Frozen Confections, Novelties, Fancy Molded Ice Creams, and Specials

17

Defects, Scoring and Grading

18

Sanitation and Quality Control

19

Refrigeration

20

Laboratory Testing

21

Sales Outlets

22

Formulas and Industry Standards

Appendixes

Preface to the Fourth Edition

This edition of "Ice Cream" is a full revision of previous editions and includes an updating of the areas that have been affected by changes and new technology. The ice cream industry has developed on the basis of an abundant economical supply of ingredients and is a high-volume, highly automated, modern, progressive, very competitive industry composed of large and small businesses manufacturing ice cream and related products. The industry underwent a difficult period of adjusting to economic changes and to the establishment of product specifications and composition regulations. The latter area has now become more stabilized and the *Frozen Desserts Definitions and Standards of Identity* are now more clearly defined, as are ingredient and nutritional labeling specifications.

The chapters that include basic information on ice cream technology remain for the most part unchanged in order to accommodate beginners in the industry and the smaller processors. In other chapters major revisions and the incorporation of new material have been made. Key classical references and information have been retained or added in order to keep intact those portions of the book which students have found most useful and helpful as reflected in my own teaching, research, and publications in the field of dairy science, and particularly in the field of ice cream production.

It is fitting that acknowledgment should be made to identify the contributions of Professor J. H. Frandsen, who died on September 21, 1962 at the age of eighty-five in Boston, Massachusetts. He was keenly interested in dairy science for more than 50 years and was deeply involved in teaching, research, extension, and editing in the many branches of the dairy industry. As a result of his invitation to me to join him as co-author on the book "Ice Cream and Related Products" this book originated.

This book is dedicated to those who have contributed to the modern knowledge of ice cream technology.

1
Development of the Ice Cream Industry

DEFINITION AND COMPOSITION

Ice cream is a frozen dairy food made by freezing a pasteurized mix with agitation to incorporate air and to ensure uniformity of consistency. The mix is composed of a combination of milk products, sugar, dextrose, corn syrup in dry or liquid form, water, and may include eggs or egg products, harmless flavorings, and added stabilizer or emulsifier—all of wholesome edible material.

Ice cream and related products are generally classified as frozen desserts, which include ice cream, frozen custard, ice milk, sherbet, water ice, frozen confections, and mellorine- and parevine-type products.

In the United States, ice cream is defined by U.S. Government standards. It must contain not less than 10% milkfat and 20% total milk solids; except in the case of bulky flavors, the fat and total milk solids must not be less than 8 and 16%, respectively. It must weigh not less than 4.5 lb/gal; it must contain not more than 0.5% stabilizer; and it must contain not less than 1.6 lb of total food solids (TS) per gallon.[1]

The composition of ice cream varies in different markets and different localities. The composition for good average ice cream is fat, 12%; milk solids not fat (MSNF), 11%; sugar, 15%, stabilizer and emulsifier, 0.3%; and TS, 38.3%. The range in composition may be fat, 8–20%; MSNF, 8–15%; sugar, 13–20%; stabilizer–emulsifier, 0–0.7%; and TS, 36–43%.

The physical structure of ice cream is a complicated physiochemical system. Air cells are dispersed in a continuous liquid phase with embedded ice crystals. The liquid phase also contains solidified fat globules, milk proteins, insoluble salts, lactose crystals in some cases, stabilizers of colloidal dimension, and sugars and soluble salts in solution. The finished product consists of liquid, air, and solid, and constitutes a three-phase system.

Ice cream is a palatable, nutritious, healthful, and relatively inexpensive food. One serving of good average composition of vanilla ice cream (1/6 qt) supplies approximately 200 cal, 3.9 g protein, 0.31 g calcium, 0.104 g phospho-

---

[1]Unless otherwise specified, the percentages for ice cream composition are by weight.

1

rus, 0.14 mg iron, 548 IU vitamin A, 0.038 mg thiamine, and 0.236 mg riboflavin.

Frozen custard (also known as French ice cream or French Custard Ice Cream) is a product similar to ice cream, except it contains not less than 1.4% by weight of egg yolk solids for plain flavors and 1.12% for bulky flavors. It may be marketed as either a soft-frozen or hardened product.

Ice cream and frozen custard contain not less than 10% milkfat and 20% total milk solids, except that in the case of bulky flavors, they must contain not less than 8% fat and 16% total milk solids, respectively. Ice cream must weigh not less than 4.5 lb/gal; it may or may not contain stabilizer and emulsifier; and it must contain not less than 1.6 lb TS/gal.

Ice milk is a frozen product that contains not less than 2% and not more than 7% fat, and not less than 11% total milk solids. It must have not less than 1.3 lb TS/gal. It may be sold as a hard or soft product.

Sherbet contains a small amount of milk products, sugar, fruit juices, and stabilizer. It must contain between 1 and 2% milkfat, and between 2 and 5% total milk solids. A sherbet must weigh not less than 6 lb/gal and have not less than 0.35% acidity, calculated as lactic acid. It must contain 2% citrus fruit, 6% berry fruits, or 10% other fruits. The acidity requirement is waived for nonfruit flavors, which do not have to contain any fruit or fruit juice.

Water ice is similar to sherbet but does not contain milk solids. Other than the milk solids (and egg ingredients other than egg white are not specified), the standards are the same as for sherbets.

Some other products not identified in federal standards may or may not be defined in state standards. Frozen confections include stick novelties and special frozen confection items. Quiescently frozen dairy confection is a product sold in the form of individual servings on a stick. It must contain not less than 13% milk solids and not less than 33% TS. Overrun must be not more than 10%.[2] Quiescently frozen confection is similar to the diary confection except it must contain at least 17% TS. It may or may not contain milk solids.

Dietary frozen dessert must contain less than 2% fat and not less than 7% total milk solids. It must weigh not less than 4.5 lb/gal and have not less than 1.1 or more than 1.45 lb TS/gal. Low-fat frozen dessert must contain less than 2% fat and not less than 7% total milk solids. It must weigh not less than 4.5 lb/gal and have not less than 1.1 or more than 1.55 lb TS/gal.

Mellorine-type products are similar to ice cream except that the butterfat has been replaced by a suitable vegetable or animal fat. The vegetable fat may include coconut, cottonseed, soybean, corn, or other plant fat. Mellorine-type products must contain not less than 6% fat from one or more specified sources, and not less than 3.5% protein of biological value at least equivalent to that of whole milk protein. They must weigh 4.5 lb/gal and contain not less than 1.6 lb TS/gal. Vitamin A must be added in such quantity that 40 USP units are present for each gram of fat.

Parevine-type products are similar to ice cream except that no dairy in-

---

[2]Overrun in ice cream manufacturing is the increase in volume of the ice cream over the volume of the mix due to the incorporation of air (see Chapter 8).

gredients are used. These have been replaced by safe and suitable optional ingredients.

Frozen yogurt is a cultured frozen product containing the same ingredients as ice cream. It contains not less than 3.25% milk fat and not less than 8.25% MSNF and has a titratable acidity of not less than 0.5%. The finished frozen yogurt shall weigh not less than 5 lb/gal.

Low-fat frozen yogurt contains not less than 0.5% or more than 2.0% milk fat.

Non-fat yogurt contains less than 0.5% fat. The specifications for these products have not become standardized at this time.

Freezer-made milk shakes contain between 3.25 and 6% milk fat, and not less than 10.0% MSNF. Freezer-made shakes meet the requirements of freezer-made milk shakes, except that they may contain less than 3.25% fat.

Ice cream or ice milk made with goat milk (goat milk ice cream or goat milk ice milk) are products prepared from the same ingredients and in the same manner as prescribed in the Code of Federal Regulations (FDA, 1981, pp. 224–231) for ice cream and ice milk, respectively, except that all milk fat and MSNF must be derived from goat milk.

Ice cream and related products are classified as frozen desserts and have product definitions and standards set forth in USDA (1980) and FDA (1981, part 135). The products involved change from time to time but include ice cream, frozen custard, French ice cream, ice milk, sherbet, water ice, and mellorine-type frozen products. Frozen dairy confections, frozen confections, dietary frozen desserts, frozen yogurt, and other products such as frozen puddings, mousses, nondairy desserts (parevine-type products), and frozen shakes do not have federal standards of identity but some are listed in USDA (1980).

HISTORICAL BACKGROUND

Although the ice cream industry as known today has been developed mainly in the United States, the product was introduced to the United States from Europe. Ice cream probably evolved from the iced beverages and water ices that were popular in Europe during medieval times. We do know that wines and fruit juices were cooled with ice and snow brought from the mountains to the court of the Roman emperor Nero in the first century. Unfortunately, no definite description exists, except that snow and ice were used to cool and possibly to freeze sweet desserts. It is conceivable that this idea originated in ancient Egypt or Babylon, where sweetmeats and other dainties may have been iced.

In the thirteenth century, Marco Polo returned to Italy from his famous journey to the Orient and brought recipes for water ices said to have been used in Asia for thousands of years. The art of making these products then moved to France, Germany, and England during the next few centuries.

Ice cream probably came to the United States with the early English colonists. In 1851, the first wholesale ice cream industry in the United States was established in Baltimore, Maryland, by Jacob Fussell.

Early plants were also established in St. Louis, New York, Washington, Chicago, and Cincinnati. The development of condensed and dry milk, the introduction of the pasteurizer and homogenizer, improved freezers, and other processing equipment accompanied a slow growth in the industry until after 1900. The ice cream soda was introduced in 1879; the ice cream cone in 1904; and the Eskimo Pie in 1921. Around 1920 the value of ice cream as an essential food was generally recognized and the product has become unusually popular since that time. The development of improved refrigeration and transportation, low-temperature storage units for the home, improved packaging, marketing through chain stores, and improved product standards have made ice cream widely available to the consumer. Modern automated and high-volume operations provide a plentiful supply of popular-sized packages, ice cream cakes, pies, stick items, novelties, and other items.

PRODUCTION AND CONSUMPTION

Ice cream production has increased rapidly in recent years in many countries of the world. Annual production in the United States has reached more than 830 million gallons of ice cream and more than 1200 million gallons of ice cream and related products, or a per capita production of approximately 21.5 qt. The states leading in ice cream production are California, Pennsylvania, Ohio, New York, Texas, Illinois, Massachusetts, Florida, Michigan, and North Carolina. Approximately 9.3% of the total U.S. milk production is used by the ice cream industry.

Other countries ranking high in annual production of ice cream and related products are Canada, over 96 million gallons or 16.5 qt per capita; Australia, over 73 million gallons or 20 qt per capita; United Kingdom, over 48 million gallons or 3.5 qt per capita; Japan, over 166 million gallons or 5.5 qt per capita; West Germany, over 85 million gallons or 5.5 qt per capita; and Italy, over 52 million gallons or 3.75 qt per capita.

The leading ice cream-consuming countries as indicated by annual per capita production are the United States, 14.6 qt; Australia, 15.6 qt; New Zealand, 16.8 qt; and Sweden, 11.8 qt.

The United States has now gained undisputed leadership among all other countries in the total production of ice cream. Available records indicate, however, that the ice cream industry grew very slowly until 1900. From 1920, when the nutritive value of ice cream was generally recognized, until 1960, growth has been unusually rapid. Since 1960, there has been a modest increase in total volume each year. Table 1.1 shows the production of ice cream and related products in the United States. The international production data are given in Table 1.2 for purposes of comparison.

Some of the factors contributing to the extensive development of the ice cream industry are

1. the perfection of refrigeration and its adaptation to the food industry,
2. improved manufacturing methods and the development of better pro-

Table 1.1. Production of Ice Cream and Related Products in the United States, 1859–1983[a]

Year	All products reported Total (1000 gal)	All products reported Per capita (qt)	Ice cream Total (1000 gal)	Ice cream Per capita (qt)	Ice milk[b] Total (1000 gal)	Ice milk[b] Per capita (qt)	Sherbet Total (1000 gal)	Sherbet Per capita (qt)	Water ices Total (1000 gal)	Water ices Per capita (qt)	Other frozen dairy products[c] Total (1000 gal)	Other frozen dairy products[c] Per capita (qt)	Mellorine-type products Total (1000 gal)	Mellorine-type products Per capita (qt)
1859	4		4											
1869	24	0.01	24	0.01										
1879	144	0.06	144	0.06										
1889	851	0.27	851	0.27										
1899	5,021		5,021											
1909	29,637	1.31	29,637	1.31										
1919	152,982	5.86	152,982	5.86										
1920	171,248	6.43	171,248	6.43										
1930	255,439	8.30	255,439	6.43										
1940	339,544	10.29	318,088	9.64	10,457	0.32	8,089	0.24			2,910	0.09		
1950	634,768	16.79	554,351	14.66	36,870	0.98	17,018	0.45	18,299	0.48	8,230	0.22	32,261	0.78
1955	819,934	19.96	628,525	15.30	90,185	2.20	37,365	0.91	28,158	0.69	3,440	0.08	45,214	1.00
1960	969,004	21.54	699,605	15.55	145,177	3.23	40,734	0.91	33,361	0.74	4,913	0.11	53,169	1.10
1965	1,130,215	23.36	757,000	15.65	230,992	4.77	45,449	0.94	37,119	0.77	6,486	0.13	51,878	1.02
1970	1,193,144	23.42	761,732	14.95	286,663	5.63	48,887	0.96	37,265	0.73	6,719	0.13		
1975	1,263,213	23.45	836,552	15.53	298,789	5.55	48,542	0.90	38,230	0.71	11,062	0.20	30,038	0.56
1979	1,212,645	21.60	811,079	14.45	296,653	5.29	45,124	0.80	32,081	0.57	12,034	0.21	15,674	0.28
1980	1,225,223	21.58	829,798	14.61	293,384	5.17	45,187	0.80	33,386	0.59	10,278	0.18	13,190	0.23
1981	1,238,712	21.61	832,450	14.52	290,992	5.08	45,732	0.80	34,344	0.60	24,003	0.42	11,191	0.19
1982	1,248,552	21.54	852,072	14.70	280,559	4.84	45,575	0.79	35,158	0.61	25,058	0.43	10,130	0.17
1983	1,292,739	22.10	878,786	15.02	295,097	5.05	47,629	0.81	39,438	0.68	21,595	0.37	10,194	0.17

Source: IAICM (1984, p.9).
[a]Data from 1859 to 1919 indicate only the estimated trend of production.
[b]Includes freezer-made milkshake beginning 1954.
[c]For 1940–1953 includes frozen custard and frosted or frozen malted milk.

Table 1.2. Production of Ice Cream and Related Products by Country[a]

Country	Year	Annual (1000 gal)	Per capita (pt)	Country	Year	Annual (1000 gal)	Per capita (pt)
Argentina	1980	11,889	3.39	Korea	1982	13,396	2.61
Australia	1983	70,730	36.58	Lebanon	1978	1,360	4.08
Austria	1981	12,153	12.92	Liberia	1978	39.5	0.18
Bangladesh	1983	2,934	0.24	Malaysia	1978	1,846	1.15
Belgium	1983	15,217	12.62	Mexico	1982	38,837	4.21
Brazil	1982	23,629	1.48	Morocco	1982	1,321	0.47
Canada	1983	98,326	32.50	Netherlands	1981	10,089	5.66
Chile	1983	5,812	3.95	New Zealand	1983	14,675	35.87
Columbia	1983	6,517	1.90	Nigeria	1980	581	0.07
Costa Rica	1981	2,593	9.07	Norway	1983	10,568	20.47
Denmark	1983	10,239	16.01	Pakistan	1983	19	1.71
Dominican Republic	1982	1,035	2.59	Peru	1980	2,008	0.86
Ecuador	1977	3,675	4.11	Poland	1982	14,700	3.25
Egypt	1983	12,005	2.10	Portugal	1983	3,571	2.86
El Salvador	1976	1,995	3.74	Singapore	1982	2,114	6.84
France	1983	52,153	7.64	South Africa	1980	16,961	4.69
West Germany	1982	107,530	13.94	Spain	1983	28,898	6.05
Greece	1982	19,600	16.09	Sweden	1982	29,421	28.26
Guatemala	1975	3,559	4.81	Switzerland	1982	13,877	17.26
Hong Kong	1978	5,501	9.37	Taiwan	1982	9,584	4.15
India	1980	113,680	1.33	Tunisia	1978	147	0.17
Indonesia	1982	433	0.02	Turkey	1982	11,044	1.83
Iran	1978	5,201	1.09	United Kingdom	1983	73,463	10.49
Ireland	1983	6,869	15.59	Uruguay	1983	1,300	3.48
Italy	1983	85,865	12.19	USSR	1982	77,665	2.30
Ivory Coast	1983	2,303	1.16	Venezuela	1982	10,652	4.73
Japan	1982	225,362	15.12	Yugoslavia	1983	111,230	3.90

Source: IAICM (1984, pp. 34–38).
[a]In some countries, production is reported only by large manufacturers and no estimates are available for the output by small establishment. In such instances, the reported figures indicate trends.

cessing equipment, including automated continuous-operation systems and in-place cleaning devices (CIP),

3.   more and improved ingredients with improved knowledge of ingredient usage,

4.   establishment of definitions and product standards,

5.   extensive advertising and merchandising programs,

6.   maintenance of product composition, nutritive and bacteriological quality, and wholesome, palatable products,

7.   continuous research and educational programs relative to ice cream making, and

8.   improved packaging and distribution methods to the consumer with improved home storage facilities.

The importance of the ice cream industry is further shown by its relation to the other branches of the dairy industry. Table 1.3 shows that approximately 9.3% of all the milk produced in the United States is utilized by the ice cream industry. Over 40% of the ice cream is made during the early summer months when there is a seasonal increase in milk production. Milk used directly in making frozen dairy products is about 12,000 million pounds. In addition, approximately 2,500 million pounds of milk derived from other manufactured

Table 1.3.   Utilization of the U.S. Milk Supply, 1980

Product	Milk used (%)	Product (unit)	Whole milk required to produce 1 unit (lb)
Fluid milk and cream	39.6	Butter (lb)	21.20
Butter	17.8	Whole-milk cheese (lb)	10.00
Cheese	26.4	Evaporated milk (lb)	2.10
Evaporated and condensed milk	1.6	Condensed milk (lb)	2.30
Ice cream and related products	9.3	Whole-milk powder (lb)	7.40
Other	5.3	Powder cream (lb)	13.50
Total	100.0	Ice cream (1 gal) when butter and concentrated milk are used	12.00
		Cottage cheese (skim milk) (lb)	15.00
		Nonfat dry milk (skim milk) (lb)	6.25
		Ice milk (1 gal)	11.00
		Sherbet (1 gal)	10.30
			2.30

Source: Compiled in part from Milk Industry Foundation (1981).

products are used, giving a total of 14,500 million pounds of milk used in the manufacture of frozen dairy products.

The economic importance of the ice cream industry has been established. The value of ice cream as a food is now realized and much scientific knowledge has been gained in the production and merchandising of ice cream.

In the past decade products related to ice cream have become important in the ice cream industry. Ice milk, sherbets, mellorine- and parevine-type products, other frozen dairy products, and water ices have been responsible for over 75% of the rise in per capita sales of all frozen desserts. Ice milk is gaining in popularity. Approximately 50% of the ice milk production is sold as a soft-frozen product, and ice milk accounts for 75% of the soft-frozen product gallonage.

The percentage of total production of ice cream and related products in 1980 for each of the products was ice cream, 67.8; ice milk, 23.9; sherbet, 3.7; water ice, 2.7; mellorine-type products, 1.1; and other products, 0.83.

Further technological advancement may be expected to demand more emphasis and research on ice cream manufacture to meet the needs of an accelerated demand for frozen dairy foods.

The ice cream industry has entered a period of adjustment caused by ingredient shortages and higher costs. Product standards have been modified and the industry has met the demands of ingredient and nutritional labeling. The trend toward natural products and a greater emphasis on quality in general has led to an increase in premium products and the development of new products. Energy conservation, waste control, and manufacturing efficiency in all its aspects present major challenges to the industry. Meanwhile, the United States continues to lead in the consumption of ice cream and related products.

2
Energy Value and Nutrients of Ice Cream

ENERGY VALUE AND NUTRIENTS

The property whereby a food produces heat and energy within the body may be expressed in terms of energy value. The unit customarily used by nutritionists for measuring human energy needs and expenditures and the energy value of foods is the kilocalorie, which is the amount of heat required to raise the temperature of 1 kg of water 1°C. (A calorie is the amount of heat required to warm 1 g of water 1°C.) Watt and Merrill (1963) cite the Atwater system (Atwater and Bryant, 1900), reviewed by a committee of the Food and Agriculture Organization of the United Nations, as being a satisfactory system for determining energy values of foods when correctly used. The system was developed working with human subjects to determine the available energy values for a wide variety of foods. The procedure is to adjust the heats of combustion of the fat, protein, and carbohydrates in a food to allow for the losses in digestion and metabolism found for human subjects, and to apply the adjusted calorie factors to the amounts of protein, fat, and carbohydrates in the food. The quantities of proteins and fat are determined by chemical analysis, and the percentage of carbohydrates is obtained by difference, the remainder after the sum of the fat, protein, ash and moisture has been subtracted from 100. (The U.S. Department of Agriculture (USDA) has published and makes available the details on derivation of the calorie factors.) The energy value of foods then represents the energy available after deductions have been made for losses in metabolism and digestion. The traditional method of evaluating the nutritive value of a food is to express its components in terms of nutrients, i.e., water, carbohydrates, fats, protein, minerals, and vitamins.

When fats, carbohydrates, and proteins are measured in a calorimeter, the fat yields 9.45 cal/g, carbohydrates yield 4.10 cal/g, and protein 5.65 cal/g. It has been estimated that 1 g of protein oxidized in the body yields only 4.35 cal, since not all the digestible food material is assimilated by the body. On the average, 2% of the carbohydrates, 5% of the fats, and 8% of the proteins are not absorbed. The actual energy value to the body derived for each gram ingested is 4, 9, and 4 cal for carbohydrates, fat, and protein, respectively.

Most authorities agree that metabolism consists of all chemical changes that nutrients undergo from the time they are absorbed into the body until they appear as excretory products. It includes the distribution of the absorbed food—building (anabolism) and breaking down (catabolism) of tissues—as well as absorption and release of energy. Digestion is a disintegration of the food into simple nutrients in the gastrointestinal tract in order to prepare them for absorption. All nutrients are equally important to the extent they are needed in a particular diet.

The energy value and nutrients of ice cream depend upon the food value of the products from which it is made (see Table 2.1). The milk products that go into the mix contain the constituents of milk, but in different amounts. Ice cream contains three to four times as much fat, and about 12–16% more protein than does milk. In addition, it may contain other food products such as fruit, nuts, eggs, candies, and sugar, which enhance its nutritive value. Ice cream contains about four times as much carbohydrate as milk. The milk solids in ice cream are usually subjected to higher heat treatments than are those of pasteurized milk; they also are subjected to lower temperatures in the freezing process; and they are stored longer before consumption. Like milk, ice cream is not a good source of iron and some of the trace minerals.

Ice cream is an excellent source of food energy, however. As has been stated, the fat content of ice cream is three to four times that of milk, and fully 50% of its total solids content is sugar, including lactose, sucrose, and corn syrup solids. The fact that these constituents are almost completely assimilated makes ice cream an especially desirable food for growing children and for persons who need to put on weight. For the same reason, its controlled use finds a place in the diet of persons who need to reduce or who do not wish to gain weight.

CALORIC CONTENT OF ICE CREAM
AND RELATED PRODUCTS

The ice cream manufacturers may often need information regarding the nutritional value of the product they manufacture. School and hospital officials and dietitians often need nutritional data when establishing diets for those whom they serve. The wide variation in the composition of ice cream and

Table 2.1. Composition of Plain Ice Cream (per 100-g Edible Portion)

Constituent	Good average ice cream	For different fat content			Ice milk	Ice cream cones	Water ice
		~10%	~12%	~16%			
Water (%)	61.7	63.2	62.1	62.8	66.7	8.9	66.9
Food energy (cal)	196.7	193.0	207.0	222.0	152.0	377.0	78.0
Protein (%)	4.1	4.5	4.0	2.6	4.8	10.0	0.4
Fat (%)	12.0	10.6	12.5	16.1	5.1	2.4	Trace
Total carbohydrate (%)	20.7	20.8	20.6	18.0	22.4	77.9	32.6
Weight per 100-cal portion (g)	50.8	51.7	48.3	45.0	65.6	26.5	128.4

related products makes it practically impossible to provide nutritional data that will apply to all products. It is, however, possible to calculate for practical use the food energy value of a given product if the composition is known.

The amount of energy normally expected to be derived from milk per gram of carbohydrates, fats, and protein is as follows: carbohydrates, 3.87 cal; fat, 8.79 cal; protein, 4.27 cal. These values are the amounts of energy released from the food nutrients as heat units or calories, and are referred to as physiological fuel values. Proteins and carbohydrates are of equal energy value per gram and fats are 2.25 times as rich in energy.

Minerals or vitamins do not furnish appreciable amounts of energy.

The type of sugar has little relation to the fuel value derived from it, and all sugars may be expected to have about the same energy value.

The lactose content of MSNF is about 52% and the protein content of MSNF is about 36%.

The total caloric value of ice cream depends on (1) the percentage of carbohydrates including lactose, added sweeteners, and sugars that may be present in fruit or flavoring; (2) the percentage of protein including milk protein or any other source of protein that may be present in nuts, eggs, or stabilizer; and (3) the percentage of fat from any source including emulsifier, egg, cocoa, or nut fat that may be in the mix.

In the field of nutrition the composition of a food is expressed as grams of constituent per 100 g of product.

The caloric value of 100 g of vanilla ice cream containing 12.5% fat, 11% MSNF, 15% sugar, and 0.3% gelatin may be calculated as follows:

Carbohydrates	$[15 + (11 \times 0.52)] \times 3.87 =$	80.19
Fat	$12.5 \times 8.79 =$	109.86
Protein	$[(11 \times 0.36) \times 0.30] \times 4.27 =$	14.09
Total		204.14

The caloric value of a serving of ice cream varies with the composition of the mix, overrun, and weight of mix per gallon. In determining the caloric value of a package or serving of ice cream it is necessary to determine the exact weight of the product contained therein. Calculations may be made readily if the weight in ounces is known since 1 oz is equivalent to 28.35 g.

PROTEIN CONTENT OF ICE CREAM

The milk proteins contained in ice cream are of excellent biological value, because they contain all the essential amino acids. Milk proteins are important sources of tryptophan and are especially rich in lysine. Proteins are essential in animal life as components of protoplasm of each living cell. Milk proteins are not only known to be complete but the assimilation of ingested milk proteins is 5–6% more complete than for other proteins in general.

Ice cream has a high concentration of MSNF, which is 34–36% milk protein.

The values for protein are calculated from determinations of the nitrogen content in the food. Early analysis of proteins showed that they have close to

16% nitrogen. The general practice then was to multiply the nitrogen content by the 6.25 conversion factor for the protein content. Instead of the 6.25, Jones (1941) recommended different conversion factors for different kinds of foods. The factor he specified for milk protein is 6.38.

MILKFAT CONTENT

Milkfat consists mainly of triglycerides of fatty acids. Webb *et al.* (1974) state that the glycerides are compounds in which one, two, or three fatty-acid molecules are combined by means of ester linkages with the trihydric alcohol; glycerol di- and triglycerides containing two and three molecules, respectively, of the same fatty acid are referred to as simple glycerides. If different fatty acids are present, they are called mixed glycerides. Milkfat contains at least 60 fatty acids. Milkfat also contains nonsaponifiable fractions and other matter such as cholesterol, lecithin, and tocopherols.

Interest in milkfat from the nutritional viewpoint is primarily for energy, essential fatty acids and fat-soluble vitamins, the proportion of saturated and unsaturated fatty acids, and the amount of cholesterol present.

Fat is the term used most often for those components in food that are insoluble in water and soluble in ethyl ether or other solvents used to extract them. Determinations by extraction method for milkfat have been well standardized.

The fatty acids are released from glycerol on saponification and the early determinations, before 1955, were based on methods that are now being replaced by more refined procedures involving gas–liquid chromatographic (GLC) methods.

Cholesterol may be determined by colorimetric or precipitation methods.

Table 2.2 shows the amount of saturated and unsaturated fatty acids and cholesterol in ice cream, ice cream cones, and ice milk.

CARBOHYDRATES IN ICE CREAM

Carbohydrates include starch, dextrine, cellulose, sugars, pectins, gums, and related substances. Carbohydrate serves as a source of heat and energy in the body. It is broken down to simple sugars under the action of specific enzymes secreted into the digestive tract and the principal end product is glucose. Sugars of several kinds may be used in the manufacture of ice cream. The commonly used sugar is sucrose, a disaccharide.[1] It may come from either cane or beet as these are identical in composition. Corn sugar, now used extensively, is predominantly glucose (dextrose) or is converted to maltose or fructose (levulose). The sugars of most fruits are sucrose, fructose, and glucose. Invert sugar, a mixture of equal amounts of the monosaccharides fructose, and glucose is used at times.

---

[1]A disaccharide is a sugar that can be reduced to two monosaccharides. A monosaccharide cannot be further reduced.

Table 2.2. Selected Fatty Acids and Cholesterol in Ice Cream and Related Items
(Per 100-g Edible Portions)

		Fatty acids			
Item	Total (g)	Total unsaturated (g)	Unsaturated oleic (g)	Linoleic (g)	Cholesterol (mg)
Ice cream	12.5	7.0	4.0	Trace	45.0
Ice cream cones	2.4	1.0	1.0	Trace	0.0
Ice milk	5.1	3.0	2.0	Trace	21.6

Lactose, milk sugar, is a disaccharide that constitutes over one-third of the solid matter in milk and approximately 20% of the carbohydrate in ice cream. It is widely recognized that lactose is unique in that it is found only in milk, whereas other types of sugars are fairly widely distributed in nature. Furthermore, liberal quantities of lactose in the diet produce a favorable medium in the intestinal tract for the establishment of growth of *Lactobacillus acidophilus*, an organism that aids carbohydrate fermentation, which in turn results in an acid condition in the intestinal contents unfavorable to protein putrefaction. It is also widely believed that lactose favors calcium assimilation and phosphorus utilization.

For calculating energy values of milk carbohydrates, the coefficient of digestibility, heat of combustion, and ingested-nutrients factor are usually given as 98%, 3.95 cal/g, and 3.87 cal/g, respectively.

MINERALS IN ICE CREAM

Certain inorganic elements are essential for growth and performance. Those needed in substantial amounts, such as calcium, phosphorus, magnesium, sodium, potassium, and sulfur, are termed major minerals or macronutrients. Those needed in small amounts, such as copper, cobalt, iodine, manganese, zinc, fluorine, molybdenum, and selenium, are termed trace minerals. The inorganic nutrients are interrelated and should be in particular proportions in the diet. Calcium and phosphorus are of vital concern since they are very closely related. Milk is considered the best source of dietary calcium. Milk and its products, including ice cream, are among the richest sources of calcium, phosphorus, and other minerals essential in adequate nutrition. Research indicates that additional amounts of lactose in the diet favor assimilation of calcium. Ice cream, which is rich in lactose, should favor assimilation of greater quantities of the calicum content of the diet, which is needed by growing children and some adults. The calcium and phosphorus content of milk and ice cream are

	Calcium (g/100 g)	Phosphorus (g/100 g)
Milk	0.118	0.093
Ice cream	0.122	0.105

The daily human requirements of calcium as recommended by the National Academy of Sciences (1974) are as follows:

Individual	g
Normal adult	0.80
Child (up to 20 yr)	1.40
Pregnant mother	1.50
Nursing mother	2.00

The ordinary mixed diet of the average American household provides the following amounts of calcium:

Daily food intake	g
Regular serving of meat, potato, and bread	0.029
Two eggs	0.101
Regular serving of fruits and vegetables	0.158
Total	0.288
One pint of milk	0.580
One average serving (1/6 qt) ice cream	0.122
Total	0.990

This provides a total above the absolute needs of adults. If children and pregnant mothers drink another pint of milk daily, their calcium intake will be abundantly sufficient.

Other indispensable mineral elements that occur in ice cream are (per 100 g edible portion) magnesium, 14 mg; sodium, 40 mg; potassium, 112 mg; iron, 0.1 mg; and zinc and iodine in small amounts. Values for minerals and ash are generally based upon actual analysis.

VITAMINS IN ICE CREAM

Vitamins can be divided into two groups: the fat soluble and the water soluble. The fat-soluble vitamins include A, D, E, and K; the water-soluble vitamins include B_1 or thiamine, B_2 or riboflavin, B_6, and B_{12}. For additional information on vitamins in milk and milk products, see Keeney (1963), Merrill and Watt (1955), Sherman (1946), and Watt and Merrill (1963).

Like milk, ice cream is a rich source of many of the essential vitamins, those food accessories without which normal health and growth cannot be maintained. A brief description of the better known vitamins may help to emphasize the importance of milk and ice cream in the diet.

Vitamin A. Often referred to as the anti-infective vitamin, it is the principal butterfat vitamin. It is the most important in building resistance to infection in the respiratory tract, in preventing night blindness, and in maintaining general good health. Ice cream is an excellent source.

Thiamine (Vitamin B_1). This vitamin is essential for growth and metabolism. A deficiency in thiamine may produce symptoms of loss of appetite and weight, general weakness, degenerative changes in the nervous system, and enlargement of the heart. Ice cream contains an average of 0.48 mg/kg, with a range of 0.38–0.65 mg/kg.

Riboflavin (Vitamin B_2). Riboflavin is a dietary essential for humans. The symptoms of riboflavin deficiency are lesions of the skin and of the eye, mouth, and tongue; abnormally red lips; lesions in the corners of the mouth; itching and burning of the eyes and increased sensitivity to light and opacity of the cornea. Ice cream contains an average of 2.3 mg/kg with a range of 2.0–2.6 mg/kg.

Vitamin B_6. This vitamin has an important role in amino acid metabolism. A deficiency may produce decreased growth rate, dermatitis, anemia, and convulsions. Ice cream contains an average of 0.68 mg/kg with a range of 0.27–1.15 mg/kg.

Vitamin B_{12}. This vitamin has the most complex structure of all vitamins. It is an essential metabolite for a wide variety of organisms. When there is faulty absorption of vitamin B_{12} from food, the human disease of pernicious anemia almost always occurs. Ice cream contains an average of 0.0047 mg/kg with a range of 0.0026–0.0078 mg/kg.

Ascorbic Acid (Vitamin C). This is the antiscorbutic factor important in prevention of scurvy. It is not stored in the body. Many fruits contain an abundant supply, especially the citrus fruits. Fruit ice cream is a fair source. Ice cream contains an average 3 mg/kg with a range of 0–11 mg/kg.

Vitamin D. Vitamin D is the antirachitic vitamin. A deficiency is accompanied by a decreased rate of growth and lowered calcium and inorganic phosphorus levels in the blood. There are only small amounts in ice cream unless milk products have been fortified with it.

Vitamin E. This is known as the antisterility vitamin since it helps to maintain normal health and the reproductive organs in laboratory animals. Its value in human nutrition is not yet fully understood. Ice cream is a fair source. It contains an average of 3 mg per kg.

Vitamin K. This vitamin has been found necessary for proper coagulation of the blood. The concentration of vitamin K is very low in milk, and it may be destroyed during pasteurization and evaporation.

Nutrient interactions that may occur among different organic compounds and mineral elements are most complex. Research has pointed to some of these interactions, which include synergism between vitamins, interrelations between minerals, including trace elements, and interactions between sugars and mineral balance as related to assimilation.

Table 2.3 shows the food value of several ice creams and related products.

Table 2.3. Approximate Food Value of Commercial Ice Cream and Related Products

Product	Fat (%)	Amount Volume	Amount Weight (g)	Cal-ories	Fat (g)	Protein (g)	Carbo-hydrates (g)	Total solids (g)	Cal-ium (mg)	Phos-phorus (mg)	Sodi-um (mg)	Vita-min A (IU)	Thia-mine (mg)	Ribo-flavin (mg)	Nia-cin (mg)	Vita-min D (IU)
Vanilla ice cream	12.0	1/6 qt	90	187	10.8	3.7	18.6	34.5	110	94.5	54	442.8	0.04	0.20	0.10	4
Chocolate ice cream	11.0	1/6 qt	90	189	9.9	3.2	22.0	37.4	120	108	47	348	0.04	0.17	0.09	4
Strawberry ice cream	9.0	1/6 qt	90	169	8.1	2.9	21.2	35.0	99	84	40	340	0.04	0.14	0.07	3
Vanilla ice milk	4.0	1/6 qt	90	136	3.6	5.1	20.8	30.6	189	142	75	151	0.07	0.27	0.14	1
Orange sherbet	1.1	1/6 qt	123	177	1.4	1.5	39.6	42.7	53	41	21	57	0.02	0.03	0.04	Trace
Orange ice	—	1/6 qt	123	177	—	0.1	43.5	45.5	1	2	Trace	17	0.01	Trace	0.02	0
Dietary vanilla ice cream	10.0	1/6 qt	90	175	9.0	4.1	19.4	33.3	151	113	59	378	0.05	0.22	0.11	4
Dietary vanilla ice milk	4.0	1/6 qt	90	133	3.6	4.4	20.7	29.7	104	123	65	151	0.06	0.23	0.12	1
Vegetable fat frozen dessert	10.0	1/6 qt	90	180	9.0	4.0	20.7	34.7	145	109	57	0	0.05	0.21	0.11	0
Chocolate coated ice cream bar	17.7	3 fl. oz	60	162	10.6	2.1	14.5	27.5	70	52	28	209	0.02	0.10	0.05	2
Twin popsicle	—	4 fl. oz	128	95	—	0.1	23.7	23.9	—	—	—	—	—	—	—	—

Note: Usual variations in composition will neither increase nor decrease the values in the table by more than 10–15%.

ICE CREAM IN THE REDUCING DIET

"Add ice cream to your regular diet and increase your weight; take ice cream as part of your regular diet and reduce your weight." Very often one sees this apparently contradictory statement, that ice cream is both a fattening food and a food that can be used to advantage in a reducing diet. This paradox clears up when it is understood that a food may be taken as a supplement to a regular diet, or as a substitute for some other food in the diet. If ice cream is consumed in fairly large amounts in addition to a diet already high in caloric values, the person will tend to put on weight. However, if ice cream is used as one of the regular foods in a diet combination and proper moderation is practiced regarding the richer desserts, there is no reason why it cannot be a part of even a slenderizing diet. A study of comparative caloric values indicates that many other desserts are far higher in calories than is ice cream. As an example, a serving of ice cream ranging in size from 1/12 to 1/6 of a quart provides approximately 96–200 cal, while an ordinary serving of lemon pie contains 450 cal.

NUTRITION LABELING

The introduction of nutrition labeling regulations for ice cream appeared in 1973. The aspects of nutritional declaration include

- a statement of nutrition information per serving;
- the serving size;
- the number of servings per container,
- the number of calories per serving,
- the amount (in grams) of protein, carbohydrates, and fat per serving;
- the percentage of U.S. recommended daily allowances (RDA) for eight mandatory nutrients and 12 additional optional nutrients.

The nutrient content of vanilla ice cream (fat, 12%; MSNF 11%; sugar, 15%; stabilizer, 0.3%; TS, 38.3%) per 100 g serving and the nutrition information for labeling are given in Table 2.4.

DIGESTIBILITY AND PALATABILITY
OF ICE CREAM

Many experiments show that homogenized milk is more digestible than milk not so treated. This is based on the fact that the homogenizer has broken the fat globules into minute particles, which can be more readily acted upon by the digestive juices than can the larger fat globules. The same holds true for the fat in ice cream mix when it is forced through the homogenizer as is now the practice in commercial ice cream plants. In addition, the high palatability of ice cream stimulates the flow of digestive juices, a valuable aid to the digestive process. These two factors, together with its sweet flavor, its smooth velvety texture, and its glistening coolness, make it an ideal food for many invalids

Table 2.4. Nutrient Content and Nutrition Information for 100-g Serving of Ice Cream

	Nutrient data	Nutrition information
Servings per container	1	1
Calories per serving	196.7	190
Protein (g) per serving	4.1	4
Carbohydrates (g) per serving	20.7	20
Fat (g) per serving	12.0	12
Mandatory nutrients	Amount	RDA (%)
Protein	4.1 g	9.0
Vitamin A	492 IU	9.0
Vitamin C	1.0 mg	2.0
Thiamine	0.04 mg	2.0
Riboflavin	0.23 mg	13.0 (13.5)
Niacin	0.1 mg	2.0
Calcium	122.0 mg	12.0
Iron	0.1 mg	2.0
Optional nutrients		
Vitamin D	4.0 IU	2.0
Vitamin B_6	0.056 mg	2.0
Vitamin B_{12}	0.48 mg	2.0
Phosphorus	122.32 mg	12.0
Magnesium	17.8 mg	4.0
Zinc	0.47 mg	3.0
Pantothentic acid	0.34 mg	3.0

suffering from throat afflictions or certain stomach ailments, when other foods do not appeal or cannot be tolerated. These qualities together with its value as a morale builder have led hospitals to use ice cream extensively in their menus.

It is safe to say that no other food product contributes so much food value in as attractive and appealing a form, or is so universally liked and distributed as ice cream.

3
Ice Cream and Related Products Classifications

Classification of the various frozen desserts considered to be related to ice cream has been done in many different ways. Early workers (Washburn, 1910; Mortensen, 1911; Frandsen and Markham, 1915) divided these products into two to ten groups, primarily depending on whether the product did or did not contain eggs; Mortensen considered commercial practices in suggesting the ten groups. Later the following classifications were used for the different groups of ice cream and frozen products: plain ice cream, nut ice cream, fruit ice cream, bisque ice cream, mousse, frozen custard, puddings, ice milk or milk ice, ices, and sherbets.

Turnbow *et al.* (1946) gave 20 commonly agreed on terms used to categorize different ice creams. They included the ten headings used by Mortensen and the following additional terms: New York or Philadelphia, lacto, soufflé, frappé, punch, frozen fruit salad, novelties (including bars and stick items), specialties (including molds, decorated items, and slices), and frosted malted milk.

More recently, other variations and changes have been made in the industry including soft serve, vegetable fat, imitation products, and frozen yogurt, and these have created other product categories. The gelato Italian-style frozen desserts that have recently gained in popularity in the United States range from frozen egg custard to fruity eggless ice cream, to sherbets and flavored ices.

The U.S. Food and Drug Administration (FDA, 1976) has identified the following products with label statement of optional ingredients: (1) ice cream; (2) frozen custard, French ice cream, and French custard ice cream; (3) ice milk; (4) fruit sherbet; and (5) water ices.

Any current grouping of ice cream products is influenced by the FDA's standards of identity, optional flavoring materials, and labeling standards in commercial practices popular at the time the grouping is made. The groupings of the kinds of ice cream may be based on commercial terms, regulatory composition requirements, or flavor labeling standards.

COMMERCIAL GROUPING OF ICE CREAM
AND RELATED PRODUCTS

This grouping includes currently popular commercial products described in commonly agreed upon terms.

Plain ice cream. An ice cream in which the total amount of the color and flavoring ingredients is less than 5% of the volume of the unfrozen ice cream. Examples are vanilla, coffee, maple, and caramel ice cream.

Chocolate. Ice cream flavored with cocoa or chocolate.

Fruit. Ice cream containing fruit, with or without additional fruit flavoring or color. The fruit, such as strawberry, apricot, or pineapple, may be fresh, frozen, canned, or preserved.

Nut. Ice cream containing nutmeats, such as almonds, pistachio, or walnuts, with or without additional flavoring or color.

Frozen custard, French ice cream, French custard ice cream. One or more of the optional egg ingredients permitted are used in such quantity that the total weight of egg yolk solids content is not less than 1.4% of the weight of the finished frozen custard or less than 1.12% for bulky flavored products.

Ice milk. A product containing 2–7% fat and 12–15% MSNF, sweetened, flavored, and frozen like ice cream.

Fruit sherbet. Made of fruit juices, sugar, stabilizer, and milk products. It is similar to an ice except that milk—whole, skim, condensed, or powdered—or ice cream mix is used in place of all or part of the water in an ice.

Ice. Made of fruit juice, sugar, and stabilizer, with or without additional fruit acid, color, flavoring, or water, and frozen to the consistency of ice cream. Usually contains 28–30% sugar, 20–25% overrun, and no dairy products.

Confection. Ice cream with appropriate flavorings plus particles of candy, such as peppermint stick, buttercrunch, or chocolate chip.

Bisque. Ice cream containing appropriate flavorings, and particles of grapenuts, macaroons, ginger snaps, sponge cake, or other bakery products.

Puddings. Ice cream containing a generous amount of mixed fruits, nutmeats, and raisins, with or without liquor, spices, or eggs. Examples are nesselrode and plum puddings.

Mousse. Whipped cream, plus sugar, color, and flavoring, and frozen without further agitation. Sometimes condensed milk is added to give better consistency.

Variegated ice cream. A plain vanilla ice cream combined with a syrup such as chocolate or butterscotch, so as to produce a marbled effect in the hardened ice cream.

Fanciful name ice cream. These products usually do not contain a single characterizing flavor, but the flavor is due to a mixture of several flavoring ingredients.

Neapolitan. Two or more distinct flavors in the same package.

New York or Philadelphia. This is usually plain vanilla with extra color for Philadelphia ice cream, and with extra fat and eggs for New York ice cream.

Soft serve ice cream or ice milk. These products are sold as drawn from the freezer without hardening.

Novelties. Quiescently frozen dairy confections and frozen confections. A novelty ice cream or frozen confection is a specially shaped and usually a low-priced package containing an individual serving, the main appeal of which consists of its shape, size, color, or convenience for eating. Examples of novelty items are Eskimo pies, and other candy- or chocolate-coated ice cream bars with or without sticks; candy- or chocolate-coated ice milk bars, with or without sticks; ice cream sandwiches—slabs of ice cream pressed between cookies, wrapped in wax paper, and hardened; pop or fudge; and other icelike mixtures frozen on sticks.

Rainbow ice cream. A product made by carefully mixing six or more different-colored ice creams as they are drawn from the freezers to give a marbled or rainbow-colored effect when the product is hardened.

Gelatin cube ice cream. An ice cream in which colored, fruit-flavored gelatin, cut into small cubes, is used in place of fruits to give color and flavor and a characteristic chewiness.

Frappé. An ice made from a mixture of fruit juices, frozen to a slushy consistency, and served as a drink.

Soufflé. A sherbet containing egg yolk or whole eggs.

Granite. Water ice frozen with very little agitation.

Frozen yogurt or lacto. Yogurt, buttermilk, or cultured sour milk with fruit and sugar, frozen like sherbet.

Fruit salad. Mixed fruits, in large pieces, in combination with a mixture of whipped cream and mayonnaise, and frozen to be served as a salad. (Mayonnaise may be omitted if desired.)

Fancy molded ice cream. Ice creams, ices, and sherbets molded in fancy shapes and composed either of one color and flavor of ice cream or a combination of colors and flavors, or specially decorated. This group includes

- Brick ice cream in one, two, or more layers, or with fancy centers.
- Sliced brick with decorative stenciled designs (individual size).
- Cakes, pies, melon molds, log rolls, sultana rolls, etc.
- Cake roll—layered ice cream on moist cake, rolled like a jelly roll.
- Individual or larger molds representing fruits, flowers, animals, other objects, emblems, and designs.
- Ice cream waffles and tarts.
- Spumoni—a combination of vanilla ice cream, chocolate ice cream or mousse, cherries, and tutti frutti ice cream, or whipped cream combined with fruits, arranged in a spumoni cup, and hardened to serve; sometimes classed as a parfait.
- Aufait—two or more layers of ice cream with pectinized fruits or preserves spread thinly between the layers; or the fruits may be stirred gently into the ice cream as it comes from the freezer, to give a marbled appearance.

Mellorine-type products. Mellorine is a product similar to ice cream in which the butterfat has been replaced by a suitable vegetable or animal fat. Such a product is illegal in over 75% of the United States. The formulas, processing, and distribution procedures for ice cream are also applicable to mellorine. In states that permit the manufacture of a mellorine-type frozen dessert, the minimum fat standards range from 6 to 10%.

In at least one state standard, vegetable fat or oil only is permitted, and in one or two states there is no standard specified but the product is permitted when properly declared. Several states require vitamin A addition of not less than 8400 USP units per gallon (with or without vitamin D concentrate) for 10.0% fat, increasing proportionately. Weight per gallon, minimum milk solids, and minimum food solids requirements are similar to those for ice cream, but the maximum stabilizer allowed ranges to 1%.

A few states have standards for a low-fat mellorine-type product. These products are known in some areas as Olarine or Mellofreeze. The minimum fat requirements for the low-fat products range from 3 to 4%, minimum total milk solids from 7.75 to 10.8%, minimum weight per gallon of 4.5 lb; minimum food solids from 1.0 to 1.3 lb/gal; and maximum stabilizer ranges to 1%. Production data for mellorine-type products are indicated in Table 1.1.

Nondairy frozen dessert. These are frozen products that do not have any dairy ingredients. The composition requirements may be similar to those for ice cream. Product standards have been developed for parevine, which is entirely nondairy.

Artificially sweetened frozen dairy foods. These products are made by replacing the regular sugar sweetener solids with nonsugar, nonnutritive, artificial sweeteners.

Other products included in state standards are

- Low-fat ice cream—milk fat 5.0–9.9%, total milk solids not less than 15%, weight 4.5 lb/gal, food solids 1.5 lb/gal.
- Nonfat frozen dessert—milk fat maximum 0.5%, total milk solids minimum 13.0%, weight 4.5 lb/gal, food solids 1.3 lb/gal.
- Dietetic frozen dessert—milk fat not less than 2.0%, total milk solids not less than 10.8%, total food solids 1.3 lb/gal.
- Frozen dietary food—milk fat 1.0–8.0%, total milk solids not less than 10.0%.
- Harmless flavoring, coloring, added protein, vitamins, and minerals are permitted. Yogurt sherbet, dietetic ice milk, and frozen dairy dessert are also included.

USDA (1980) contains technical composition data on a wide range of frozen dairy dessert products. These standards can be changed at any time by legislative action or by regulatory authority.

LABELING REQUIREMENT GROUPING

The International Association of Ice Cream Manufacturers (IAICM) in developing guidelines for the purpose of fulfilling the labeling provisions of the ice cream standards of the FDA for all ice cream, French ice cream, and ice milk, has grouped these products into three categories depending on the nature of the characterizing flavor as follows:

Category 1—Those which contain no artificial flavor.

Category 2—Those which contain both natural and artificial flavor and in which the natural flavor predominates.

Category 3—Those which are flavored exclusively with artificial flavor or with a combination of natural and artificial in which the artificial predominates.

The IAICM made a further grouping of products in determining predominance of flavor as follows:
(1) Vanilla.
(2) Fruit: (a) citrus, (b) berry and cherry, (c) other fruits.
(3) Nut.
(4) Two or more distinct flavors in the same package.
(5) Neapolitan.
(6) Fanciful-name ice cream.
(7) Variegated product.
(8) Cherry vanilla.
(9) Confectionary.
The standards provide that ice cream may be flavored with any one of the ten classes of optional flavoring ingredients specified for the above grouping of products. This grouping is necessary to provide information necessary to meet flavor labeling standards.

In addition to the labeling requirement involving the flavor categories, there are general nutrition labeling requirements (U.S. Government, 1973) and ingredient labeling requirements for frozen desserts. The nutrition labeling regulation of the FDA (FDA, 1976) gives the preamble, rationale, and interpretations of these regulations (see appendix).

REGULATORY TYPE OF CLASSIFICATION

For regulatory purposes, legislative and administrative officials are finding it desirable to establish a different type of classification. Any classification based upon methods of processing (such as "agitation while freezing"), upon the kind of ingredients (such as bakery goods), or upon shape is without much meaning from a regulatory enforcement point of view. Some regulatory officials have found it convenient to use a classification based on the concentration of some of the constituents, e.g., milk fat, egg yolk solids, and stabilizer. Table 3.1 suggests the form of such a classification arranged in the order of decreasing richness of product. This classification is easy to interpret and should be simpler to enforce; it includes all products that are generally prepared by ice cream manufacturers and is broad enough to include almost any combinations that may become popular. Its chief disadvantage is the fact that it does not suggest names for particular combinations of ingredients, processing techniques, or shapes. The legal specifications for ice cream in various states usually include the following requirements: (1) a minimum percentage of fat, (2) a minimum weight per gallon and (3) a maximum percentage of stabilizer. In addition, one or more of the following may be included: a minimum percentage of milk solids, a minimum weight of food solids per gallon, a minimum percentage of total solids, or a minimum percentage of MSNF. In fruit and nut ice cream, a reduction is usually allowed in the fat and milk solids resulting from the addition of flavoring materials to fruit-, nut-, and chocolate-flavored ice cream. This often amounts to at least 2% fat and 4% milk solids.

Table 3.1. Classification of Frozen Dairy Foods Based upon the Concentration of Certain Constituents

Group	Distinguishing characteristics	Suggested regulatory limitations
I Frozen custard	High in egg yolk solids, which are cooked to a custard before freezing Medium to high in milk fat and MSNF With or without fruit, nuts, bakery products, candy, liquor, or spices With or without agitation while freezing	Not more than: 0.5% edible stabilizer 50,000 bacteria/g Negative **E. coli** test Not less than: 1.4% minimum egg solids content for plain and 1.12% for bulky flavors of custard 10.0% milk fat 20.0% total milk solids 1.6 lb food solids per gal of finished product
II Plain ice cream	Medium to high in milk fat and MSNF With or without egg products With or without agitation while freezing Without visible particles of flavoring material With the total volume of color and flavor less than 5% of the volume of the unfrozen ice cream	Not more than: 0.5% edible stabilizer 50,000 bacteria/g Negative **E. coli** test Not less than: 10.0% milk fat 20.0% total milk solids 1.6 lb food solids per gal of finished product
III Composite ice cream or bulky flavors	Medium to high in milk fat and MSNF With or without egg products With or without agitation while freezing With the total volume of color and flavor material more than 5% of the volume of the unfrozen ice cream or with visible particles of such products as cocoa, fruit, nut meats, candy, bakery products, liquor, or spices	Not more than: 0.5% edible stabilizer 50,000 bacteria/g Negative **E. coli** test Not less than: 8.0% milk fat 16.0% total milk solids minimum 1.6 lb food solids per gal of finished product

IV Ice milk	Low in milk fat With or without egg products, chocolate, fruit, nut meats, candy, liquor, or spices With or without agitation while freezing	Not more than: 0.5% edible stabilizer 50,000 bacteria/g Negative **E. coli** test Not less than: 3.3% milk fat—2.0% minimum, 7% maximum 14.0% total milk solids—11% minimum 1.3 lb food solids per gal of finished product
V Sherbet	Low in MSNF Tart flavor Sweetener, water, harmless fruit, or fruit juice flavoring, coloring	Not more than 50,000 bacteria/g Negative **E. coli** test Not less than: 0.35% acidity as determined by titrating with standard alkali, and expressed as lactic acid 4.0% total milk solids—2.0% minimum, 5.0% maximum 6.0 lb minimum weight per gal 1.8 lb food solids per gal of finished product Citrus fruit flavors 2%, berries 6%, and other fruits 10%
VI Ice	No milk solids Tart flavor Sweetener, water, harmless fruit, or fruit juice flavoring, coloring	Sanitary requirements same as for sherbet
VII Imitation ice cream (mellorine- and parevine- type products)	Proper labeling No minimum requirements, to not less than 10% food fat No minimum requirements to not less than 20% food solids	Sanitary requirements same as for ice milk

The term frozen dairy foods is a general term and includes ice cream, soft-frozen products, ice milk, sherbet, and ices.

Frozen custard represents the more expensive type of ice cream, including such products as parfait. It may be sold as fancy molded, molded novelty (such as candy coated), "soft," or bulk frozen custard.

Plain ice cream includes the wide range of commercial ice creams, even to the high-fat ice creams and those containing small amounts of egg yolk solids. A mousse containing no fruit or nuts would be included as a plain ice cream. These products may be fancy molded, novelties, or bulk ice cream.

Bulky flavored ice cream is either ice cream in which the total volume of coloring and flavoring material is more than 5% of the volume of the unfrozen product, or ice cream containing visible particles of such products as cocoa, fruit, nutmeats, candy, and bakery products. It may have a high fat content, contain a small amount of egg yolk solids, and be fancy molded, novelty, or bulk composite ice cream. It includes such ice creams as chocolate, fruit, nut, candy, bisque, and puddings.

Ice milk may be fancy molded, novelty, or bulk ice milk.

Sherbet may be fancy molded, novelty, or bulk sherbet, and includes such products as lacto.

Ices may be fancy molded, novelty, or bulk ices. This group includes such products as punch, granite, and some stick novelties.

Imitation ice cream includes products such as those made with vegetable fat and containing milk constituents but not meeting ice cream standards. This product obviously cannot be marketed where its use is illegal.

Soft-frozen products usually refer to ice milk served in a soft condition with a lower fat content than that required for ice cream. Ice cream, custard, sherbet or imitation ice cream may be served as soft frozen products.

The term "bulk" refers to ice cream such as is commonly purchased by retailers for repackaging, and served directly to the consumer in cones or dishes.

Packaged ice cream refers to ice cream in containers in the kind and size of which it reaches the consumer.

FEDERAL ICE CREAM STANDARDS

The FDA standards for ice cream and related products are set out in full in FDA (1976) (see Appendix).

In calculating butterfat, the order permits (regardless of the amount of actual sugar present) a reduction in the case of chocolate or cocoa 1.5 times the weight of the unsweetened chocolate or cocoa, and 1.4 times the weight of unsweetened fruits or nuts.

Frozen custard standards are the same as ice cream, except that there is a 1.4% minimum egg yolk solids content for plain and 1.12% for bulky flavors.

Ice milk standards permit no reduction for bulky flavors. Bulk can be colored or flavored.

Sherbet and water ice standards permit natural and artificial flavors. The minimum fruit contents of sherbets and ices are citrus 2% (including cold-pressed citrus oil), berries 6%, other fruits 10%.

Labeling requirements specify that the flavor name on ice cream must be in the same type size as the name of product and must be easily read. If artificial flavoring is used, this must be declared on the label, e.g., "artificially flavored vanilla." If both natural and artificial flavors are used, with natural predominant, e.g. the label should read "vanilla and artificial vanilla flavor." If both are used and the artificial flavor is predominant, the label should read "artificial vanilla flavor." Thus only ice cream carrying 100% of the true flavor or fruit can be designated by that flavor term without using the words "artificial flavor." The same holds true for the ice milk except when artificial color is used—this must also be included on the label.

Artificial coloring or flavoring in sherbets and water ices must be declared on the label. If natural flavors are added to fruit sherbets this must also be declared, e.g., "flavoring added" or "with added flavoring" or "[name of] flavoring added."

The final FDA order forbids the use of mild alkalies to adjust the acidity and the use of mineral salts to adjust salt balance (see Appendix).

Concentrated fruit is suitable for use in ice cream.

Caseinates are permitted by the standards, but they may not count toward the 20% total milk solids. (Sodium, calcium, potassium, and ammonium caseinates may be used.)

The optional stabilizers are agar-agar, algin (sodium alginate), calcium sulfate, gelatin, gum acacia, guar seed gum, gum karaya, locust bean gum, oat gum, gum tragacanth, carrageenan, lecithin, psyllium seed husk, sodium carboxymethylcellulose.

Monoglycerides, diglycerides, or both from the glycerolysis of edible fats are listed as optional ingredients used as emulsifiers in an amount not more than 0.5%. This new description of the source of mono- and diglycerides is more limited than in the provisional order.

Polysorbate 65 and 80 are recognized as suitable optional ingredients at levels not to exceed 0.1% in all of the standardized products except water ices.

4
Composition and Properties

Ice cream is composed of a mixture of food materials such as milk products, sweetening materials, stabilizers, flavors, or egg products, which are referred to as ingredients. The wide variety of ingredients that may be used to produce different kinds of ice cream is apparent from the classifications discussed in Chapter 3. Furthermore, any one kind of ice cream may be made by combining the ingredients in any of several different proportions. However, the effect of these ingredients upon the finished product is due to the constituents of the ingredients. An ice cream mix is the unfrozen blend of the ice cream ingredients and consists of all the ingredients of ice cream with the exception of air and flavoring materials. The composition of ice cream is usually expressed as a percentage of its constituents, e.g., percentage of milkfat, MSNF, sugar, egg yolk solids, stabilizer, and total solids.

The composition of ice cream varies in different localities and in different markets. The best ice cream composition for a manufacturer to produce is often difficult to establish. After consideration is given to legal requirements, quality of product desired, raw materials available, plant procedures, trade demands, competition, and cost, there is a choice of a product of minimum, average, or high milk solids composition. Some plants may choose to manufacture only one of these products, others two, and still others all three, i.e., an economy brand product, a good average composition product as a trade brand, and a deluxe high-quality product.

It may be inadvisable for a small manufacturer to produce more than one brand of ice cream. If only one composition is manufactured, it is highly important that every effort be made to produce the best product possible.

In ice cream, the percentage of milkfat varies more than any other constituent. The milkfat content may vary from 8 to 24%, depending upon such factors as state or city requirements, grade, price, and competition. As the fat content of ice cream is increased, the MSNF must be decreased so as to avoid "sandiness" (i.e., the crystallization of milk sugar or lactose in the finished ice cream). Table 4.1 suggests compositions that avoid sandiness and permit recognition of particular local preferences as to sugar content, fat content, etc., of commercial ice creams and related products. These local preferences and the quality of the ingredients, as well as the technique of manufacture, are fully as

Table 4.1. Approximate Composition (%) of Commercial Ice Cream and Related Products

Product	Milkfat	MSNF	Sugar	Stabilizers and emulsifiers	Approximate TS
Economy ice cream	10.0	10.0–11.0	15.0	0.30	35.0–37.0
	12.0	9.0–10.0	13.0–16.0	0.20–0.40	
Trade brand ice cream	12.0	11.0	15.0	0.30	37.5–39.0
	14.0	8.0–9.0	13.0–16.0	0.20–0.40	
Deluxe ice cream (premium–super premium)	16.0	7.0–8.0	13.0–16.0	0.20–0.40	40.0–41.0
	18.0–20.0	6.0–7.5	16.0–17.0	0.0–0.20	42.0–45.0
	20.0	5.0–6.0	14.0–17.0	0.25	46.0
Ice milk	3.0	14.0	14.0	0.40	31.4
	4.0	12.0	13.5	0.40	
	5.0	11.5	13.0	0.40	29.0–30.0
	6.0	11.5	13.0	0.35	
Sherbet	1.0–3.0	1.0–3.0	26.0–35.0	0.40–0.50	28.0–36.0
Ice	—		26.0–35.0	0.40–0.50	26.0–35.0
Mellorine	6.0–10.0	2.7 (Protein)	14.0–17.0	0.40	36.0–38.0
Frozen yogurt	3.25–6.0	8.25–13.0	15.0–17.0	0.50	30.0–33.0
	0.5–2.0	8.25–13.0	15.0–17.0	0.60	29.0–32.0
	<0.5	8.25–14.0	15.0–17.0	0.60	28.0–31.0
Dietary frozen dessert	<2	Not less than 7% TMS	11.0–13.0 or more	0.50	18.0–20.0

important as the composition in determining the best ice cream for that locality.

Table 4.2 gives federal composition requirements for frozen desserts.

CHARACTERISTICS OF A
SATISFACTORY COMPOSITION

Some of the characteristics that merit consideration are cost, handling properties (including mix viscosity, freezing point, and whipping rate of the mix), flavor, body and texture, food value, color, and general palatability of the finished product. In developing a formulation to fulfill the needs of any particular situation, numerous factors must be considered. These include the personal preferences of company management or customer demands for flavor, body and texture, and color characteristics of the finished product; for example, natural flavor or flavor fortified with artificial flavoring material; smooth, chewy-to-heavy, or coarser texture; higher overrun or more cooling body and texture characteristics; or increased milk to intensify color in various products. Other factors might include meeting composition standards; the nature of the competition; type of manufacturing operation; source, availability, and cost of dairy and nondairy ingredients; volume of operation; and desired quality of ingredients.

Although the methods of processing and freezing influence the characteristics of the mix and the finished product, the effect of constituents supplied by the ingredients is also important. Therefore, the role of each constituent (fat, MSNF, sweetener solids, egg solids, stabilizers, emulsifiers, total solids, salts, optional ingredients, flavors, and colors) is important in contributing to the characteristics of the ice cream.

THE ROLE OF THE CONSTITUENTS

Basic Ingredients

When commercial ice cream was first being introduced in this country, the ingredients were cream, fluid milk, sugar, and stabilizer. Later, condensed milk, nonfat dry milk, and butter became popular ice cream ingredients. Technological developments and changes in marketing and economic conditions have since encouraged the development and use of many other products.

A wide range of ingredients for ice cream is now available from various sources. These ingredients may be grouped as dairy products and nondairy products. The dairy products are most important as they furnish the basic ingredients of milkfat and MSNF, which have essential roles in good ice cream. Some dairy products provide fat, some provide MSNF, others supply both fat and MSNF, and still others supply bulk to the mix. The nondairy products include sweetener solids, stabilizers and emulsifiers, egg products,

Table 4.2. Federal Composition Requirements for Frozen Desserts

Product	Minimum fat (%)	Maximum fat (%)	Minimum protein (%)	Minimum TMS[a] (%)	Weight (lb/gal)	Minimum TS (lb/gal)	Minimum acidity (%)	Egg yolk solids (%)
Ice cream[b]								
Plain flavor	10	—	—	20.0	4.5	1.6	—	<1.4
Bulky flavor	8	—	—	16.0	4.5	1.6	—	<1.12
Ice milk[c]	2	7	—	≥11.0	4.5	1.3	—	<1.4
Sherbet	1	1–2	—	2–5 TMS	6.0	—	0.35	—
Water ice	—	—	—	—	6.0	—	0.35	—
Dietary frozen dessert	—	<2	—	7	4.5	1.1–1.45	—	—
Mellorine-type product[d]								
Plain flavor	6	—	2.7	—	4.5	1.6	—	—
Bulky flavor	4.8	—	2.2	—	4.5	1.6	—	—

Source: USDA (1976).
[a] TMS: total milk solids.
[b] Frozen custard, French ice cream, and French custard ice cream have the same solids requirements, except they must contain not less than 1.4% egg yolk solids (plain flavor) or not less than 1.12% egg yolk solids (bulky flavors).
[c] In bulky flavors, when milkfat content is increased in increments of 1% above the 2–7% levels, MSNF may be reduced by a like amount, but the TMS must remain not less than 11%.
[d] Vegetable or animal fats other than butterfat may be used.

flavors, special products, and water. The basic ingredients in frozen dairy foods are milkfat, MSNF, sweetener solids, stabilizers and emulsifiers, flavorings, and water. The functional properties imparted by these different basic ingredients from which the mix is formulated are quite varied.

Milkfat

The role of milkfat as a constituent of ice cream has been reviewed by various workers (see, for example, Arbuckle and Cremers, 1954; Cremers, 1954; Cremers and Arbuckle, 1954; Keeney, 1958, 1962; King, 1950, 1955; Klosser and Keeney, 1959; Klotzek and Leeder, 1963; Reid and Mosely, 1926; Valaer and Arbuckle, 1961). Milkfat is an ingredient of major importance in ice cream. The use of the correct percentages is vitally essential not only to balance the mix properly, but also to satisfy legal standards. Studies cited tend to show consistently that the fat particles concentrate toward the surface of the air cell during the freezing process in ice cream. This perhaps accounts, in part, for milkfat imparting a rich characteristic to the flavor. Milkfat does not lower the freezing point. It tends to retard the rate of whipping. High fat content may limit consumption, will have a high caloric value, and will increase the cost. The fat content of commercial ice cream is usually 10–12%. The best source of milkfat is fresh cream. Other sources are frozen cream, plastic cream, butter, butter oil, and condensed milk blends. More recent sources of fat include the butterfat mix products, condensed sweetened cream, specially heat-treated milkfat, and fractions of milkfat. Milkfat is associated with a small amount of phospholipids of which lecithin is one of the most important in contributing to its properties. Doan and Keeney (1965) stated that milkfat contributes a subtle flavor quality, is a good carrier and synergist for added flavor compounds, and promotes desirable tactual qualities. It is the characteristics noted by these workers that account for the superior flavor qualities of frozen dairy foods made from fresh milkfat compared with those made from vegetable fat.

Milk Solids Not Fat

MSNF is the solids of skim milk, and consists of protein (36.7%), milk sugar (lactose; 55.5%), and minerals (7.8%). It is high in food value, is inexpensive, and while not adding much to the flavor of ice cream, does enhance its palatability. The lactose adds slightly to the sweet taste largely produced by added sugars, and the minerals tend to have a slightly salty taste, which rounds out the flavor of the finished product. The proteins in MSNF help to make the ice cream more compact and smooth, and thus tend to prevent a weak body and coarse texture. Therefore, as much MSNF as can be added is desirable—except that an excess of MSNF may result in a salty, overcooked, or condensed-milk flavor. MSNF increases viscosity and resistance to melting, but also lowers the freezing point. Variations over the usual range of concentration have no pronounced effect on whipping ability, but variations in the quality of the MSNF do have an important influence on it.

MSNF content is varied inversely with fat content in order to maintain the proper mix balance and to ensure good body, texture, and storage properties.

However, one problem that occurs is that the high concentration of lactose, which may crystallize under certain conditions, can cause a sandiness in texture. Because of the many factors that may affect lactose crystallization, it is difficult to give a statistically certain limit to the percentage of MSNF that should be used in an ice cream mix. However, as a rule of thumb, the MSNF should be no more than 15.6–18.5% of the total solids in the mix, depending on whether the turnover will be slow or rapid.

To calculate the range of the maximum MSNF content of a mix, subtract from 100 the sum of the percentages of all the other solids in the mix, and then divide by a factor of 6.4 (15.6%) and 5.4 (18.5%). For example, for a mix with 10% fat, 15% sugar solids, and 0.3% stabilizers, the highest percentage MSNF for expected rapid turnover would be

$$\frac{100 - (10.0 + 15.0 + 0.3)}{5.4} = \frac{74.7}{5.4} = 13.83\%$$

For the same mix, the highest percentage MSNF for expected slow turnover would be

$$\frac{100 - (10.0 + 15.0 + 0.3)}{6.4} = \frac{74.7}{6.4} = 11.67\%$$

Sweetening Value. Sweetening value means the sweetening effect of added sugars, and is expressed as the weight of sucrose necessary to give an equivalent sweet taste. For many years sucrose was the only sweetening agent added to ice cream; consequently, it has been used as a standard in comparing the sweetening effect of other sugars. However, during the last 30 years there has been an increasing tendency to obtain the desired sweetness by blending sucrose with other sugars. This tendency has been due to insufficient supplies of sucrose, to the gradual improvement in quality of other more economically priced sugars, and to a desire to increase the total solids of some ice creams without exceeding the limit of desirable sweetness of flavor.

It is now accepted that the desired optional sweetening agent can be obtained only by using some sucrose in the blend. The percentage of the sweetening agent that can be obtained from other sources is influenced mainly by (1) the desired concentration of sugar in the mix, (2) the total solids content of the mix, (3) the effect on the properties of the mix, such as freezing point, viscosity, and whipping ability, (4) the concentration in the sugar source of substances other than sugar (e.g., the undesired flavor of honey or the undesired color of molasses), and (5) the relative inherent sweetening power of the sugars other than sucrose.

Sweetener Solids

The sugars used to give ice cream its sweet flavor are called sweetening agents, or simply sweeteners. The sweeteners for ice cream can be either sucrose (cane or beet sugar) alone or sucrose in combination with some corn product. The sugar may be used in dry or liquid form. While a sweet ice cream is generally desired by the public, sweeteners should be used in moderation, not only for optimum palatability, but also for handling properties. Although it is commonly agreed that the best ice cream is made from sucrose, approximately 45% of the sucrose can be replaced by corn sugar for economy, handling, or storage reasons. Many good sugar blends are now commercially available: A great deal of interest has been shown in low-conversion corn syrup solids, because they increase the solids content without sacrificing product properties or sweetness. Blends of sucrose and medium- or high-conversion corn solids have also been used advantageously.

The main function of sugar is to increase the acceptance of the product, not only by making it sweeter but more especially by enhancing the pleasing creamy flavor and the delicate fruit flavors. Lack of sweetness produces a flat taste, while too much tends to overshadow desirable flavors. The total amount of sugar may vary from 12 to 20%, while 14–16% seems most desirable. The sugars used as a source of sweetening increase the viscosity and the TS concentration of the mix. This improves the body and texture of the ice cream provided the TS content does not exceed 42% or the sugar content does not exceed 16%. Above these limits, the ice cream tends to become soggy and sticky. These sugars, being in solution, depress the freezing point of the mix. This results in slower freezing and requires a lower temperature for proper hardening. In addition to their effect on the quality of the ice cream, they are usually the cheapest source of TS in the mix.

Egg Yolk Solids

Egg yolk solids are high in food value but greatly increase the cost of ice cream. They impart a characteristic delicate flavor, which aids in obtaining a desirable blending of other flavors, but even slight off flavors in egg products are easily noticeable in the ice cream.

They have a pronounced effect in improving the body and texture, have almost no effect on the freezing point, and increase the viscosity. Egg yolk solids, regardless of their source, improve whipping ability, presumably due to lecithin existing in a lecithin–protein complex. They are especially desirable in mixes of low TS concentration and in mixes where the fat is obtained from such ingredients as butter and butter oil.

Stabilizers

Stabilizers are used to prevent the formation of objectionable large ice crystals in ice cream and are used in such small amounts as to have a negligible influence on food value and flavor. They are of two general types: (1) gelatin stabilizers, which come from animal sources (such as calfskin, pork-skin, and bones), and which supply certain desirable amino acids; and (2) vegetable stabilizers, such as sodium alginate, carrageenan, agar-agar, CMC (sodium carboxymethylcellulose), and gums such as tragacanth, karaya, and oat gum. All stabilizers have a high water-holding capacity, which is effective in smoothing the texture and giving body to the finished product. Thus, their effect on flavor is indirect. They increase viscosity, have no effect on the freezing point, and with a few exceptions tend to limit whipping ability. Their most important function is to prevent coarsening of texture under temperature fluctuations in retail cabinets.

The amount of stabilizer to use varies with its properties, with the solids content of the mix, with the type of processing equipment, and with other factors. The amount used may be in the range 0–0.5%, but generally is from 0.2 to 0.3%.

Stabilizers extensively used in frozen dairy foods include sodium and propylene glycol alginates, CMC, guar gum, locust bean gum, carrageenan (Irish moss extract), gelatin, and pectin. The alginates have an immediate stabilizing effect upon addition to the mix. CMC produces a chewy characteristic in the finished product. Gelatin produces a thin mix and requires an aging period. Pectin is used in combination with the gums as a sherbet or ice stabilizer.

The use of stabilizers (1) improves smoothness of body, (2) aids in preventing ice crystal formation in storage, (3) gives uniformity of product, (4) gives desired resistance to melting, and (5) improves handling properties. The problems that come from using excessive amounts of stabilizers include (1) undesirable melting characteristics and (2) soggy or heavy body. Commercial stabilizer products are usually blends of the various stabilizing materials in the proportions necessary to give the desired characteristics in the frozen product.

Emulsifiers

Emulsifiers are used in the manufacture of ice cream (1) to produce a finished product with a smoother texture and stiffer body, (2) to reduce the whipping time, and (3) to give the mix a uniform whipping quality. The use of emulsifiers results in air cells that are smaller and more evenly distributed throughout the internal structure of the ice cream. While egg yolk solids may produce similar results, their effect is not so pronounced.

The emulsifying ingredients commonly used in the ice cream industry are mono- and diglycerides of fat-forming fatty acids. One or the other, or both, may be used in a mix. The total amount of emulsifiers by weight may not exceed 0.2%. The use of two polyoxyethylene-type emulsifiers—sorbitan tristearate and polysorbate—has been authorized as safe in frozen dairy foods, but only up to a 0.1% limit. The excessive use of emulsifiers may result in slow melting, and body and textural defects.

Total Solids

TS replace water in the mix, thereby increasing the nutritive value and viscosity, and improving the body and texture of the ice cream. This is especially true when the increase in TS is due to added dextrine (prosugars), sweet cream buttermilk solids, or eggs. Egg yolk solids, like sweet cream buttermilk solids, improve the whipping ability and shorten the freezing time. Increasing the percentage of TS decreases the percentage of frozen water and frequently permits a higher overrun while maintaining the minimum of 1.6 lb of food solids per gallon of ice cream. During hot weather one disadvantage is that the increase in calorie content associated with TS somewhat reduces the cooling effect of the ice cream. A heavy, soggy product results when the TS content is too high, i.e., above 40–42%.

Water and Air

Water and air are important constituents of ice cream, but can easily be overlooked. Water is the continuous phase, which is present as a liquid, a solid, or as a mixture of the two physical states. The air is dispersed through the water–fat emulsion, which is composed of liquid water, ice crystals, and solidified fat globules. The interface between the water and air is stabilized by a thin film of unfrozen material. The interfaces of the fat are covered by a layer of fat-emulsifying agent.

Water in the ice cream mix comes from fluid dairy products, or from added water. The water from milk, having passed through the mammary gland, may be expected to be clean. The water from other sources, must come from a supply where purification is assured.

In the manufacture of ice cream, the overrun, or the increase in volume of ice cream over the volume of mix used, is due to the incorporation of air. The amount of air in ice cream is important because it influences quality, is involved in meeting legal standards, and influences profits. Maintaining a uniform amount of air is important in quality and product control. Some freezers use air filters to maintain air quality.

Studies have been conducted on gases other than air in ice cream. Researchers have developed a method of injecting into the mix during the freezing process liquid nitrogen (N_2) at atmospheric pressure and at a temperature well below that of milk. Others have described a process and apparatus for injecting a mixture of nontoxic, inert gas into ice cream mix. Still others have added finely shredded solid carbon dioxide (CO_2) to ice cream during the manufacturing process to replace the air with CO_2 instead of air. They claim an improved, very acceptable product.

Optional Ingredients

Several special ingredients are used for the various effects they have in the preparation of the mix and on the finished products. Ordinary salt is sometimes used in ice cream. This is usually unnecessary, except in certain flavors such as custards and nut ice creams. Some believe that a small amount of salt ($\leq 0.1\%$) improves the flavor of ice cream. Perhaps this is a carryover of earlier times when ice cream formulations contained a lower percentage of MSNF and thus less natural milk salts. In any case, a salty flavor should be avoided.

The caseinate derivatives, especially sodium caseinate, are effective in increasing the whipping rate and influencing the whipping properties.

The mineral salts, including citrates and phosphates, and calcium and magnesium salts, affect mix and finished-product qualities. Mineral salts are usually used in limited amounts, and affect handling properties and appearance of the product.

The citrates and phosphates are good casein solvents and increase the hydration of the casein. They also impart stability to the mix during heat-treatments and processing.

Calcium salts may decrease the stability of the protein, but also give the mix and finished product a creamy, rich appearance. Calcium sulfate in small quantities affects the dryness and stiffness of the frozen product as it is drawn from the freezer.

Specially prepared low-lactose milk solids are available for increasing the TMS without causing an excessive lactose content. These products contain the milk protein and mineral salts and impart their nutritive value and properties to the product.

Importance of Flavor

Flavor is generally considered the most important characteristic of ice cream. It is easily confused with taste, which includes the "feel sensation" of body and texture as well as the true flavor. The flavor of ice cream is the result of blending the flavors of all the ingredients, some of which may not be sufficiently pronounced to be recognizable, although each actually contributes to the final effect. This makes it difficult to predict the effect of a certain ingredient upon the flavor of the ice cream. Furthermore, the desirability of a particular flavor, or more properly "blend of flavors," depends upon the individual doing the tasting. The subjectivity involved in flavors explains why a certain blend of flavors is less popular at some times than at others.

Flavor has two important characteristics: type and intensity. Flavors that are delicate and mild are easily blended and tend not to become tiresome even when very intense, while harsh flavors soon become tiresome even in low concentrations. As a general rule, therefore, delicate flavors are preferable to harsh ones; but in any case the flavor should be only intense enough to be easily recognized and delicately pleasing to the taste.

THE BALANCED MIX

A balanced mix is one in which the proportions of the constituents and ingredients will produce a fine and generally satisfactory ice cream—an ice cream in which the defects, if any, cannot be further corrected by any change in the composition or ingredients of the mix.

Defects such as rancid flavor, feed flavor, or uneven color cannot be corrected by changing the concentration of the constituents. Therefore, they do not indicate a poorly balanced mix. However, other defects, such as (1) lack of flavor—insufficient concentration of flavoring, (2) lacks of richness—insufficient concentration of fat, (3) sandiness—too high concentration of MSNF, or (4) weak body—low total solids or low stabilizer, may be corrected by

changing the composition of the mix. These defects do, therefore, indicate that
the mix is incorrectly balanced.

Conditions That Limit the Balancing of a Mix

It should, however, be remembered balancing is done to give desirable
results under certain limited conditions of processing and handling the mix or
even of handling the finished ice cream. For example, a mix may be properly
balanced for a finished ice cream that is to have a rapid turnover, but might
cause sandiness if the ice cream were to be stored for any length of time.
Another mix may be properly balanced for freezing in a batch freezer but not in
a continuous freezer. A mix may also be thrown out of balance by changing the
source of the constituents. For example, if the fat in the mix is obtained from
butter, the mix may need the addition of egg yolk solids to improve its
whipping ability and to give it the proper balance, but if the mix is made with
sweet cream, the egg yolk solids would not be necessary. A knowledge of the
role of each constituent together with its advantages and limitations is
necessary in selecting a desired composition and in properly balancing a mix.
Usually an ice cream mix that is properly balanced for average commercial
conditions will have between 36 and 42% TS and between 20 and 26% TMS
(obtained by adding the percentage of fat to the percentage of MSNF). This
does not apply to a mix for ice milk, sherbet, or ice. Furthermore, there has
been a tendency to improve the nutritive value of ice cream by increasing the
concentration of MSNF and reducing the fat, sugar, and flavor concentrations.
(Calculations for balancing mixes are given in Chapter 8.)

For easy references the advantages and limitations of ice cream's constituents are summarized in Table 4.3.

MIX PROPERTIES

The ice cream mix represents a complex colloidal system, many of whose
properties have not been fully investigated. In the mix, some of the substances
occur in true solution (the sugars—including lactose, and the salt constituents—including milk salts), others are in colloidal suspension (milk
proteins, stabilizers, insoluble sweetener solids, and possibly some of the milk
mineral phosphates), and others are in coarse dispersion (the fat globules).

Some substances are in true solution because of their small molecular or
ionic size and their strong affinity for water.

The substances in colloidal suspension typically have particles with an
opposite electrical charge to that of the solvent, and the mutual attraction
keeps them together in suspension. The electric charges on the particles also
keep them apart from each other, which helps to maintain the suspension, as
do the collisions between particles in suspension with those of the solvent.
Occasionally, the substances in suspension may not have sufficient attraction
for the solvent to remain in suspension. Different substances also have differing affinities for water. Some particles have so little affinity for water that if
there is no charge on the particle precipitation occurs. Suspensions of these are
called hydrophobic colloids. On the other hand, substances with high degrees

Table 4.3. Advantages and Limitations of Various Ice Cream Constituents

Constituent	Advantages	Limitations
Milk fat	Increases the richness of the flavor Produces a characteristic smooth texture Helps give body to the ice cream	Cost Fat slightly hinders, rather than improves, whipping High fat content may limit the amount of ice cream consumed High caloric value
MSNF	Improves the texture Helps to give body A higher overrun without snowy or flaky texture A comparatively cheap source of solids	A high percentage causes sandiness The condensed-milk flavor may be objectionable May cause salty or cooked flavor
Sugar	Usually is the cheapest source of solids Improves the texture Enhances the flavor	Excessive sweetness Lowers whipping ability Longer freezing time required and ice cream requires a lower temperature for proper hardening
Stabilizers	Very effective in smoothing the texture Very effective in giving body to the product	Excess body and melting resistance
Egg yolk solids	Very effective in improving whipping ability Produces a smooth texture Flavor	Excessive amounts may produce foaminess on melting Egg flavor not relished by some consumers Cost
TS	Smoother texture Better body More nutritious Ice cream not as cold	Heavy, soggy or pasty body Cooling effect not high enough
Flavor	Increases acceptability	Harsh flavors less desirable Intense flavors quickly satisfy desire
Color	Improves attractiveness Aids in identifying flavor	

of affinity for water may remain in suspension even with no electrical charge. Such suspensions are called hydrophilic colloids.

Colloidal suspensions are very sensitive to slight changes and since ice cream is so complex, many factors have an impact on mix properties.

Substances in coarse dispersion or suspension do not stay uniformly dispersed, but settle or rise depending on their specific gravity relative to the suspending medium.

It is useful to describe the nature of ice cream mix as essentially an oil-in-water type of emulsion: the dispersed phase is the milkfat; the continuous phase is aqueous serum consisting of calcium caseinate–calcium phosphate micelles, serum proteins, carbohydrates, and mineral salts. On the basis of particle size, the serum phase is a mixture of a colloidal suspension and a true solution. This complex emulsion can withstand the stress of freezing, mechanical agitation, and concentration. Aeration is remarkable considering the inherent instability of the fat globules, casein micelles, and lactose under these conditions.

Mix properties of practical importance include stability, density, acidity, surface tension, interfacial tension, viscosity, absorption, freezing point, and whipping rate.

Mix Stability

Mix stability refers to the resistance to separation of the milk proteins in colloidal suspension and the milkfat in emulsion. Instability results in separation of the protein particles as coagulated or precipitated material from the mix, fat or whey separation, or syrup separation in the mix upon aging.

Homogenization, mix acidity, dehydrating salts, ratio of fat to MSNF, heat-treatment, freezing, aging time, and the extent to which the water in the mix is bound all affect mix stability.

Hydration. The most stable mix particle is the hydrophilic suspension (Fig. 4.1a) because it is charged and hydrated; the next most stable is the hydrophilic or hydrophobic suspension (Fig. 4.1b), in which the particle is not hydrated but is charged; less stable is a hydrophilic suspension (Fig. 4.1c), in which the particle is hydrated but has no charge; least stable is a suspension where the particle is neither hydrated nor carrying a charge (Fig. 4.1d). The particle that is neither hydrated nor charged results in unstable mixes.

Factors affecting the hydration of milk proteins include temperature, previous heat-treatment, salts, acidity or alkalinity, and homogenization.

Colloidal substances in ice cream mixes become more strongly hydrated at low temperatures, but possibly greater affinity of the protein for water is produced through chemical changes in the protein molecule as a result of heat-treatment. Calcium salts may be expected to cause a greater depressing effect on the hydration of proteins than sodium or potassium. The hydrating effect of citrates or phosphates for casein is shown in the following double decomposition reaction:

calcium caseinate + sodium citrate $\rightleftarrows$ sodium caseinate + calcium citrate
calcium caseinate + sodium phosphate $\rightleftarrows$ sodium caseinate + calcium phosphate

Any charge that shifts the reaction to sodium caseinate would be expected to increase the hydration of the casein. (Hydration is at a maximum at pH

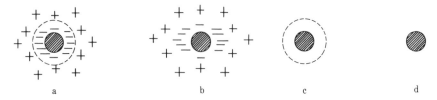

Fig. 4.1. (a) Hydrophilic suspension, with particle charged and hydrated; (b) hydrophilic or hydrophobic suspension, with particle charged but not hydrated; (c) hydrophilic suspension, with particle hydrated but not charged; (d) suspension with particle neither charged nor hydrated.

6.2–6.4.) Two-stage homogenization may be expected slightly to increase the bound water, while there is a slight decrease in single-stage homogenization.

Emulsion Stability. Mix stability is dependent on emulsion (fat) and colloid (protein) stability. Ice cream is homogenized in order to reduce the fat to fine particles with a high degree of dispersion. The fat globules in homogenized mix are surrounded by an interfacial layer, which may be hydrated and is thick with respect to the dimensions of fat globules. The interfacial layer consists mainly of complexed milk protein and has been reported to be 0.3 μm thick. An increase in internal liquid cohesion stabilizes the fat emulsion against partial churning in the freezer and increases the resistance to foam destruction when the mix is extended into the lamellae during shipping.

The state of dispersion of butterfat in ice cream reveals the forces that tend to drive the fat globules apart—the shattering, shearing, or explosive effects of the homogenizing valve and the mutual repulsion of the globules due to their electric charges. The forces that tend to bring the globules together are the collisions of the globules as they emerge from the valve of the homogenizer, the Brownian movement of the small globules, the cohesion of the absorption layers surrounding the globules, the interfacial tension between globules in close proximity, and concentration of the fat in the serum.

High temperatures increase the electric charge on the fat globules, thus decreasing clumping, and citrates and phosphates increase the negative charge, thereby also decreasing clumping. Low temperatures and calcium salts increase the positive charge and thus cause or increase clumping.

In ice cream it is desirable to retain, as far as possible, the original fine dispersion of the fat, and the extent to which and form in which milkfat globules may aggregate are closely linked to the behavior of the fat globule surface. Making the fat globule surface partly or totally hydrophobic may be regarded as the first stage in the "demulsification" of the milkfat.

The second stage takes place when the fat globules are in a partially solidified state, containing the crystalline and liquid fractions of the fat in an optimum ratio. If clumping is to occur, a certain amount of the liquid fat has to be squeezed out of the fat globules. The liquid fat remains attached to the outer surface of the globule membrane, and when two or more globules approach each other closely enough the liquid fat fuses.

At low temperatures, when only small quantities of liquid fat are present, no clumping takes place. Freezing alters the fat globule membrane and during subsequent thawing, the globules join together in clumps and liquid fat is spread between the outer surface of the membrane and the plasma, which renders the fat hydrophobic.

Optical methods with special immersion media are used to identify the fat globules in the internal structure of ice cream. Fat globules can be detected dispersed in the unfrozen material, around the air cells individually, and in chainlike arrangements. There is a relationship between the degree to which the fat globules are grouped in chainlike arrangements and clusters (which is affected by the freezing and whipping process of the ice cream mix) and different percentages of fat and overrun content.

One of the factors affecting the stability of fat in ice cream is the process of freezing. The fat globules begin to agglomerate due to the agitation and concentration of freezing; when observed with the microscope, the agglomerates begin to look like bunches of grapes. The rate of agglomeration and coalescence is a function primarily of the degree of agitation, but also is affected by such factors as protein stability, melting point of the fat, temperature of the freezer, emulsifier, stabilizer, sugars, and salt content.

Dryness in ice cream is directly correlated with emulsion instability, and the greatest dryness and stiffness is obtained in ice cream where the maximum amount of fat clumping has taken place short of actual churning. As ice cream is manufactured under lower freezing temperatures and with longer agitation periods, a greater degree of fat destablilization is exhibited.

To summarize recent research, dryness and stiffness are primarily due to the agglomeration of the butterfat globules. It has been shown that this agglomeration of fat results in a slower meltdown, due perhaps to its greater resistance to flow. In the light of recent findings, we may consider fat agglomeration during freezing as being beneficial, particularly in the case of the continuous freezer.

If agglomeration is carried too far, as might be the case with the extended agitation received in the soft-serve freezer, the result will be eventual churning, with the production of visible butter chips. The negative charges carried by the fat globules, which cause them to repel each other, are lost or overcome during the agitation. An ideal ice cream would be one in which all of the fat is agglomerated but in which none has churned out as visible butter chips. Ice cream in this condition would possess optimum properties of texture, body, dryness, and stiffness as well as an improved apparent richness.

The agitation of colder and stiffer ice cream mix causes more rapid churning, contrary to the belief held by some that a longer initial freezing time leads to increased churning. In fact, at the higher temperatures associated with longer initial freezing, churning takes place much more slowly.

Certain emulsifiers tend to destabilize the butterfat, thus accelerating churning. Fat emulsion destabilization is indicated when there is a poor meltdown, i.e., the ice cream does not melt to a smooth consistency but retains much of its original shape or structure even after it has been exposed to room temperature. The reduction of freezing temperature results in a drier product with a greater amount of destabilized fat, and consequently an increased tendency toward the churning of the fat; a similar problem exists in the soft-serve industry, where a dry stiff product is desired.

Results of a survey of commercial ice cream have shown that ice cream sandwiches manufactured under conditions regulated to extrude a dry product have approximately three times the amount of destabilized fat as ice cream frozen under conditions where dryness is not of particular importance.

The factors affecting fat stability in chocolate ice cream include homogenization, pressure and temperature, type of chocolate product, acidity, emulsifier, corn syrup solids, and calcium and phosphate salts.

Density of Mixes

The specific gravity or density of ice cream mix varies with composition. The specific gravity may be measured by a hydrometer or by weighing a known volume of mix at a known temperature on a gravimetric balance. We can also calculate the specific gravity for a mix at 60°F (15.6°C) by the formula

$$\frac{100}{[\text{fat } (\%)/0.93] + [\text{sugar, MSNF, stabilizer } (\%)/1.58] + \text{ water } (\%)}$$

Wolff used a value of 1.601 for the solids other than fat, which will give a value approximately 0.0026 higher than the 1.58 factor. Investigations indicate that specific gravity of the mix may vary from 1.0544 to 1.1232.

Acidity of Mixes

The normal acidity of mix varies with the percentage of MSNF it contains and may be calculated by multiplying the percentage of MSNF by the factor 0.018. Thus, a mix containing 11% MSNF would have a normal acidity of 0.198%. The normal pH of ice cream mix is about 6.3.[1] The acidity and pH are related to the composition of the mix—an increase in MSNF raises acidity and lowers the pH. The acidity and pH values for mixes of various MSNF content are given in Table 4.4.

If fresh dairy products of excellent quality are used, the mix can be expected to have a normal acidity. The normal or natural acidity of ice cream mix is due to the milk proteins, mineral salts, and dissolved gases. Developed acidity is caused by the production of lactic acid by bacterial action in dairy products. When the acidity is above normal it indicates that developed acidity is present in the dairy products used in the mix. A high acidity is undesirable as it contributes to excess mix viscosity, decreased whipping rate, inferior flavor, and a less stable mix, resulting in "cook on" or possible coagulation during the pasteurizing and processing procedure.

Influence of Mineral Salts

The influence of various mineral salts on the properties of ice cream has been studied by many investigators. In the past, these studies have concentrated on the effects of such materials on acid standardization of the ice cream mix.

The use of various mineral salts in ice cream has also been considered from the standpoint that some of these materials help to control churning and separation of the fat in the mix during the freezing process and impart the desired stiffness, smoothness, or other characteristics to the finished ice cream, claims made by industry representatives. Studies on the effects of sodium and magnesium phosphates, calcium and magnesium oxides, and sodium bicarbonate have shown that they tend to improve the flavor, body and texture, and general characteristics of the finished product.

Calcium and magnesium oxides or carbonates are recommended in preference to the sodium products because sodium's strong wetting effects counteract

---

[1] A neutral substance (i.e., neither acidic nor alkaline) would have a value of 7.0, with decreasing values indicating increasing acidity.

Table 4.4.   Acidity and pH Values for Various Compositions

MSNF (%)	Approximate acidity[a] (%)	Approximate pH
7	0.126	6.40
8	0.144	6.35
9	0.162	6.35
10	0.180	6.32
11	0.198	6.31
12	0.206	6.30
13	0.224	6.28

[a] As lactic acid.

and nullify most of the beneficial reaction it might have on the protein. Sodium citrate and disodium phosphate are effective protein stabilizers. Such materials as calcium and magnesium oxides and carbonates help control the properties of the mix.

Studies have been done on the effect of sodium citrate, disodium phosphate, tetrasodium pyrophosphate, and sodium hexametaphosphate on the churning of butterfat in soft ice cream. All salts used were chemically pure. In practice, the usage levels are 0.05, 0.10, 0.15, and 0.20%, but the 0.10% level was selected as a medium level of usage and higher amounts were avoided because of possible off-flavors and high mix viscosity. A combination of 50% tetrasodium pyrophosphate and 50% of the other salts was also tried. Results indicate that the use of phosphate salts might or might not increase fat stability, but in no case do they decrease it.

Disodium phosphate, sodium tetrapyrophosphate, sodium hexametaphosphate, and sodium citrate have been studied for their possible effect on controlling the churning defect of soft-serve ice cream. The mineral salts were used at the 0.1 and 0.2% level and compared with a control that did not contain any added salt. The compounds were blended with the stabilizer before mix preparation. Without exception the ice cream samples containing one of the salts showed less fat destabilization than the control sample drawn after the same length of time in the freezer. It seems most likely that these buffering salts influence fat emulsion stability through some mechanism involving the milk proteins. The effects of these salts on acidity, with the possible exception of the pyrophosphate, were so small that they would not conceivably be used as neutralizing agents.

The use of emulsifier materials on protein and fat globule stability control through the use of mineral salts is important in influencing the handling characteristics of ice cream. The beneficial effects on flavor, body, texture, and handling characteristics of the products studied, as a result of mineral salts at the 0.02 and 0.04% levels as compared to the control, were evident not only to the professional observers but to others as well.

Mix Viscosity

Rheology is a branch of physics concerned with the composition and structure of flowing and deformed materials, and has application to the many materials possessing components with rheological behavior. Published data on the rheological characteristics of ice cream mix and ice cream are mainly tabulations of these values in research results expressing the effect of the various mix constituents on product properties. The flow properties are expressed in terms of viscosity, and considerable attention has been given to the factors affecting mix viscosity, including rheological methods for studying the physical properties of the oil–water interface in ice cream.

Viscosity, the resistance of a liquid to flow, is the internal friction that tends to resist the sliding of one part of the fluid over another. It has long been considered an important property of the ice cream mix, and a certain level of viscosity seems essential for proper whipping and for retention of air. The viscosity of a mix is affected by:

- Composition—viscosity is influenced more by the fat and the stabilizer than by the other constituents.
- Kind and quality of ingredients—those carrying the fat are especially important. Also, heat and salts (such as calcium, sodium, citrates) greatly affect the viscosity due to their effect on the casein and other proteins.
- Processing and handling of the mix—the steps in processing that have the greatest effect are pasteurization, homogenization, and aging.
- Concentration—TS content.
- Temperature.

Although much has been written about the causes and effects of viscosity, there has been no final answer to the question of how much is desirable and how it can be accurately measured. A high viscosity was believed essential at one time, but for fast freezing (rapid whipping) in modern equipment a lower viscosity seems desirable. In general, as the viscosity increases, the resistance to melting and the smoothness of body increases, but the rate of whipping decreases. Viscosity is now considered a phenomenon that frequently accompanies rather than causes good whipping, body, and texture. Therefore, the mix should be properly balanced (in regard to composition, concentration, and quality of ingredients) and then properly processed to produce the desired whipping ability, body, and texture. Under these conditions a desirable viscosity is assured.

Viscosity may be measured in three ways: (1) by time required to flow under a fixed pressure through a pipette; (2) by measuring the force required to move two layers of liquid past each other; or (3) by measuring the fall of a ball through a column of liquid.

Viscosity may be expressed in absolute or relative values. The absolute unit of measurement commonly used is a centipoise. The absolute viscosity of water at 68°F is 1.005 cP. Ice cream mix has apparent viscosity, i.e., a thickened condition that disappears with agitation, and basic viscosity, that which remains after the apparent viscosity disappears. The basic viscosity of ice cream mix may range from 50 to 300 cP.

Relative values may be expressed as ratios with values obtained for water. Viscosity values of ice cream mix are valuable in indicating whether there are any factors which may be influencing the mix unduly.

It has not been demonstrated that there is a significant correlation between mix viscosity and the body and texture characteristics of ice cream.

Data indicate that ice cream should be considered a viscous system rather than a plastic. The absolute viscosity of ice cream at 100% overrun is 20 billion centipoises at $-8.0°C$. Lowering the temperature a few degrees may double or triple this value.

Surface Tension

Surface tension is a force resulting from an attraction between surface molecules of a liquid that gives surfaces filmlike characteristics. The greater the attraction between the molecules, the higher the surface tension value, and the less the attraction between the molecules of the liquid, the lower the surface tension value.

The unit of measurement of surface tension is the dyne. The du Nouy apparatus is commonly used to determine the surface tension of ice cream mixes. This apparatus measures the force required to pull a platinum ring with a circumference of 4 cm free from the surface of the liquid.

Investigation of the surface tension of ice cream is limited. Studies indicate that increasing the surface tension above that of the freshly made mix made from fresh ingredients is difficult, although the surface tension may be readily decreased by the addition of products such as emulsifiers. Mixes with lower surface tension values caused by the addition of emulsifier to the mix have shown excessive rates of whipping, fluffy, short body characteristics, and susceptibility to the shrinkage defect.

The normal range of surface tension values for ice cream mix is 48–53 dynes.

Interfacial Tension and Absorption

Interfacial tension is the force involved at the interface between two liquids, liquid and gas, or liquid and solid. The surface tension and interfacial tension are related, because the conditions that produce stress on the surface of a liquid may also produce stress in the bounding surface at the interface. The surface tension and interfacial tension values vary inversely.

Absorption involves dissolved substances at the interface. Substances absorbed at the interface may form an absorption film and lower the interfacial tension. In case of dilution the concentration of the absorption film decreases except when the absorption is of a nonreversible character.

Freezing Point

The freezing point of ice cream is dependent on the soluble constituents and varies with variation in composition. It has been demonstrated that the freezing temperature can be calculated with considerable accuracy and can be determined in the laboratory with special apparatus.

An average mix containing 12% fat, 11% MSNF, 15% sugar, 0.3% stabilizer, and 6.17% water has a freezing point of approximately 27.5°F. The freezing point of mixes with high sugar and MSNF content may range to 26.5°F while for mixes with high fat, low MSNF, or low sugar content it may range to 29.5°F.

The initial freezing point of the average ice cream mix is approximately

27–28°F and essentially reflects the freezing point lowering due to total sugar content of the mix. When latent heat is removed from water and ice crystals are formed, a new freezing point is established for the remaining solution since it has become more concentrated in respect to the soluble constituents. A typical freezing curve for ice cream shows the percentage of water frozen at various temperatures (Fig. 4.2).

The calculation of the freezing point of ice cream mixes and the quantities of ice separated during the freezing process are in close agreement with experimental values.

Whipping Rate

Sodium caseinate improves whipping properties and affects air cell and ice crystal distribution to an extent hardly expected of any other commonly used ice cream constituent.

A theoretical explanation of mix whipping ability based on the cohesion and strength of the lamellae includes the importance, relationship to viscosity, surface tension, strength of lamellae (walls around the air cells), effect of constituents and their heat treatments, flavoring materials, processing methods, and equipment. The rate of whipping is dependent upon (a) the efficiency of the whipping mechanism; (b) viscosity of the partly frozen mix; and (c) the completeness with which air, once incorporated, is held.

High whipping rate describes the property to whip rapidly to a high overrun. It is now definitely known that differences in whipping ability cannot be explained on the basis of viscosity. The present hypothesis is that whipping ability is based on tensile strength and strength of the lamellae. Whipping ability is improved by high processing temperatures, proper homogenization, and aging the mix for 2–4 hr.

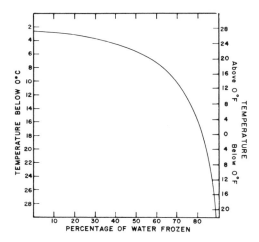

Fig. 4.2. A typical freezing curve for ice cream showing the percentage of water frozen at various temperatures. Courtesy of Doan and Keeney (1965).

Smaller fat globules and less clumping give increased whipping ability. Mixes made with butter, butter oil, or frozen cream have a less satisfactory dispersion of fat and poorer whipping ability. Egg yolk solids, regardless of their source, and fresh cream buttermilk solids improve whipping ability, presumably due to lecithin existing as a lecithin–protein complex. Emulsifiers, which are described later, also improve whipping ability. Usual variations in concentration of MSNF have no pronounced effect on whipping ability, but qualitative variations in MSNF are important. Sugar decreases the whipping ability except when added after homogenizing and then it increases whipping ability. Finally, the construction and operation of the freezer itself determine whether the maximum whipping ability of a given mix is obtained.

Rate of whipping is determined by measuring the overrun at 1-min intervals while the mix is being frozen in a batch freezer. Normally, within 3-1/2 min after the freezing process is started, the mix is frozen and within 7 min an overrun of 90% is obtained. In mixes possessing a high whipping rate the 90% overrun may be reached within 5 min. Mixes requiring 8 min or more to reach 90% overrun are considered to have a low whipping rate.

5

Ice Cream Ingredients

The essentials for the manufacture of high-quality ice cream are good ingredients mixed and balanced so as to produce a satisfactory composition, together with intelligent processing, freezing, and hardening of the product. All of these factors are important and should be carefully controlled by the ice cream maker.

The selection of good ingredients is, without doubt, the most important factor in successful ice cream manufacture.[1] A clean, fresh, creamy flavor in ice cream can be secured only by the use of products that have been carefully produced and handled. In general, the more the product has been handled and the longer it is held in storage, the less desirable are the flavor and other properties imparted to the ice cream.

OPTIONAL INGREDIENTS

The wide choice of ingredients available from various sources may be grouped by source as shown in Table 5.1. The optional ingredients most widely used may influence the ingredients choice along with the factors previously mentioned.

The FDA (1976) definitions and standards of identity for frozen desserts specify optional dairy ingredients, optional caseinates, and other safe and suitable non-milk-derived ingredients. The source groups may include dairy ingredients, sweetening ingredients, caseinates, emulsifiers, water, egg products, stabilizers, mineral salts, coloring, flavor-characterizing ingredients, and other optional ingredients.

Proposed Ingredient Declaration Grouping

A further proposed grouping for dairy sweetener and egg ingredient declaration is as follows:

---

[1]Stabilizers and flavoring are discussed in Chapters 6 and 7, respectively.

Table 5.1. Essential and Optional Ingredients for Ice Cream

Dairy Ingredients	Sweetening ingredients
Cream	Sugar (sucrose) or sugar syrup
Dried cream	Dextrose
Plastic cream (concentrated milkfat)	Invert sugar (paste or syrup form)
Butter	Corn syrup, dried corn syrup, glucose
Butter oil (anhydrous fat)	syrup, dried glucose syrup
Milk (cow's milk)	Maple syrup, maple sugar
Concentrated milk	Honey
Evaporated milk	Brown sugar
Sweetened condensed milk	Malt syrup, maltose syrup, malt extract
Superheated condensed milk	Dried malt syrup, dried maltose syrup,
Dried milk	dried malt extract
Skim milk	Refiners syrup
Concentrated skim milk	Molasses (other than blackstrap)
Evaporated skim milk	Lactose
Condensed skim milk	Fructose
Superheated condensed skim milk	
Sweetened condensed skim milk	
Sweetened condensed part-skim milk	**Caseinates**
Nonfat dry milk	
Sweet cream buttermilk	Casein prepared by precipitation with
Condensed sweet cream buttermilk (when	gums
adjusted with water to ≥8.5%; acidity	Ammonium caseinate
should be ≤0.17%	Calcium caseinate
Dried sweet cream buttermilk (when ad-	Potassium caseinate
justed with water to ≥8.5%; acidity	Sodium caseinate (may be added in liquid
should be ≤0.17%)	or dry form, but must be free of excess
Skim milk that has been concentrated and	alkali—may be added to ice cream mix
from which part of the lactose has been	containing ≥20% TMS
removed by crystallization	
Skim milk in concentrated or dried form	
that has been modified by treating the	
concentrated skim milk with calcium	**Egg products**
hydroxide and disodium phosphate	**(added before pasteurization)**
Concentrated cheese whey (contribute	
25% by weight of total MSNF)	Liquid eggs Egg yolk
Dried cheese whey (contribute ≤25% by	Frozen eggs Frozen egg yolk
weight of total MSNF)	Dried eggs Dried egg yolk

Skim milk, concentrated skim milk, and nonfat dry milk may be declared as "skim milk."

Milk, concentrated milk, and dried milk may be declared as "milk."

Bacterial cultures may be declared by the word "cultured" followed by the name of the substrate, e.g., "made from cultured skim milk or cultured buttermilk."

Sweetcream buttermilk, concentrated sweetcream buttermilk, and dried sweetcream buttermilk may be declared as "buttermilk."

Cheese whey, concentrated cheese whey, and dried cheese whey may be declared as "whey."

Cream, dried cream, and plastic cream (sometimes known as concentrated milkfat) may be declared as "cream."

Butter oil and anhydrous butterfat may be declared as "butter."

Sugar (sucrose) shall be declared as "sugar," and invert sugar may be declared as "sugar."

Table 5.1. Continued

Stabilizers or thickening agents	Water
Agar-agar	May be added or evaporated from the mix

Agar-agar
Algin—sodium alginate
Propylene glycol alginate
Calcium sulfate
Gelatin
Gum acacia
Guar seed gum
Gum karaya
Locust bean gum
Oat gum
Gum tragacanth
Carrageenan
Salts of carrageenan
Furcellaran
Salts of furcellaran
Lecithin
Psyllium seed husk
Sodium carboxymethyl cellulose (≤0.5% of weight of finished ice cream)

Water

May be added or evaporated from the mix

Mineral salts

Sodium citrate, disodium citrate
Disodium phosphate
Tetrasodium pyrophosphate
Sodium hexametaphosphate or any combination of these (0.2% by weight of the finished ice cream)
Calcium oxide, magnesium oxide
Calcium hydroxide or any combination of these (0.4% of the weight of the ice cream)

Coloring

Natural and artificial colorings may be added

Emulsifiers

Monoglycerides or diglycerides (≤0.2% of finished product)
Polyoxyethylene (20)
Sorbitan tristearate polysorbate (80) (≤0.1% by weight of finished product)
Microcrystalline cellulose (≤1.5% by weight of finished product)
Dioctyl sodium sulfosuccinate (0.5% of weight of stabilizers)

Acids—Ices and Sherbets

Citric acid
Tartaric acid
Malic acid
Lactic acid
Ascorbic acid
Phosphoric acid or any combination in such quantity as seasons the finished food

Sweeteners derived from corn may be declared as "corn sweeteners."

Dried whole eggs, frozen whole eggs, and liquid whole eggs may be declared as "eggs."

Dried egg whites, frozen egg whites, and liquid egg whites may be declared as "egg whites."

Dried egg yolks, frozen egg yolks, and liquid egg yolks may be declared as "egg yolks."

COMPOSITION OF MILK

Since milk is the source of the dairy products used as ice cream ingredients it is important to have an understanding of its composition and properties.

Milk is composed of water, milkfat, and MSNF. The TS content of milk includes all the constituents of milk except water. The MSNF constituents are those found in skim milk and include lactose, protein, and minerals. These solids are also referred to as skim milk solids, and serum solids (SS). The composition and physical properties of milk are shown in Tables 5.2 and 5.3, respectively.

The composition of milk is influenced by numerous factors. For example, the MSNF content varies with the fat content of milk. A 0.4% change in MSNF for each 1% change in fat may be used in a general way to determine the MSNF content of milk at the various fat levels.

Milk is produced in the mammary gland from constituents supplied through the blood. Some constituents may pass through the mammary system and into the milk by filtration, but most of them are secreted or produced by the mammary gland. As a result, certain of the constituents of milk, including milkfat, casein, and lactose, are found in major amounts only in milk.

Milk is a structurally complex physiochemical system. The degree of dispersion of the constituents in milk includes true solution (lactose), colloidal suspension (casein), and coarse dispersion (milkfat). Table 5.4 gives the particle size of milk constituents and of those constituents occurring in ice cream.

The water present in milk is similar to any other water except it has passed through the mammary gland, and it is reasonable to assume it has a high

Table 5.2. Approximate Composition of Milk

Constituents	Mean (%)	Normal variation (%)
Water	87.1	82.10–89.44
Fat	3.9	2.60–8.37
Protein	3.3	2.44–6.48
Lactose (milk sugar)	5.0	2.41–6.11
Ash (minerals)	0.7	0.56–0.97
MSNF	9.0	7.20–11.90
TS	12.9	10.56–17.90

Table 5.3. Physical Properties of Milk

Property	Value
Acidity (%)	0.16 ± 0.02
pH	6.6 ± 0.2
Surface tension (dynes)	55.3
Specific gravity	1.032 ± 0.004
Freezing point (°C)	-0.55
Boiling point (°C)	100.17
Specific heat at	
0°C	0.920
15°C	0.938
40°C	0.930
Coefficient of expansion at	
10°C	0.9975
15.6°C	0.9985
21.1°C	1.0000
Viscosity (cP)	1.6314
Electrical conductivity (mho)	45–48×10^{-4}

Table 5.4. Particle Size and State of Dispersion of the Constituents of Milk and Ice Cream[a]

1 nm (1/100 μm)	10 nm	100 nm	1 μm	10 μm	100 μm	1 mm (1000 μm)
Electron microscope	Ultramicroscope		Microscope			Visible
Passes filters and membranes		Pass filters but not membranes	Passes neither filters nor membranes			
Molecular movement		Brownian movement		Slow Brownian and gravitational movement		
	Sedimentation and oil globule rise extremely slowly		Sedimentation and oil globule rise			
High osmotic pressure	Low osmotic pressure		No osmotic pressure			
True solution	Colloidal suspension		Coarse suspension			
			Milk constituents			
Lactose and soluble salts	Whey protein albumin, globulin	Calcium caseinate		Fat globules		
		Colloidal phosphates				
			Ice cream constituents			
Lactose, sucrose corn sugar and soluble salts	Whey protein, albumin, globulin	Casein	Fat globules		Ice crystals Flavoring particles	
	Stabilizers, colloidal phosphates					

[a] 1 μm = 1/25,000 in.

degree of purity. Water provides bulk and acts as a dispersion medium for the other constituents holding them in solution, colloidal suspension, or emulsion.

Milkfat is found only in milk. It occurs in milk in the form of tiny globules held in suspension in the state of emulsion. Normal milk contains about 2.5 billion fat globules per milliliter. The fat globules vary in size from 0.8 to 20 μm in diameter (Fig. 5.1), depending on the breed of cow and stage of lactation. Fat globules tend to cluster together. This property is responsible for rapid creaming, viscosity, and body characteristics in various manufactured dairy products. The fat globules have on their surface a layer of colloidal substances composed of protein and lecithin. This layer is commonly referred to as the fat globule membrane.

Milkfat is composed of various fatty acids and may contain other materials.

The fatty acids of milkfat exist in combination with glycerol, $C_3H_8O_3$, as glycerides. Glycerol molecules combine with fatty-acid molecules according to the reaction

$$1 \text{ glycerol } + \text{ 3 fatty acid} \Rightarrow 3H_2O + 1 \text{ fat}$$

When the three molecules of fatty acid are the same, a single glyceride is formed. When the three molecules of fatty acid are of more than one kind, a mixed glyceride is formed. Milkfat probably contains both simple and mixed glycerides, but the mixed glycerides predominate. Obviously, a very large number of different combinations of glycerol and fatty acids may exist, since milkfat is a mixture of fats. Variations in its properties depend upon the proportion and properties of the various fat components present.

Substances associated with milkfat include related compounds such as the phospholipids lecithin and cephalin; the sterols cholesterol and ergosterol; the carotenoids carotene and xanthophyll; and the vitamins A, D, and E. In phospholipids, part of the fatty acids present is replaced by phosphoric acid and a nitrogen base. Lecithin is one of the best known phospholipids. The nitrogen base in lecithin is choline, which is a part of the vitamin B complex. Milk contains about 0.075% lecithin and cephalin, and milkfat about 0.6% lecithin. Cholesterol is the principle sterol in milk. Milk contains about 0.015% cholesterol. Ergosterol, $C_{28}H_{43}OH$, is the precursor of vitamin D and carotene is the precursor of vitamin A.

The protein components of milk are casein and whey. The major proteins of casein are α-, β-, and γ-casein. The immune globulin, α-lactalbumin, β-lactoglobulin, serum albumin, and some minor proteins comprise the whey protein.

Casein comprises approximately 80% of the total protein in milk and occurs only in milk. In the pure state casein is white, odorless, and tasteless. It occurs in milk in a colloidal state, and may be removed by filtration through a porcelain filter. Casein particles in milk can be observed with an ultramicroscope or by use of a dark-field attachment. The particle size of casein ranges from 1 to 100 nm, with an average size of 40–50 nm. Casein is found in milk in combination with calcium as calcium caseinate. It is precipitated by enzymes, alcohols, heat, various salts, and by acids at a pH of 4.6. A temperature of approximately 270°F is required to coagulate the casein of a high-quality milk.

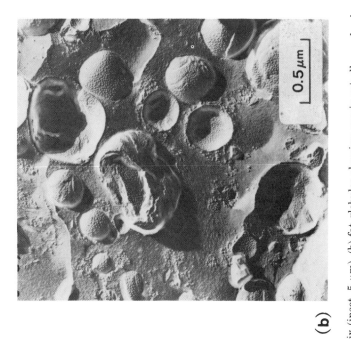

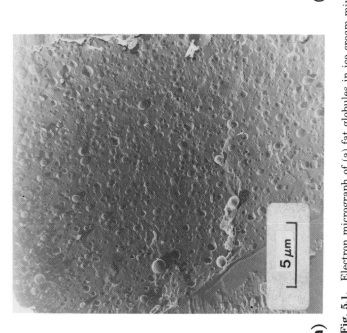

(a)

(b)

Fig. 5.1. Electron micrograph of (a) fat globules in ice cream mix (inset, 5 μm), (b) fat globules showing casein micelles and subunits attached (inset 0.5 μm). From K. G. Berger, A.W. White, G. Lyons & Co. Ltd., personal communication (1977).

The whey protein particles range in size from 1 to 20 nm, with the average size about 10 nm. These proteins are not precipitated with acid or with rennin but they are readily precipitated by heat at temperatures about 170°F. These proteins resemble casein in chemical composition.

Lactose or milk sugar is in solution in milk. Lactose, which is found only in milk and is one of its major constituents, is a disaccharide composed of two monosaccharides, glucose and galactose, linked together. Lactose is a carbohydrate and, at favorable temperatures, part of the lactose is converted into lactic acid by the action of bacteria usually present in milk, thus souring the milk.

The lactose content of milk does not vary widely, averaging about 4.9%. It reduces Fehlings solution, forming cuprous oxide, Cu_2O. Lactose is optically active, having a specific rotation of 52.53°. It may occur in three forms, two anhydrous and one a monohydrate. In solution lactose exists in two forms, α- and β-lactose. There is an equilibrium between the forms; approximately 60% of the lactose is in the β form, although the exact percentage depends on the temperature of the solution.

Crystalline lactose exists in three forms, α-lactose hydrate, $C_{12}H_{22}O_{11}H_2O$; α-lactose anhydride, $C_{12}H_{22}O_{11}$; and β-lactose anhydride, $C_{12}H_{22}O_{11}$. Lactose is 17–25% as sweet as sucrose, and 25 and 33% as soluble as sucrose at 32 and 212°C, respectively. The crystals of lactose occur in many forms. The crystalline forms of α-lactose anhydride have appeared in as many as nine different stages in the development of the same crystal pattern.

Milk ash occurs in milk as mineral salts. Minerals in milk include calcium, phosphorus, potassium, magnesium, iron, chlorine, copper, and traces of other materials. These minerals, in the form of citrates, phosphates, or oxides, are important in influencing the behavior of milk that is subjected to manufacturing procedures. Milk minerals are also of considerable importance as nutrients. The mineral constituents in the form of salts in milk are given in Table 5.5 and the average values of the minerals themselves are given in Table 5.6.

A large number of trace elements are present in milk from cows receiving

Table 5.5. Percentage of Mineral Constituents as Mineral Salts of Milk

Grouping	%
Sodium chloride, NaCl	10.6
Sodium bicarbonate, $NaHCO_3$	2.4
Potassium chloride, KCl	9.0
Potassium sulfate, K_2SO_4	1.7
Monopotassium phosphate, KH_2PO_4	10.4
Dipotassium phosphate, K_2HPO_4	9.4
Dicalcium phosphate, $CaHPO_4$	6.5
Tricalcium phosphate, $Ca_3(PO_4)_2$	7.8
Tripotassium citrate, $K_3C_6H_5O_7$	6.5
Trimagnesium citrate, $Mg_3(C_3H_5O_7)_2$	7.4
Tricalcium citrate, $Ca_3(C_6H_5O_7)_2$	17.2
CaO combined with casein	5.7
Sulfur combined with casein, albumin, and globulin	3.0
Phosphorus combined with casein, albumin, and globulin	2.4
	100.0

Table 5.6.   Average Amount
of Minerals in Milk

Constituent	Amount (mg/ml)
Calcium	123
Magnesium	12
Phosphorus	95
Sodium	58
Potassium	141
Chlorine	119
Sulfur	30
Citric acid	160

normal rations. These elements, measured in micrograms per liter, include aluminum, 460; arsenic, 50; barium, quantitative; boron, 270; bromine, 200; chromium, 15; cobalt, 0.6; copper, 130; fluorine, 150; iodine, 43; iron, 450; lead, 40; lithium, quantitative; manganese, 22; molybdenum, 73; nickel, 0; rubidium, quantitative; selenium (nonseleniferous), 40; selenium (seleniferous), up to 1270; silicon, 1430; silver, strontium, tin, titanium, and vanadium, quantitative; and zinc, 3900.

The mineral content of milk is less variable than most of the other constituents. The ash content of mixed milk averages approximately 0.7% and ranges from 0.65 to 0.75%, while the average mineral salts content is about 0.9%.

There are also in milk considerable numbers of other inorganic and organic substances in small percentages or traces, some apparently unimportant and others highly important because of effects they produce out of all proportion to the concentration in which they occur. These other minor constituents of milk are gases, enzymes, nonprotein nitrogenous substances, flavoring substances, phospholipids, sterols, carbohydrates other than lactose, vitamins, and pigments. Since ice cream has a high concentration of milk solids, the minor constituents of milk may be expected to occur in amounts in proportion to the amount of milk constituents used in the mix.

The gases carbon dioxide, nitrogen, and oxygen are found dissolved in milk in the approximate percentages by volume of 4.5, 1.3, and 0.5%, respectively. The gas content may readily change depending on the treatment given the milk.

The enzymes in milk may be produced by the mammary glands during the secretory process or by bacteria in the milk. The enzymes that occur are phosphatase (alkaline and acid), lipase, esterase (A, B, and C), oxidase, protease, amylase, catalase, aldolase, carbonic anhydrase, salolase, rhodonase, and lactase. Enzymes are proteins and are inactivated by high temperatures.

The literature indicates that there are approximately 19 vitamins normally present in fresh milk, including vitamins A, B_{12}, D, E, K, ascorbic acid, nicotinic acid, riboflavin, and thiamine. Vitamins and references are discussed in more detail in Chapter 2.

Other constituents of milk include the nonprotein nitrogenous substances, such as ammonia N, urea N, creatine, and α-amino N. The flavoring substances other than the main constituents include carbonyl compounds, lactones, methyl sulfides, and similar compounds. Lecithin, cephalin, and sphing-omyelin are the phospholipids present in milk, in the concentration range 0.028–0.037%. The phospholipid content of dairy products used as ingredients in ice cream has an important role in influencing processing and product qualities in ice cream manufacture.

The cholesterol content of milk may range from 120 to 140 ppm. Cholesterol is usually thought to be associated with fat, but it has been reported that 18% of the cholesterol is associated with the proteins.

The carotenes and riboflavin are the major pigments in milk.

MILK PRODUCTS USED IN ICE CREAM[2]

Sources of Fat

Both butterfat and MSNF of the milk products used in the mix contribute to the flavor of ice cream. The butterfat is more important in this respect because the full, rich, and creamy flavor that ice cream should have comes mostly from the butterfat of the mix. The MSNF, on the other hand, has a more indirect effect on flavor. The proteins help give the ice cream body and a smooth texture. The milk sugar adds to the sweet taste largely produced by the added sugars, and the milk salts tend to carry a slightly salty taste, which rounds out the flavor of the finished ice cream.

Whole milk is very desirable as a source of fat as well as of MSNF. Only milk of clean flavor and odor, with a low acidity ($\leq$0.2%), should be used. A combination of milk and sweet cream is probably the best source of fat for ice cream. Fresh whole milk is seldom used because in many markets it is too expensive a source of fat and MSNF.

Fresh sweet cream is the most desirable concentrated source of butterfat for use in the mix. Other concentrated milk products do not impart the same clean, rich, creamy flavor that a good-quality sweet cream does. Cream containing 40% fat should not exceed 0.15% acidity and should be free from off-flavors and -odors. A butterfat test should be made on each purchase so that buyers are assured of receiving the full amount of fat for their money. However, sweet cream is relatively expensive as a source of fat, fluctuates considerably in quality and price, and has the added disadvantage of being difficult to secure in good quality at certain seasons of the year in some markets.

Frozen cream is stored by many companies during the months of surplus and low price. In storing frozen cream only the very best fresh cream should be used. It should be pasteurized at 165–175°F for 15 min to inhibit the development of off-flavors. Neither milk nor cream should come in contact with exposed iron or copper, (which may occur when the tin has worn off separator parts or utensils, or when bronze fittings or bronze pumps are used). Copper, iron, and bronze from these sources dissolve in the cream, producing a tallowy

---

[2]Table 5.7 gives the composition and weight of the ingredients used in ice cream mix.

and metallic flavor during storage of the frozen cream. Storage rooms should be about $-10°F$, and the cream should be held no longer than 6 months. While the storing of frozen cream is ordinarily economical, the flavor of such cream after storage is never quite equal to that of good fresh cream. Rancid, fishy, oily, and tallowy flavors are likely to develop in frozen cream. Local regulations may or may not permit the use of cream containing added antioxidants.

When storing cream for use in ice cream, the addition before freezing of 10% by weight of cane sugar is desirable. This cream retains its flavor better, melts more quickly and with less fat separation, and produces a mix with higher whipping ability. However, the addition of sugar ties up additional capital in stored sugar. Moreover, if such cream happens to develop off-flavors there is increased difficulty in finding an outlet for it. Cream stored with 10% added sugar has improved keeping qualities.

Frozen cream may be used to provide all the cream needed in a mix providing the temperature of heating the cream before freezing exceeded 170°F and the copper content was low. Some recommend the use of about 60% frozen cream and 40% fresh cream.

Plastic cream is used to some extent in ice cream when a concentrated source of fat is desired. Plastic cream is essentially a very rich cream (80% fat) and is similar in consistency to butter at ordinary temperatures. It is prepared by separating cream of a lower fat content (25–35%) using a special separator bowl. The product is stored and handled commercially like butter. Mixes made with plastic cream as a source of fat may show some oiling off and possess slightly lower whipping properties, similar to mixes made with frozen cream, butter oil, or butter. Usage rates at levels providing all the fat in ice cream are feasible only when the very best quality plastic cream is available.

Unsalted butter (sweet butter) is next to sweet cream in importance as a source of fat. The advantages of butter are that it is a comparatively cheap source of fat, can be transported at low cost, can be stored for months with little deterioration in quality, and is nearly always available in fairly uniform quality. If the butter is of good quality, from 50 to 75% of the fat of the mix can be secured from this source. The unsalted butter should be of a grade that will score 92 or higher on the USDA grading system (scale 0–100) and preferably should be made from sweet cream. Off-flavors—ripened cream, neutralizer, stale, rancid, and tallowy, which are found in butter of low quality—will carry over directly into the mix.

Studies show that the use of butter in place of cream as a source of fat in ice cream mixes produces less desirable freezing properties; the differences are due to the presence of lecithin in the cream mixes.

Anhydrous milkfat (butter oil) is a relatively new source of fat for ice cream mix. The method of preparation involves heating cream or butter to a temperature of approximately 212°F to drive the water out and to precipitate the milk solids. Gravity separation and centrifugal methods of manufacture have also been outlined in recent literature on the technology of anhydrous milkfat.

Other ingredients providing fat include concentrated sweetened cream, special heat-treated milkfat, butter–sucrose and butter–sucrose–powder mix products, and dried cream.

Several papers have appeared in the literature on concentrated sweetened

Table 5.7. Ice Cream Ingredients—Approximate Composition, Weights per Gallon, and Density

Ingredient	Fat (%)	MSNF (%)	Sugar (%)	TS (%)	Moisture (%)	Weight per gallon (lb)	Density
Water	0.00	0.00	0.00	0.00	—	8.33	1.000
Skim Milk	0.00	8.60	0.00	8.60	—	8.63	1.036
Milk	3.00	8.33	0.00	11.33	—	8.60	1.032
	4.00	8.79	0.00	12.79	—	8.60	1.032
	5.00	9.10	0.00	14.10	—	8.60	1.032
Cream	18.00	7.31	0.00	25.31	—	8.45	1.014
	20.00	7.13	0.00	27.13	—	8.43	1.020
	25.00	6.68	0.00	31.68	—	8.39	1.007
	30.00	6.24	0.00	36.24	—	8.35	1.002
	35.00	5.69	0.00	40.69	—	8.31	0.997
	40.00	5.35	0.00	45.35	—	8.28	0.994
frozen[a]	50.00	4.45	0.00	54.95	—	8.20	0.984
plastic	80.00	1.80	0.00	81.80	—	7.95	0.954
Dried cream	65.00	34.34	0.00	99.34	0.65	—	—
Concentrated sweet cream	43.00	7.50	30.00	80.50	19.50	9.60	—
Butter, unsalted	82.50	0.50	0.00	83.00	18.05	7.92	0.951
Butter oil	99.00	0.00	0.00	99.00	1.00	7.50	0.900
Evaporated milk canned	8.00	20.00	0.00	28.00	—	8.90	1.068
bulk	10.00	23.00	0.00	33.00	—	9.20	1.044
Sweetened condensed whole milk	8.00	23.00	42.00	73.00	—	10.87	1.305
Condensed skim, unsweetened	0.00	32.00	0.00	32.00	—	9.40	1.128
Condensed skim, sweetened	0.50	30.00	42.00	72.00	—	11.00	1.321
Condensed skim milk	0.00	20.00	0.00	20.00	—	8.98	1.078

	Fat	MSNF	Sugar	Total solids	Other		Density
Condensed whole milk	0.00	27.00	0.00	27.00	—	9.25	1.110
	0.00	30.00	0.00	30.00	—	9.35	1.122
	8.00	22.00	0.00	30.00	—	8.99	1.079
	10.00	26.00	0.00	36.00	—	9.00	1.080
Condensed whole milk (blend)	19.00	21.00	0.00	40.00	—	8.90	1.068
Nonfat dry milk (skim milk powder)	0.00	97.00	0.00	97.00	—	—	—
Whole milk powder	26.00	72.00	0.00	98.00	—	—	—
Plain condensed whole milk	8.00	20.00	0.00	28.00	—	8.90	1.068
Anhydrous milkfat	99.90	0.00	0.00	99.90	0.10	—	—
Butter–powder mix	44.00	46.00	0.00	90.00	10.00	—	—
Butter–powder–sucrose mix	44.00	26.00	0.00	80.00	20.00	—	—
Dry buttermilk solids	5.00	91.00	0.00	96.00	—	—	—
Dry whey solids	0.00	93.00	0.00	93.00	—	—	—
Granulated sugar	0.00	0.00	100.00	100.00	—	7.50	0.900
Corn sugar	0.00	0.00	92.00	92.00	—	7.50	0.900
Invert sugar syrup	0.00	0.00	71.50	71.50	—	11.25	1.350
Corn syrup	0.00	0.00	82.00	82.00	—	11.98	1.438
30DE	0.00	—	—	79.45	—	11.81	1.417
36DE	0.00	—	—	79.86	—	11.81	1.417
42DE	0.00	—	—	80.30	—	11.81	1.417
high-fructose, 42	0.00	—	—	71.00	—	11.23	1.348
high-fructose, 55	0.00	—	—	77.00	—	11.55	1.386
high-fructose, 90	0.00	—	—	80.00	—	11.74	1.409
Honey	—	—	—	82.30	—	11.98	1.438
Maple syrup	—	—	—	68.00	—	11.14	1.337
Maple syrup	—	—	—	92.00	—	7.50	0.900
Dried egg yolk	58.00	0.00	0.00	98.00	—	—	—
Whole eggs	10.50	0.00	0.00	26.30	—	8.58	1.030
Cocoa powder	23.00	0.00	0.00	95.50	—	—	—
Chocolate liquor	49.00	0.00	0.00	94.00	—	—	—

aMay contain 10% sugar.

cream and its uses in ice cream. In one study concentrated sweetened cream prepared from milk was held 15 sec at 180°F, cooled to 130°F, and separated to obtain 76% fat. To 65.8 lb of this warm cream was added 8.5 lb of freshly prepared condensed skim milk containing 51.8% solids and 26 lb of sucrose. This blend was heated to 200°F for 15 sec, cooled to 170°F, and flashed into an unheated pan under a vacuum of 26 in., all in a continuous operation. Here it was held 1 hr, the vacuum broken, and the product packaged in plastic bags. Another study showed that concentrated sweetened cream as a source of fat in ice cream manufacture had better storage properties than did frozen cream or butter.

Butterfat mix products have been defined as a blend of butter or anhydrous milkfat with either sucrose alone or a blend of sucrose and MSNF. The butterfat mix products have been imported into the United States and distributed under a cost structure that has created extensive interest.

One study shows that the storage life of butterfat mix at 0°F is 9–12 months and the amount used to replace fresh cream varies with the user from less than 50 to 100%, with most plants using the product staying below the 50% level.

The composition of four types of butterfat mix products is as follows: the fat–sucrose blend with butter or with butter oil as the source of fat; and fat–sucrose–MSNF blend with butter or with butter oil as the source of fat. The effects of the butterfat mix blends on the properties of ice cream have been studied. Results indicate that some of the products examined are of poor quality and that butterfat mix blends must be of good quality if usage rate levels of 50% replacement of cream are to produce satisfactory results.

The use of special heat-treated milkfat (230–302°F) and high-melting-point anhydrous milkfat in the ice cream mix has been found to impart an acceptable flavor and desirable keeping qualities.

A small quantity of dry cream is manufactured in the United States and this product is used in ice cream only for special requirements.

Skim Milk and Buttermilk

Fresh skim milk should be used in the mix whenever available at reasonable prices, because it is a cheap source of MSNF. It should have a low acidity and a clean flavor. Skim milk when purchased should be bought on the basis of a definite MSNF content in order to guard against dilution with water. A hundred pounds of skim milk will normally contain about 8.7 lb MSNF.

When water is used in place of skim milk a larger portion of condensed skim milk or nonfat dry milk is necessary in order to supply the needed MSNF. Fresh spray process nonfat dry milk solids or fresh condensed skim milk may be successfully used under these conditions. Unless these products are of the best quality, this practice usually results in a slightly cooked or "serum solids" off-flavor in the finished ice cream.

Sweet cream buttermilk is obtained by churning cream that has not developed noticeable acidity, i.e., cream of the same quality as that used in ice cream or retail market cream. A larger supply of sweet cream buttermilk will be available when better methods of storage are developed and continuous churning is more widely practiced. Sweet cream buttermilk has beneficial effects on the whipping ability of the mix and contributes a richness of flavor. The use of sweet cream buttermilk, either as such or in condensed or powdered form, is especially desirable in ice cream of low fat content or in ice cream made with butter. Sweet cream buttermilk can supply nearly 20% of the MSNF of the mix; if a larger proportion is used, there is danger of a slight undesirable flavor. The fat content of condensed sweet cream buttermilk will be about 3–4% and should, of course, be considered in calculating the ice cream mix. The lecithin content of buttermilk ranges from 0.1 to 0.2%.

If a high-quality, good-flavored dry buttermilk is used, it can supply all the MSNF of the mix without affecting taste or texture. Ziemer *et al.* (1962) made a survey of commercial buttermilk powders that showed pronounced variations in fat, moisture content, and flavor. After less than 6 weeks of storage a majority of powders were unacceptable in flavor. Some powders retained good flavor quality for more than a year. In a comparison of mixes made of spray-dried buttermilk, condensed buttermilk, and nonfat dry milk it was found that fresh dry buttermilk could be used in ice cream without adding to or detracting from the flavor. No flavor difference could be attributed to heat-treatment of the fluid buttermilk (145–185°F), and no differences were noted in the ice creams that contained dried versus concentrated buttermilk as the source of solids.

Nonfat dry milk is a frequently used concentrated source of MSNF. There are three forms of nonfat dry milk on the market: spray process powder, drum-dried powder, and flakes, each containing over 90% MSNF. The spray process powders are more soluble than the drum-dried. The skim milk flakes have the advantage of not lumping when added to the mix. A good powder should be of fine flavor, light in color, free from darkened particles, fluffy, and easily soluble. A poor powder often is yellow in color and granular. Nonfat dry milk should be bought only in such quantities as can be used before the product develops off-flavors, and preferably should be kept in cold storage. Buying in large quantities and storing at room temperature as frequently practiced is unwise, because skim milk powders and flakes have a tendency to become stale and impart old or storage flavors to ice cream. Modern forms of nonfat dry milk are known as instant powders because of their ability to disperse easily and quickly in water without forming lumps.

It is recommended that the ice cream manufacturer specify extragrade powder for use in ice cream according to the specific grading regulations of the American Dry Milk Institute (1965). Extragrade powder will be of good quality with good storage qualities. Low, medium, and high heat-treated powder can be used in ice cream with good results. The desirable effects of medium and high heat-treated powders on mix properties, body and texture, and melting and storage characteristics of the finished product merit the consideration of the ice cream manufacturer in the development of the most effective formulation.

The use of MSNF in ice cream and related products has numerous advantages. It has excellent keeping qualities and refrigeration is not required. MSNF is hygroscopic and proper protection is necessary or it will absorb moisture. It has been found to keep best when kept in cool, dry storage and when packed in tight containers to prevent moisture absorption (Hall and

Hedrick 1966). MSNF may be successfully stored for 2 or 3 months under good conditions (Price and Whittier 1931). The use of MSNF provides an economical source of solids with low handling costs. It is a product of uniform composition and gives minimum variation in quality and composition of the finished ice cream. MSNF is always available and affords a constant source of milk solids to meet the needs of the ice cream manufacturer.

Considerable amounts of MSNF are being used currently in the manufacture of ice cream and other frozen dairy foods. Extensive studies have been reported in the literature showing that MSNF may be successfully used in the manufacture of very good quality ice cream (Arbuckle 1948, 1966; Braatz 1969; Dahle et al. 1931; Hall and Hedrick 1966; Hedrick et al. 1964; Price and Whittier 1931; Reid et al. 1940).

It has been shown that either low-heat or high-heat MSNF can be satisfactorily used as the sole source of MSNF in ice cream and ice milk (Hedrick et al. 1964).

Early work (Williams and Hall 1931) recommended the use of dry milk solids that had been preheated before drying at 181.4°F in preference to dry milk solids that had been preheated before drying to 145.4°F. A preference test showed that the majority of consumers preferred ice cream made from dry milk solids preheated to 181.4°F to ice cream containing condensed milk preheated to the same temperature. Results of more recent studies (Arbuckle 1969) of the use of low-, medium-, and high-heat MSNF conclude that the flavor characteristics of the ice cream from mixes in which low-heat MSNF was used were slightly more desirable than those made from high-heat MSNF. However, these results also indicate that ice cream from mixes in which high-heat MSNF was used was superior in mix whipping properties, body and texture characteristics, resistance to heat shock, and storage and melting properties. Valuable effects of the heat-treatment given MSNF in its processing are indicated in these observations.

MSNF may be used to supply all the nonfat solids, all the nonfat solids not supplied by the milk and cream, or only a part of the nonfat solids provided by the milk and cream. The amount of MSNF generally varies inversely with the fat content of the mix and ranges from 7.5 to 8% in an 18% fat ice cream mix to 14% in a 4% ice milk mix.

Powdered Whole Milk

Up to the present time, powdered whole milk has not been widely used in ice cream mix because off-flavors develop fairly rapidly in storage, even though Tracy (1945) stated that powdered whole milk was becoming available and that both powdered whole milk and powdered ice cream mix could be used successfully and advantageously by ice cream manufacturers.

Condensed Milks

Plain condensed skim milk is used more frequently than any of the other condensed-milk products. The keeping quality of condensed skim milk is only a little better than that of cream; hence, the product should be used while fresh and sweet. It should be shipped and stored under refrigeration. Condensed skim milk varies from 25–35% in MSNF.

Superheated condensed skim milk is made by heating the already condensed product to a high temperature, which increases the viscosity at ordinary temperature. Its use in ice cream improves whipping ability. The superheated product when used in ice cream should have that viscosity that will result in the best body, plasticity, and meltdown characteristics in the finished ice cream. It should be free from visible curd specks and not have a pronounced cooked flavor. Formerly, superheated condensed milk and skim milk were used quite extensively. Since superheated products cost more than plain condensed products and are not always of the desired uniformity, they are now used mostly by manufacturers who omit stabilizers.

Condensed whole-milk blend is perfectly satisfactory for use in ice cream. It has not been in general use in the past but more recently is being used extensively as an ingredient in the manufacture of ice cream. It is easily transported and handled in bulk form and for many plants supplies the main source of both fat and MSNF. Such a product is prepared to contain approximately 18–19% fat and 20–21% MSNF as specified by the ice cream manufacturer. Then the ice cream mix of the desired composition is readily composed by the addition of sugar and stabilizer.

Sweetened condensed whole milk or skim milk is sometimes used as a concentrated source of MSNF. The added sugar (40–44%) improves the keeping quality over that of plain condensed milk. The sweetened condensed milk is thick and viscous, and hence not so easily handled as the plain condensed. A defect in this milk is the tendency toward crystallization of the milk sugar (lactose) into large crystals. Sweetened condensed milk should be smooth in texture, never sandy. In judging the quality of a condensed-milk product, attention should be centered on flavor—a pronounced cooked flavor will show up in the finished ice cream. Condensed milk should also be free from excessive amounts of copper or iron. These taints will appear as a metallic flavor, which in storage may develop into a tallowy or oxidized fat flavor. The acidity test should also be applied to condensed milk products. When diluted so as to contain the same MSNF concentration as skim milk, the acidity should be approximately that of fresh skim milk (about 0.18%).

The effects of the use of concentrated milk products on the properties of ice cream have been reported by Tracy and Hahn (1938), who concluded that superheated condensed milk will result in mixes with higher viscosity, have better whipping properties, produce more resistant body and greater melting resistance in the finished ice cream, and that the flavor of the ice cream will be less desirable compared with that of ice cream made with condensed milk.

Whitaker and Hilker (1938) stated that any benefit caused by the superheated condensed milk is not the result of increased viscosity, but the effect of the higher heat-treatment on milk constituents.

Special Commercial Products

Special commercial products are sometimes used as constituents of ice cream mix. These products include sodium caseinate, delactosed milk products, modified MSNF, certain mineral salts, or a combination of some of these materials. The functions of these products vary, depending upon their composition and purpose. The products are designed mainly to improve whipping qualities, storage properties, resistance to heat shock, body and texture, to increase the solids content, or to adjust mix acidity.

Sodium caseinate is available for use in a nondesiccated and in a dry form. The amount of the nondesiccated product used ranges from 2.5 to 5% by weight of mix and 0.5 to 1.0% of the dehydrated product. These products must be free from excess alkali when used as ice cream ingredients. The use of sodium caseinate may produce a slight undesirable flavor in the finished ice cream, decrease the mix viscosity significantly, increase the mix acidity about 0.01% for each percentage of sodium caseinate used, improve the texture, and increase the rate of melting in the finished ice cream, but the greatest influence of sodium caseinate is in improving the whipping properties of the mix.

The manufacture and use of sodium caseinate in ice cream has been reported by Bird *et al.* (1935) and Arbuckle *et al.* (1944).

Low-lactose milk products have been used in high-solids ice cream either to replace a portion of the regular milk solids or to supplement the MSNF without the occurrence of sandiness during storage or without the usual lowered effect on the drawing temperature during the freezing process. Approximately 25% of the MSNF in a high-solids ice cream can be obtained from a low-lactose skim milk, or 10–12% when a dehydrated low-lactose product is used. The use of low-lactose products may increase the mix acidity as an increase in the mix protein content results from their use. There is also an increase in mix viscosity during storage and an improvement in texture and storage quality of the finished ice cream when delactosed products are used. There is little influence on whipping properties or rate of melting.

The preparation of low-lactose skim milk for use in ice cream has been described by Webb and Williams (1934) and Tracy and Corbett (1939). The former were able to increase the MSNF to 13% without occurrence of sandiness and with improved body and texture. The latter workers recommended the use of 9% regular milk solids and 4% low-lactose solids for superior flavor, body and texture, and storage properties.

MSNF products such as Nutrimix are used to increase the nonfat solids content 1–3.5% with improved body and texture and without the occurrence of sandiness. Such products may also be used to replace a portion of the regular MSNF. The use of special processed nonfat solids products reduces the acidity of the mix, but has little effect on the viscosity and whipping properties of the mix or the melting properties of the ice cream. The usual effect on flavor is desirable and the body, texture, and keeping qualities are improved by the use of the special processed nonfat milk solids.

The use of several of the special commercial products formerly used in ice cream is not now permitted by federal standards.

Evaporated milk differs from condensed milk in that it has received a sterilization heat-treatment and this process imparts a noticeable cooked and caramelized color, which is undesirable in most ice cream. Malted milk imparts a typical flavor, which limits its use.

Dry whey solids contain the nonfat solids portion of milk except the casein. The composition of whey solids is listed as fat, 1%; lactose, 72%; lactalbumin, 12%; minerals, 11%; moisture, 4%. This compares with fat, 1%; casein, 25%; lactose, 25%; lactalbumin, 11%; minerals, 8%; moisture, 3% for MSNF.

A review of laboratory and commercial experience (Leighton 1944; Potter and Williams 1949) shows that whenever MSNF is supplied in part or entirely in dry form to make ice cream, dry whey can be used to replace it up to a point where the lactose:water ratio of the ice cream mix is approximately 10.4:100. In most mixes this is about 25% of the MSNF or 3% of the total mix weight. The use of vegetable gum stabilizer helps prevent sandiness and when extragrade whey powder is used at these levels, the flavor is satisfactory. Approximately 25% of the MSNF in the mix could be provided by whey solids without objectionable effects on the flavor and with improved body and whipping quality at a reduced cost. The approximate composition of nonfat whey solids is 13.4% protein (lactalbumin), 76.1% lactose, and 10.5% mineral salts. This compares with 35.8% protein (approximately 27.1% casein and 8.7% lactalbumin), 54.4% lactose, and 9.8% mineral salts for MSNF.

Other sources of MSNF are not used very extensively in ice cream, but they may serve valuable needs under special conditions.

Dried ice cream mix is available and may be reconstituted by adding 5 parts of water to 3 parts of the dried mix. It may be frozen immediately after reconstitution with good results.

Results of Potter and Williams (1949) indicate that the composition (%) of dried ice cream mix should be within the following range:

Butterfat:	27–30
MSNF:	27–28
Sugar:	39.5–44
Stabilizer:	0.6–1
Moisture:	<3

A reconstituted ice cream mix testing 10.94% butterfat, 10.56% MSNF, 15.09% sugar, 0.38% stabilizer, and 63.03% water may be obtained from a dried mix of the following composition, when it is reconstituted at the ratio of 1 part of dried mix to 1.65 parts of water:

Butterfat:	29.0
MSNF:	28.0
Sugar:	40.0
Stabilizer:	1.0
Moisture:	2.0

Mineral Salts

Mineral salts are used as an ingredient of ice cream mix for the purpose of improving the properties of the mix and the characteristics of the finished product. These salts are used in small amounts and have many and varied effects. They may improve the appearance, affect the gloss, dryness, or stiffness of soft-serve products, or influence creaminess, handling properties, mix stability, flow through processing equipment, whipping properties, storage

Table 5.8. Approximate Composition (%) of Products That Provide MSNF
for Ice Cream

Product	Water	Fat	Protein	Lactose	Sucrose	Ash
Evaporated milk	73.00	8.30	7.50	9.70		1.40
Plain condensed milk	70.00	8.50	7.80	11.90		1.80
Skim milk	90.5	0.1	3.60	5.10		0.70
Condensed skim milk	71.00	0.50	8.80	12.70		2.00
Sweetened condensed whole milk	27.47	9.28	7.42	13.35	40.60	1.88
Sweetened condensed skim milk	29.00	0.06	10.32	15.60	42.27	2.25
Condensed buttermilk	72.00	1.95	10.61	13.01		3.33
Condensed whey	48.10	2.40	7.00	38.50		4.00
Sweetened condensed whey	28.50	1.70	5.00	28.50	38.00	2.80
Dried whole milk	2.00	27.00	26.50	38.00		6.05
Nonfat dry milk	3.23	0.88	36.89	50.52		8.15
Dry buttermilk	3.90	4.68	35.88	47.84		7.80
Dry whey	6.10	0.90	12.50	72.25		8.90
Dried malted milk	3.29	7.55	13.19	72.40[a]		3.66
Whey	93.2	0.30	0.90	5.10		0.50
Sodium caseinate	4.0	1.50	94.00			4.00

[a]Lactose, maltose, dextrin.

properties, resistance to heat shock, and the flavor, body, texture, and appearance of the finished products.

Table 5.8 gives the approximate composition of the main sources of MSNF in ice cream.

The relationship between salt balance and stability to heat coagulation of the milk components has long been realized. The importance of the effects of the mineral salts has been recognized in the acceptance of the mineral salts as optional ingredients in the frozen-dessert standards and specifications. The mineral salts recognized as optional ingredients for frozen desserts are listed in Table 5.1. A review of the effects of the various salts is given in Chapter 4.

Calcium sulfate is included as an optional ingredient and is typical of specific effects salts may produce. Calcium sulfate's rate of use is 0.08–0.16%, and should be added to the mix before the pasteurization process. The use of calcium sulfate increases the acidity of the mix, produces a dry, stiff ice cream from the freezer, and reduces the rate of melting but has little effect on other properties of the mix or finished ice cream, which may be influenced by the kind of stabilizer used.

SOURCES OF SWEETENER SOLIDS

Many kinds of sweeteners are used in ice cream (see Table 5.9). They include cane and beet sugar, corn sweeteners, maple sugar, honey, invert sugar, fructose, molasses, malt syrup, brown sugar, lactose, and refiners syrup.

From 25 to 50% or more of cane or beet sugar may be replaced by corn sugar with good results. The use of a combination or blend of sugars in either dry or liquid form is a popular practice—such blends are usually 70% sucrose and 30% corn sweetener. The desired sugar concentration in ice cream is 15–16% on a sucrose basis. The different kinds of sugar do not produce equal sweetening effects although sweetness can neither be exactly defined nor measured. Leighton (1942) stated that the zone of satisfactory sweetness in ice cream was 13–16% sugar content, and that sweetness in ice cream is dependent upon the concentration of sugar in the water of the mix and that decreasing the water in the mix is equivalent to increasing sweetness. He further stated that sugars are important as an ingredient in ice cream other than for their sweetness because of the physical properties of the sugars and their effect upon the freezing point of the mix. In addition, they depress the freezing point of the mix, produce a thinner mix with a slower whipping rate, and produce an ice cream with a smoother body and texture with faster melting qualities. Sugar blends may be expected to affect mix and finished product qualities in accordance with the proportion of the kind of sugars in the blend.

Relative Sweetness

Dahlberg and Penczek (1941) studied the relative sweetness of sugars, the effects of one sugar on another, their concentration, and temperature. Since there is no chemical test for sweetness there is not complete agreement on the relative sweetness value of the various sweetners. An approximate relative sweetening value of sugars and other substances (using sucrose as a basis with a value of 100) is given in Table 5.10.

Effect on Freezing Point

Sugars do not dissociate in solution and the freezing point of their solution can be computed by the known concentration of the solution and the molecular weight (see Fig. 5.2). With given weights and volumes of solvent, the effect on the freezing point will be inversely proportional to the molecular weight, i.e., the higher molecular weights will cause the least lowering of freezing point, while the sugars with the low molecular weights will cause the greatest lowering of freezing point. The molecular weights of some sweetener solids are given in Table 5.11.

Tharp (1982) gave formulas for calculating the freezing point based on the differences in molecular weight of carbohydrates and other dissolved material. He stated that the freezing of any multicomponent system (such as a frozen-dessert mix) is somewhat more complex than the simplicity of the calculations may suggest.

For the years 1950, 1960, 1972, 1975, 1980, and 1981, Tharp gave the following data for the freezing point of ice cream (based on typical mix compositions): 27.70, 27.00, 27.17, 27.07, 26.47, and 25.77°F, respectively. It appears that changes in the amount of sweetener solids included in the mix formulation were mainly responsible for the freezing-point variation.

Table 5.9. Sources of Sweetening Agents in Ice Cream

Product	Physical appearance	Type of sugar	Sugar (%)	Amount equal to 1 lb sucrose (lb)	Maximum total sugar supplied (%)	TS (%)	Weight per gallon (lb)
Sugar							
granulated sugar	Dry crystals	Sucrose	100	1.00	100	100	7.5
dextrose	Dry crystals	Glucose	80	1.25	35	92	—
Dried corn syrup solids	Dry crystals	Dextrose, maltose	47	2.10	35	96.5	—
Liquid sugar	Liquid	Sucrose	67	1.50	100	67.0	11.1
(80–20 blend)[a]	Liquid	Sucrose, dextrose	68	1.58	100	68.0	11.2
Sucrose 67 Brix, corn syrup 42 DE	Liquid	Dextrose, maltose	67	1.50	35	83.0	9.5
Corn syrup[b]							
low-conversion, 36 DE	Liquid	Dextrose, maltose	52	1.90	25–50	80	11.8
regular-conversion, 42 DE	Liquid	Dextrose, maltose	60	1.66	25–50	80.0	11.8
intermediate-conversion, 52 DE	Liquid	Dextrose, maltose	68	1.47	25–50	81.0	11.8

high-conversion, 62 DE	Liquid	Dextrose, maltose	80	1.25	25–50	81.0	11.8
High maltose	Liquid	Maltose, dextrose	63	2.00	25–50	80.0	11.8
Invert sugar syrup[c]	Liquid	Dextrose, levulose	95	1.05	33	74	11.5
Honey[e]	Liquid	Dextrose, levulose, sucrose	75	1.40	30[d]	—	—
High fructose							
42	Liquid	Dextrose, fructose	71	1.40	25–30	71	11.23
55	Liquid	Dextrose, fructose	77	1.30	50	77	11.55
90	Liquid	Dextrose, fructose	80	0.70	50–100[f]	80	11.74
55 and 36 DE (1–1)	Liquid	Dextrose, fructose	78	1.30	78–100[g]	78	11.77

[a] The usual liquid sugar (67%) employed by ice cream makers.
[b] The usual commercial syrup of 43° Baumé.
[c] Assuming 95% complete inversion with a 74% sucrose solution.
[d] Assuming a mild-flavored honey, less if strong flavored.
[e] Higher percentage may lower freezing point.
[f] Low-calorie frozen dessert.
[g] Economy brand.
Note: Approximate data to serve as a guide for calculating mixes. DE stands for dextrose equivalent, which is a measure of reducing-sugar content calculated as dextrose and expressed as a percentage of the total dry substance. For pure dextrose, DE = 100. Corn syrups and corn syrup solids are available in the DE range 28–62.

Table 5.10. Relative Sweetness of Ice Cream Ingredients[a]

Fructose	173
Invert sugar (glucose and fructose)	127
Sucrose	100
Glucose (dextrose)	74
Corn syrup	
high-conversion (62 DE)	68
medium-conversion (52 DE)	58
low-conversion (42 DE)	50
low-conversion (32 DE)	42
Xylose (wood sugar)	40
Galactose	32
Maltose	32
Rhamnose	32
Lactose	16
Saccharin	200–700
Dulcin	70–250
Hexahydric alcohol	50
Sucaryl	30–50

[a]Sucrose as basis, 100.

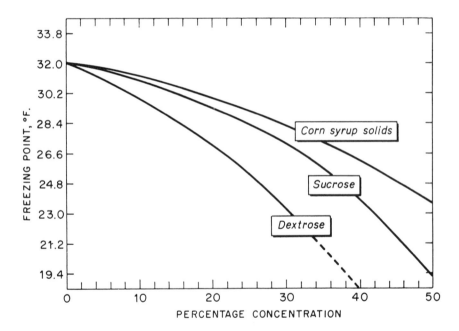

Fig. 5.2. Freezing point variation with differing sugar concentrations. Courtesy of American Maize Products Co.

Table. 5.11.   Approximate Molecular Weights
of Sweetener Solids

Sucrose	342
Lactose	342
Maltose	342
Dextrose	180
Fructose	180
Fructose-90	182
Fructose-55	185
Fructose-42	190
Corn syrup	
enzyme-converted	258
62 DE	298
52 DE	360
42 DE	428
36 DE	472
32 DE	540
28 DE	568

Sucrose

Sucrose, commonly known as granulated sugar, comes from cane sugar and beet sugar and is the most widely accepted source of sugar. Cane sugar contains approximately 99.9% TS. It is highly soluble and has a specific gravity of 1.595. Although sucrose depresses the freezing point, its concentration in ice cream is limited only by its sweetening effect (see Fig. 5.2). It has been found that a 2% increase in sucrose content of a mix lowers the freezing point approximately 0.4°F. Sucrose may be used as the sole source of added sweetener solids in ice cream with excellent results. It is not satisfactory as the only source of sugar in ices and sherbets since it may crystallize out at the surface. This defect in ices and sherbets can be avoided by using 1 part of dextrose to 3.5 parts of sucrose. Sucrose is a disaccharide, and when hydrolyzed a molecule of sucrose combines with a molecule of water and breaks down into glucose and fructose (levulose). This sugar may be used in a dry or liquid form (liquid sugar contains approximately 67% sucrose).

Corn Sweeteners

Corn sweeteners of three major types are available for use in ice cream: refined corn sugar (dextrose), a dry crystalline product; dried corn syrup (or corn syrup solids); and liquid corn syrup. The use of corn syrup solids in ice cream has been reported by Corbett and Tracy (1939), Corn Industries Research Foundation (1958), Drusendahl (1963), Nieman (1960), Tharp (1961), Trempel (1962), Tracy and Edman (1940), and Wolfmeyer (1963).

Corn syrup solids or corn syrup impart a firmer and heavier body to the finished ice cream, provide an economical source of solids, and improve the shelf life of the finished products. The sweetness comes from dextrose, i.e., D-glucose. Commercially, the term glucose is incorrectly applied to a variety of products that contain some dextrose. A combination of corn syrup and corn syrup solids is used with sucrose as a sweetening agent for ice cream because it is cheaper, improves body, texture, and flavor characteristics, and extends the shelf-life of the finished product.

Many good sugar blends are now available. There has been much interest in blends of the low-conversion corn syrup solids products, because they help increase solids and maintain product properties and sweetness. Similarly, blends of sucrose with medium- or high-conversion corn syrup solids have also been used advantageously. High-fructose corn syrups (42, 55, and 90%) have an important role as an ice cream sweetener.

The values sometimes used as a guide in estimating the freezing point depression for these products are given in Table 5.12.

Dextrose, or refined corn sugar, is a white crystalline or granular sugar obtained by the hydrolysis of corn starch. Dextrose is a monosaccharide, containing approximately 99.8% sugar solids. Mack (1927) recommended the use of dextrose in high-fat mixes for more desirable body, texture, and melting characteristics. Dextrose is now quite extensively used in ice cream and is considered necessary in sherbets and ices to inhibit the crystallization of sucrose on the surface. Since it is only about 80% as sweet as sucrose, 1.25 lb of dextrose is needed to obtain the sweetening effect of 1.0 lb of sucrose. Dextrose lowers the freezing point more than does sucrose because its molecular weight is lower. This effect on the freezing point limits the amount of dextrose that can be used to about 25% of the total desired sugar. Usually dextrose is more economical than sucrose as a source of sweetness. Dextrose has a slightly greater tendency than cane or beet sugar to become lumpy when exposed to or stored in slightly moist air.

Dried corn syrup solids are produced by dehydration of corn syrup and are available in two forms—a white powder and a coarser granular material. The

Table 5.12.   Guide to Estimating the Freezing Point Depression
of Various Sweeteners[a]

Sweetener	Sucrose equivalence value (SE)	Freezing point equivalence factor
Sucrose	100	1.00
Lactose	100	1.00
Maltose	100	1.00
Dextrose	180	0.55
Fructose	180	0.55
90%	187	0.53
55%	185	0.54
42%	180	0.55
62 DE	114	0.58
52 DE	95	1.05
42 DE	79	1.27
36 DE	72	1.39
32 DE	63	1.59
28 DE	58	1.67
Dextrin (C18–C40)	67	1.47

[a] The sucrose equivalence value is based on the molecular weight of sugar. The freezing point equivalence factor for freezing point depression of a sweetener is based on the molecular weight relative to that of sucrose. The percentage of the sweetener is multiplied by the appropriate freezing point equivalence factor to give the freezing point depression.

chemical composition of corn syrup solids is identical with that of the syrup from which they were made (see Table 5.13). They contain the sugars dextrose and maltose together with dextrine (prosugar), but usually contain no starch. They are white granular solids and about equal to cane sugar in their tendency to become lumpy when exposed to moist air. They usually have been more economical than cane sugar, but because of their lower sweetening effect it requires about 2.1 lb of Frodex or corn syrup solids to produce the sweetness obtained from 1.0 lb of sucrose. The dextrins they contain actually raise the freezing point slightly. These dextrins also increase the total solids of the mix and supply some stabilizing effect against coarseness. The effect on the freezing point and smoothness seems to give corn syrup solids an advantage over dextrose not only in sherbets and ices but also in ice creams of low TS concentration. Usually not more than 25–35% of the total sweetener is supplied by corn syrup solids.

Corn syrup, frequently incorrectly called "glucose," is made either by acid hydrolysis or by enzyme hydrolysis of corn starch. It contains no sucrose, but does contain a variable amount of dextrose and maltose with some impurities depending upon the degree of refining used in its manufacture. It may be considered as a source of dextrose. While its sugar content and also TS content vary considerably, it is usually safe to assume that 1.5 lb of corn syrup will replace 1.0 lb of sucrose. The effect on the freezing point is similar to that of corn syrup solids.

The four major types of corn syrups used in ice cream based on degree of conversion are (1) low-conversion, 28–38 DE; (2) regular-conversion, 38–48 DE; (3) intermediate-conversion, 48–58 DE; and (4) high-conversion 58–68 DE. The high-conversion syrups are further classified as acid conversion and acid enzyme syrups, depending on the method of manufacture.

Other Sweeteners

A maltose syrup containing approximately 45% maltose has been introduced for use in ice cream manufacture. It is bland in flavor and is sweeter than the lower-DE syrups.

Malt syrup may contain approximately 70% maltose. Dried maltose syrup, malt syrup, or malt extract, with properties similar to those imparted by maltose, may be used. Malt products carry a typical malt flavor and may impart it to ice cream depending on usage rates.

Maple and Brown Sugars

Maple sugar and brown sugar (which is raw or muscovado sugar obtained from the juice of sugar cane by evaporation and draining of molasses) contain characteristic flavoring materials, which limits their use in ice cream. For example, only 6% of maple sugar in the mix will produce a good maple flavor. Furthermore, these sugars are usually more expensive than other sources of sweeteners.

Both maple sugar and brown sugar are very high in sucrose. Maple sugar

Table 5.13. Approximate Carbohydrate Composition of Corn Syrup and Corn Syrup Solids (Dry-Substance Basis)[a]

	Saccharides (%)							
	Mono-	Di-	Tri-	Tetra-	Penta-	Hexa-	Hepta-	Higher
Low (32 DE)	11.5	10.2	9.2	8.6	7.5	6.2	5.3	41.5
Regular (42 DE)	18.5	13.9	11.6	9.9	8.4	6.6	5.7	25.2
Intermediate 52 (DE)	27.5	17.2	13.1	9.9	7.7	5.7	4.7	14.2
High-conversion (62 DE) (acid or enzyme)	38.8	28.1	13.7	4.1	4.5	2.6	—	8.2[b]
High-fructose								
42 DE	94	—	—	—	—	—	—	6.0
55 DE	97	—	—	—	—	—	—	3.0
90 DE	99	—	—	—	—	—	—	1.0

[a]Courtesy, Corn Industries Research Foundation, Inc.
[b]Includes heptasaccharides.

has about 10% moisture, 86% sucrose, and 4% invert sugar; whereas maple syrup has about 45% moisture, 52% sucrose, and 3% invert sugar.

Honey

Honey is composed of about 74.5% invert sugar, 17.5% moisture, 2% sucrose, 2% dextrin, and 3.8% miscellaneous matter. It is used in ice cream principally to make honey-flavored ice cream, at the rate of 9 lb honey and 8 lb sucrose to produce the desired sweetness and flavor. Honey may not blend well with other flavoring, and the addition of other flavors to honey ice cream is not recommended. Tracy *et al.* (1930) found considerable variation in the color and composition of honey, depending on the source of the bees' food.

Fructose is a white crystalline powder (DL-1 levulose) produced in commercial quantities. It was approved as an ice cream sweetener in the 1970s. Its empirical formula is $C_6H_{12}O_6$, with a molecular weight of about 180. It seems to have potential as a sweetener in dietetic ice cream, because of the high relative sweetness value. Fructose gained stature as a safe and suitable ingredient in the mid-1970s. At that time its cost was $0.70–0.75/lb, but its production cost has dropped markedly since that time.

Saccharin, the first nonnutritive sweetener to be used commercially, is not a sugar, but a product derived from coal tar. It has a sweetening effect up to 550 times that of sucrose. However, its use has been drastically reduced because it has been linked to the occurrence of cancer in laboratory animals. The status of nonnutritive sweeteners has changed greatly within the past few years, since they have been in the group of dietetic or dietary frozen desserts. It is generally recognized that a dietetic or dietary frozen dessert is prepared from the same ingredients and in the same manner as ice cream, ice milk, or nonfrozen dairy desserts except that the optional sweetening ingredients are replaced entirely by a low-caloric or noncaloric sweetening agent.

SUGAR-SAVING SUGGESTIONS

In times of sugar shortage the following suggestions should be helpful to the ice cream manufacturer in stretching an allotment of cane and beet sugar:

1. Use more of other sources of sugar such as corn sugar and corn syrup solids. As already noted, these products can be used to replace as much as 25–35% of the sugar required in the formula. Many ice cream makers are coming to believe that a finer quality of ice cream is produced when part of the sucrose is replaced by corn syrup solids. Maple sugar, maple syrup, honey, and sorghum, when available and not too high priced, can also take the place of a limited amount of cane or beet sugar in the mix.

2. Reduce the sugar content in the ice cream by replacing part of it with milk solids. Research carried on by the USDA revealed the fact that sweetness of ice cream depends upon the concentration of sugar in the water of the mix. Therefore, if part of the free-water content of the mix is absorbed by the addition of milk solids, there will be less volume of water to dissolve the sugar,

and this higher concentration will taste sweeter. It was found that a saving of as much as 20% of sugar can be made without lowering the degree of sweetness of the ice cream.

3. Invert up to 35% of the cane or beet sugar required in the mix. Since invert sugar tastes sweeter, its use in time of sugar scarcity is recommended even though some additional labor and expense is involved in the inversion process.

Syrups

Sugars in the form of syrups may also be used. This form of sweetener is coming into general use as liquid sugar products, because of their favorable handling and price advantages. These products sometimes contain two or more sugars. Sucrose can be purchased as a liquid product containing 67% sucrose solids, and blends of sucrose with corn sweeteners are available in various combinations.

The TS concentration of sucrose syrups is usually measured by "degree Brix," which assumes all the solids to be sucrose. This is a safe assumption for practical purposes. Corn syrup, and many others, are often labeled with a Baumé reading. This reading is based on the specific gravity of the syrup and therefore is also a measure of the TS concentration.[3] However, it does not indicate the kind or amounts of the various sugars and dextrins present in the syrup. Baumé and Brix are not the same (see Table 5.14). Baumé readings must be converted into specific gravity terms before the TS concentration can be calculated (see Table 5.15).

Baumé readings and percentage total solids should not be called "sweetness" or "percent sweet" and should not be confused with the sweetening effect, which depends upon the kinds and concentration of sugar present.

Blended syrups are used in the manufacture of ice cream in many areas. A typical commercial blend is one containing 70% sucrose (66.5°Brix) and 30% corn syrup. This blend has approximately 70% solids.

Refiners' Syrup or Liquid Sugar

Refiners' Syrup and liquid sugar are trade designations for the colorless sucrose syrup used by ice cream manufacturers. As yet, deliveries of liquid sugar are made only in tank cars and tank trucks, and so its use has been restricted to ice cream manufacturers having facilities for this type of delivery.

Hydrolyzed Cereal Solids

Hydrolyzed cereal solids is a newer food grade ingredient that increases the solids but adds little sweetness or flavor and has little effect on the freezing

---

[3]Specific gravity is the ratio of the density of a liquid compared to the density of water at 39°. It is given by $145/(145 - d)$, where d is the Baumé hydrometer reading at 68°F.

Table 5.14. Relation of Baumé Reading to Brix Reading (Sucrose Syrup)

Degrees Baumé	Degrees Brix	Weight (lb/gal)	Sugar (lb/gal)	Water[a] (lb/gal)
33.0	61.0	10.78	6.58	4.20
33.5	62.0	10.83	6.71	4.12
34.0	63.0	10.88	6.85	4.03
34.5	63.9	10.92	6.98	3.94
35.0	64.9	10.97	7.12	3.85
35.5	65.9	11.02	7.26	3.76
36.0	66.9	11.07	7.41	3.66
36.5	67.9	11.13	7.56	3.57
37.0	68.9	11.18	7.70	3.48
37.5	68.9	11.23	7.85	3.38
38.0	70.9	11.28	8.00	3.28
38.5	71.9	11.33	8.15	3.18
39.0	72 9	11.39	8.30	3.09
39.5	73.9	11.44	8.45	2.99
40.0	74.9	11.49	8.61	2.88

[a]One U.S. gallon of water at 68°F. weighs 8.322 lb.

Table 5.15. Approximate Physical Constants of Corn Syrups

Baumé	Specific gravity	Solids (%)	Weight (lb/gal)	Solids (lb/gal)
Low-conversion corn syrup—32 DE				
42	1.4049	77.64	11.700	9.084
43	1.4184	79.59	11.813	9.402
44	1.4322	81.53	11.928	9.725
45	1.4463	83.51	12.045	10.059
46	1.4605	85.49	12.163	10.389
Regular-conversion corn syrup—42 DE				
42	1.4049	78.30	11.700	9.161
43	1.4184	80.27	11.813	9.482
44	1.4322	82.25	11.928	9.811
45	1.4463	84.25	12.045	10.148
46	1.4605	86.26	12.163	10.492
Intermediate-conversion corn syrup—52 DE				
42	1.4049	78.94	11.700	9.236
43	1.4184	80.94	11.813	9.561
44	1.4322	82.96	11.928	9.895
45	1.4463	84.98	12.045	10.236
46	1.4605	87.03	12.163	10.586
High-conversion corn syrup—62 DE				
42	1.4049	79.59	11.700	9.312
43	1.4184	81.62	11.813	9.642
44	1.4322	83.67	11.928	9.980
45	1.4463	85.72	12.045	10.325
46	1.4605	87.80	12.163	10.679

point. It may be used at the rate of 2–5% of the mix for body-building properties.

Analysis shows that it contains a maximum of 5% moisture, has a DE of 10–20, and a pH of 4.5–5.5. The carbohydrate of the 10–13 DE product consists of 1% dextrose, 4% disaccharide, 5% trisaccharide, 4% tetrasaccharide, 4% pentasaccharide, and 82% hexasaccharide and above.

Invert Sugar

Invert sugar is a mixture of equal parts of glucose and fructose resulting from the hydrolysis of sucrose and is generally obtained in the form of a syrup. It is sweeter than sucrose and the increased sweetness obtained by hydrolyzing a given weight of sucrose is sufficient to justify the inversion process at a time of sugar scarcity. Even though this invert sugar syrup contains from 25 to 30% water, 1 lb of invert sugar syrup will produce almost as much sweetening as 1 lb of sucrose. However, it is similar to dextrose in depressing the freezing point and therefore should be used to supply not more than 35% of the total sugar in the mix.

Invert sugar may be prepared by the following procedure: Heat 26 lb of water to 180°F and add 74 lb of sucrose slowly, to avoid having much undissolved sugar present at any one time. When the syrup is at 180°F shut off the heat and add 36.3 ml hydrochloric acid (40%, sp. gr. 1.20) with suitable stirring to distribute it evenly. There will be a temperature rise due to the chemical action. After the acid has acted 15 min, cool promptly. When the temperature is down to about 140°F, add sodium bicarbonate at the rate of 1-1/3 oz/100 lb of syrup to neutralize the acid and then continue cooling. This procedure will give approximately 95% complete inversion (Sommer 1951; Coulter and Thomas 1943).

Lactose

Lactose, the sugar that is found only in milk, is not as sweet as sucrose and is much less soluble. When the water portion of the mix contains as much as 9% lactose, the lactose may separate out in crystals large enough to be discernible and produce an undesirable sandy feel in the mouth. This property definitely limits the concentration of lactose to be used in ice cream. The source of lactose is the MSNF of dairy products, and about 54% of these solids is lactose. Therefore, the maximum concentration of lactose that can be safely used also establishes the maximum concentration of MSNF.

This maximum concentration of MSNF to avoid sandiness varies somewhat with conditions under which ice cream is produced and stored. For instance, if ice cream is frozen at the higher temperatures generally prevailing in batch freezers, if excessive amounts of corn syrup solids are used in the mix, if there is much fluctuation in storage temperatures, and if the ice cream is likely to be held in the customer's cabinet for longer periods (14 days or more) before it is consumed, such ice cream may be considered as being subjected to rather severe conditions and any or all of these unfavorable factors are likely to produce sandiness. Where such conditions have to be met, experiments have proved that the maximum concentration of lactose (and therefore of MSNF) that can safely be used is less than for ice cream that is produced and stored under more favorable conditions.

The ratio of fat to MSNF for the proper blend under practical use was given in Table 4.1. The properties of the formulated mix should be such that the mix has the proper viscosity, stability, and handling properties. The finished ice cream should meet the conditions that prevail in the plant where it is to be produced. Properties of various sweetness are given in Table 5.9.

SOURCES OF EGG YOLK SOLIDS

Fresh eggs are seldom used in ice cream except in rich ice creams, such as puddings. The cost of fresh eggs is generally such that they can be economically used only in ice cream retailing at higher than average prices.

The use of egg yolk solids produces the following beneficial effects:

- Increased rate of whipping, particularly for slow whipping mixes.
- Firmer ice cream at a given drawing temperature.
- Less change in percentage overrun while unloading the freezer.
- Improved appearance while ice cream is melting.
- Slightly improved texture.
- Increased food value.

The disadvantages are the cost of the egg yolks and the fact that frequently they may be slightly off-flavored.

Frozen and powdered egg yolk are used by many ice cream makers because the egg yolk solids improve the whipping ability of the mix. Usually not more than 0.5% of egg yolk solids in the mix is needed for this purpose. Egg yolk solids are especially desirable in mixes in which butter or butter oil is used as a main source of fat. Investigations have shown that egg yolks improve the rate of whipping more if they are sweetened with 10% sugar before they are frozen.

It is necessary to use egg products in custard-type ice cream and the amount is usually equivalent to the yolks from 4–5 doz eggs per 100 lb of mix: 1 doz eggs yields approximately 1.2 lb edible portion or 0.5 lb of yolks, 1 lb of dried yolks requires approximately 4 oz of eggs (see Table 5.16). The manufacturer of

Table 5.16. Approximate Data on Egg Products to Serve as a Guide in Calculating Mixes

Egg product	Weight (lb/dozen)	Eggs/lb of egg product	Egg yolk solids (%)	Egg fat (%)	TS (%)
Fresh eggs (edible portion)	1.17	10.0 to 10.6	20.0	10.5	26.3
Egg yolk	0.50	24	50.5	33.3	50.5
Egg white	0.67	18	—	0.2	13.8
Dried whole egg	0.33	36	55.0	40.0	94.0
Dried egg yolk	0.25	48	94.0	62.5	94.0
Dried egg white	0.083	144	—	1.4	96.0

ice cream can justify the use of egg products from the standpoint of quality improvement and improved handling properties in mixes made from butter and nonfat dry milk solids, regardless of whether the mix is frozen by a continuous or batch freezer. The use of eggs also improves mixes made of fluid dairy products when a batch freezer is used. The value of using eggs under other conditions is more questionable and must be justified by the policies of the individual plant.

Frieschknect (1945) reported that egg solids give smoothness, improved whipping properties, increased quality and food value, and resistance to melting. He reported results of experiments using approximately 0.2, 0.4, 1.3, and 2.1% and concluded that eggs could be used at the rates of 0.5–1.5%. Masurovsky (1945) stated that in American-type ice cream about 0.5% egg solids are used.

Arbuckle (1948) studied the use of egg solids in ice cream and concluded that at least 0.5% egg yolk solids produced desirable results. Egg whites were used as a source of solids at the rate of 0.5% and found to have little effect on mix and finished-product properties. The milk solids were replaced with whole-egg solids by Arbuckle (1969) in the successful formulation of a parevine-type frozen dessert.

FOOD ADDITIVES

If a substance is found by the FDA to be safe for its intended use in a food product, it is put into the generally recognized as safe (GRAS) category. Use limits and restrictions are also specified for such substances (see Chapter 22).

Flavorings, stabilizers, emulsifiers, sweeteners, and acid materials are some of the substances classified as additives for ice cream. Approximately 150 natural flavorings are classed as GRAS and about 650 artificial flavors are being considered. A survey reported by Hall and Oser (1970) includes over 70 substances and the usage rate (ppm) as used in ice cream flavors.

New products are continually being considered for the GRAS list, and for this reason it is not possible to give a complete list of food additives used in ice cream at this time.

Hall (1971) made a comprehensive analysis of the reasons for the GRAS list review and stated that by law any ingredient is a food additive and must be covered by a food additive regulation unless it is generally recognized as safe under the conditions of its intended use. He states that the reasons for review are as follows:

- The information on which the original GRAS determinations were made might now be outdated.
- Conditions of use have changed.
- New data on toxicity and metabolism are available.
- Nearly 300 substances have been dropped from use, and the usage of others has shifted to replace them.
- Some new materials are in use.

FUNCTIONAL INGREDIENTS

Advances in biotechnology have introduced many new ingredients that will influence the formulation and composition of frozen dessert products of the future.

Among these are whole milk retentate, lactose-reduced dairy products, whey protein concentrate, modified whey solids, low-calorie fats, sucrose fatty acid polyesters (SPE), bulking agents, polydextrose, cellulose, malto dextrins, aspertame, and other high-intensity sweeteners. The use of these ingredients in combination and with conventional ingredients may be expected to influence product development trends.

6
Stabilizers and Emulsifiers

In 1915 Frandsen used the word *stabilizer* to designate a group of substances that at that time were generally referred to as holders, colloids, binders, and fillers (Frandsen and Markham 1915). The primary purposes of using stabilizers in ice cream are to produce smoothness in body and texture, to retard or reduce ice crystal growth during storage, and to provide uniformity of product and resistance to melting. Stabilizers function through their ability either to form gel structures in water or to combine with water as water of hydration.

An emulsifier is a substance that will produce an emulsion of two liquids that do not naturally mix. The function of an emulsifying agent in the manufacture of ice cream lies mainly in improving the whipping quality of the mix, producing a smooth texture, giving a dry stiff product at the time it is drawn from the freezer, and obtaining more control during the various manufacturing processes.

Excellent ice cream can be made (and considerable amounts are made) without the use of a stabilizer or emulsifier. Since milk and milk products contain natural stabilizing and emulsifying materials (milk protein, fat, lecithin, phosphates, and citrates) mixes of certain composition and processing treatment may be stabilized by the effect of these natural materials.

THE USE OF STABILIZERS

It is known that the water in ice cream is never completely frozen. When the temperature rises some of the ice crystals melt; conversely, when temperatures drop more water is refrozen into ice crystals. This fluctuation in temperature and slow freezing results in texture changes. Stabilizers absorb or hold some of the water freed by melting, thereby preventing the formation of large ice crystals if refreezing occurs.

The amount and type of stabilizer needed in ice cream varies with the conditions; the composition or kind of mix; the ingredients used; processing times, pressures, and temperatures; storage periods; and many other factors. Usually 0.1–0.5% stabilizer is used in the ice cream mix.

Mixes with higher fat or higher TS (40%), chocolate mixes, or ultrahigh-temperature (220°F or above) pasteurized mixes require less stabilizer. Mixes with lower TS (37%), high-temperature–short-time (HTST) pasteurization (175°F, 25 sec) mixes, or ice cream expected to endure long storage periods require more stabilization. When modified whey solids are used as an ingredient in the mix, the gum-type stabilizers with microcrystalline cellulose seem best to provide the desired body and texture, meltdown, and storage and handling characteristics.

KINDS OF STABILIZERS

Among the stabilizer substances that are permitted and used in the making of ice cream are agar; algin (sodium alginate); propylene glycol alginate; gelatin; gum acacia; guar seed gum; gum karaya; locust bean gum; oat gum; gum tragacanth; carrageenan; salts of carrageenan; furcelleran; salts of furcelleran; lecithin; pectin; psyllium seed husk; and CMC (sodium carboxymethylcellulose). Algin derivatives and CMC have gained important places as basic stabilizing materials for ice cream.

Most stabilizers used in ice cream are of natural origin, but some are chemically modified natural products, such as propylene glycol alginate and sodium carboxymethyl cellulose, which are polysaccharides from botanical sources. Gelatin, on the other hand, is an animal protein. Proprietary stabilizers contain a combination of various stabilizers and include emulsifiers. These combinations may be even more effective than the stabilizer material used alone. Other materials that perform valuable functional effects when used in conjunction with stabilizers include microcrystalline cellulose, calcium sulfate, and other salts.

There are many early references in the literature on the use of stabilizers in the manufacture of ice cream and related products.

The first report of gelatin being used in ice cream seems to have been Alberts (1905), and it was the only material used extensively until after World War I. Pectin and carrageenan were used somewhat later. Sodium alginate as an ice cream stabilizer was introduced in the 1930s and studied by Mack (1936). During one period it became the most widely used of all stabilizer materials for ice cream.

A product containing a mixture of an emulsifier and a stabilizer (monoglyceride and gelatin), which gave superior whipping properties, was introduced to the industry and studied by Lucas (1941). In 1945 the use of carboxymethyl cellulose (CMC) was evaluated by Josephson and Dahl (1945) as a stabilizer for ice cream.

The mono- and diglycerides of edible fatty acids and polyoxyethylene sorbitan monooleate or tristearate in the late 1940s and early 1950s were introduced for use in stabilizer–emulsifier products to produce a mix with good whipping properties and a dry, stiff finished ice cream.

The change to different mix pasteurization methods after HTST standards were approved in 1953 also led to a change in stabilizers. The HTST system required about 25% more stabilizer and a material with cold-water solubility.

Under these conditions guar gum and propylene glycol alginate were developed as stabilizers.

CMC in combination with these gums, with locust beam gum, and with carrageenan has been used successfully in ice cream stabilization for a number of years.

During the period 1965–1975, when the trend was to ultrahigh pasteurization (200°F or above) and to sterile mixes, there was need for still further application of emulsifier–stabilizer technology to meet the demands of the industry.

Moss (1955) stated that, compared to ice cream that does not contain a stabilizer, properly stabilized ice cream will have a heavier body, will not taste as cold, and will melt down to a creamier consistency.

Doan and Keeney (1965), noting that in many food applications stabilizers are used as thickening, suspending, and emulsifying agents, explained that all stabilizers increase the viscosity of the unfrozen portion, which restricts molecule migration to crystal nuclei, thereby limiting crystal size. The ability of stabilizers to bind or hold relatively large amounts of water also plays a role in maintaining a smooth texture.

Glickman (1963) stated that it is fairly well agreed that the basic role of hydrophilic gums in stabilizer products is to reduce the amount of free water in the mix by binding it as water of hydration or by immobilization within a gel structure. This is theoretically accomplished by an ideal gum or gum combination without reacting or disturbing the physiocochemical equilibrium of the mix components so as to introduce artificial viscosity characteristics in the mix. It is the ability of small percentages of gum to absorb and hold large amounts of unbound water that produces good body, smooth texture, slow meltdown, and heat shock resistance in the resulting products.

Shipe et al. (1963) found that the effect of stabilizers on the freezing characteristics of ice cream are associated with changes in viscosity and the rate of migration of solutes through dialyzing membranes. Migration of the solute is believed to influence the rate of crystallization.

Klose and Glickman (1968) reviewed the use of stabilizers in ice cream and concluded that most of the other gums have at one time or another been used as ice cream stabilizers, but for reasons of price or functionality have been generally replaced by alginates, CMC, and guar and locust bean gum. They classified gums as natural, modified, and synthetic. They grouped natural gums by source as tree exudates, seeds and roots, seaweed extract, and other sources; modified gums as cellulose derivatives, starch derivatives, microbial fermentations, and other sources; and synthetic gums as vinyl polymers, acrylic polymers, and ethylene oxide polymers.

Potter and Williams (1950) listed the following factors as important considerations in selecting a stabilizer: (a) ease of incorporation into the mix; (b) effect on the viscosity and whipping properties of the mix; (c) type of body produced in the ice cream; (d) effect on meltdown characteristics of the ice cream; (e) ability of the stabilizer to retard ice crystal growth; (f) quantity required to produce the desired stabilization; and (g) cost.

Leighton (1941) reported favorable results in studies using gelatin, algin, and monoglycerides. Turnbow et al. (1946) described the merits of gelatin as a stabilizer as having the peculiar property of absorbing water and forming a gel when the temperature and concentration factors are favorable, enabling it to retard the formation of large ice crystals in frozen ice cream. His usage rates were 0.18–0.25%, depending on ice cream composition. Mack (1936) reported the early successful use of sodium alginate in ice cream. Stebnitz and Sommer (1938) conducted a study on the effects of sodium alginate on the properties of ice cream and reported favorable results. Josephson *et al.* (1943) reported the successful use of CMC in ice cream at the usage rate 0.15–0.20%.

Dahle (1946) discussed the use of various stabilizers in ice cream and gave usage rates for the stabilizers available at that time: gelatin, 0.30–0.50% for 250–150 Bloom strength, respectively (see below); sodium alginate, 0.22–0.3%; carrageenan, 0.08–0.12%; CMC, 0.15–0.18% pectin, 0.15%; and psyllium seed, 0.15–0.2%

Glickman (1963) stated that CMC met immediate acceptance after it was introduced as an ice cream stabilizer, but results were best when CMC was used together with one or more other stabilizers.

Rothwell and Palmer (1965) indicated that the trend in prepared stabilizers was the use of a blend of stabilizing materials.

Furcelleran is extracted from red marine algae. It is quickly soluble in hot (175°F) water or hot milk products and will thicken or gel depending on concentration and temperature. The recommended usage rate in ice cream is 0.015–0.055%, and in sherbets, is ≤0.4% of mix weight or less.

Redfern and Arbuckle (1949) and Bayer (1965) evaluated a number of commercial stabilizers in ice cream and found that most produced desirable results.

Tallman (1958), Moss (1955), and Sperry (1955) considered stabilizers for HTST and continuous processing. Moss stated that mixes processed by HTST pasteurization required 25% more stabilizers. He further stated that special mixes and chocolate mixes required carefully balanced blends of locust bean gum plus carrageenan, CMC plus carrageenan, or all three. He noted that stabliziers that performed satisfactorily in mixes prepared by the batch system did not always do so in HTST systems.

Steinitz (1958) formulated a prepared stabilizer mixture of various gum combinations by suspending them in a mixture of propylene glycol and glycerol monostearate for use in a liquid form for continuous sytems. CMC was later suspended in alcohol and glycerine for adding to the mixes during processing with rapid dispersion.

Milk Proteins

Milk proteins have a stabilizing property depending on the heat-treatment they have received to form a stabilization structure throughout the liquid mix. This property is evident when superheated condensed milk is used as an ingredient or when the mix has been exposed to ultrahigh temperature (220°F or higher). There are, however, definite changes in the milk protein: the changes seem to be greatest beginning at 265°F, but no method of treating milk protein has been discovered that will improve its stabilizing properties to the extent that no stabilizer is required.

Gelatin

Gelatin, the first of the commercial stabilizers, is still used. Its advantages lie in its ability to form a gel in the mix during the aging period as well as during the freezing process, and even after the frozen product is placed in the hardening room. Its peculiar gel structure and its great affinity for water prevent the formation of large ice crystals in ice cream and contribute to smoothness in texture and firmness in body of the frozen product. Although not a complete protein, its amino acids do contribute slightly to the food value. It is generally thought less satisfactory than vegetable stabilizers for sherbets and ices because it has a tendency to produce too high an overrun, which is often associated with poor body and texture in these products.

The amount of gelatin used depends on many factors, such as the source of the gelatin; whether from calf or pork skins or bone material; its gel strength as measured by the Bloom Test; its viscosity value; and the composition of the mix. In general, the amount to use is approximately the amount required to produce a meltdown (in the evenly melted ice cream) of about the same consistency as aged 40% sweet cream (usually between 0.25 and 0.5% for a 250 Bloom gelatin).

An ice cream mix stabilized with gelatin usually requires about 4 hr of aging to develop complete stabilizing properties, while other stabilizing materials do not require an aging period.

Tests for Gel Strength.   Several tests have been developed to determine gel strength and to serve as guides to the amount to be used in the mix. Among these are the Bloom Test for Gel Strength, the Dahlberg Test (see Chapter 20), and the Protein–Nitrogen Content Test developed at University of Illinois. In a general way it may be said that, other factors being equal, the gelatin that carries the greatest gel strength per unit of cost is the one to select. Good-quality gelatin should have low bacteria count and should be practically odorless and colorless (or, if made from calf products, of light amber color). A modified gelatin is composed of gelatin and a monoglyceride or a monostearate. It stabilizes the fat emulsion and improves the whipping quality of the mix and the texture of the finished product.

The Bloom Test for Gel Strength has been adopted by the Edible Gelatin Manufacturers Association as a standard for grading gelatin on the basis of gel strength. The test therefore serves as a general guide to the value of a gelatin in ice cream, but it is not an absolute quality guide. It requires special equipment, careful temperature control, and other special conditions, and is used primarily by gelatin manufacturers.

The gel strength is determined by means of a Bloom Gelometer, which measures resistance to deformation under the specified conditions of the test. For example, a Bloom test of 200 means that a weight of 200 g is required to depress the surface of a 6-2/3% gelatin gel through a distance of 4 mm.

Gelatins on the market for use in ice cream range from 125 to 275 Bloom, with a 200-Bloom gel commonly preferred for ice cream manufacture.

Various more practical tests have been developed to evaluate gelatin specifically for ice cream plants.

Sodium Alginate

Sodium alginate and a modified form sold under a trade name are rather widely used vegetable stabilizers. Their basic stabilizing agent, algin, is extracted from giant ocean kelp growing on the shores of California and Japan. The commercial product seems to consist almost entirely of sodium alginate with small amounts of sugar and sodium citrate added to assist its solubility and to standardize its stabilizing properties. This product improves whipping ability and leaves a slightly cleaner flavor in the mouth—two distinct advantages. It dissolves properly only when added to the mix at about 155–160°F, which may be a disadvantage in certain methods of processing. A slightly smaller amount of sodium alginate is needed to give the same stabilizing effect as gelatin. Usage rates range from 0.18 to 0.25%, depending on ice cream composition.

Sodium alginate combined with phosphate salts is a rather widely used vegetable stabilizer for ice cream, as is propylene glycol alginate, which gives favorable results with HTST mix processing.

Other Stabilizers

Carrageenan. This is extracted from carrageen (Irish moss), a seaweed growing on the coast of Massachusetts, France, and Ireland. These products are comparable in stabilizing value to a 250 Bloom gelatin, and (it is claimed) can be added to the mix as easily as gelatin.

It is used in combination with other gum stabilizers and aids in the prevention of wheying off at the rate of approximately 0.02% of the weight of the mix.

Agar. A product extracted from red algae growing on the Pacific coast, agar has been recommended in combination with gums or gelatin for use as a stabilizer in sherbets and ices. Although it swells and absorbs large quantities of water and thus prevents coarseness in the finished product, it is not easily dispersed in the mix and tends to produce a crumbly body. It is also high in cost.

CMC. CMC, the trade name for sodium carboxymethyl cellulose, forms the basis of stabilizers that are now being accepted by the ice cream industry. It has high water-holding capacity and is easily dissolved in the mix—two qualities of a fine stabilizer—and also acts as an emulsifier. Used in slightly smaller quantities than gelatin, it does not form as firm a gel as gelatin and some of the vegetable stabilizers but seems to have merit for use in ice cream, and especially in sherbets and ices.

CMC has been found to give the best results when used together with one or more other stabilizers, preferably carrageenan, locust bean gum or guar gum. The useful characteristics imparted to ice cream are a chewy body, smooth texture, and improved whipping properties. The amount of CMC needed in ice cream varies from 0.15 to 0.20% of the mix; the levels usually recommended are 0.16% for ice cream, 0.18% for ice milk, 0.2% for sherbets, 1% for fruit purees, and 0.75% for chocolate syrups.

Pectin. Pectin is a carbohydrate obtained mainly from citrus fruit, and is used as an ingredient in the syrups and fruits used in making aufaits and rippled effects in ice cream. It is also effective in sherbets and ices. However, it is not very satisfactory as a stabilizer for ice cream. Purified sugar beet pectin forms a weaker and less brilliant gel than citrus pectin, and is used more commonly in sherbets and ices. The usage level is about 0.5% of the mix.

Locust Bean Gum. Locust bean gum (carob) is a product imported from Europe and is mainly grown in Cyprus. It is an ingredient of stabilizers that are prepared for use in sherbets and ices. Its principal advantage in these products is that it inhibits overrun. Since it has a tendency to cause curdling of the milk protein, its use in ice cream is limited unless used in combination with carrageenan. Its concentration range is 0.1–0.3% of the mix for ice cream and ≤0.5% of the mix for sherbets and water ices.

Guar Gum. Guar gum is a complex carbohydrate obtained from a legume grown in India. Its use in ice cream is fairly recent and it is often used in combination with carrageenan. Guar gum is readily soluble in cold solutions and is used as a stabilizer for mixes undergoing either HTST or continuous pasteurization. Its concentration range is 0.2–0.3% of the mix for ice cream.

Other Gums. Other gums such as tragacanth, arabic, karaya, or India gum are exudates from incisions made in the bark of certain trees and plants growing usually in the warmer regions of the earth. They find their chief use as ingredients in stabilizers for ices and sherbets and in the so-called ice cream improvers. The mucilaginous extracts from some plant seeds (quince and psyllium) are less widely used.

Egg Yolk Solids. Egg yolk solids have emulsifier properties and improve the whipping properties of the mix and the body and texture of the ice cream. Lecithin acts as an emulsifier and is contained in egg yolk solids. Levels of 0.5% of the mix produce noticeable effects.

Ice Cream Improvers. These are used by some manufacturers to improve the body and texture of ice cream. Some of these improvers consist mainly of the gum type of stabilizer (one or a mixture of two or more gums) and are sold under various trade names. Other improvers contain an enzyme such as rennin (rennet extract) or pepsin, capable of coagulating casein. Partial coagulation of the casein by these enzymes affects the body and texture of the ice cream. Therefore, care must be taken to check the coagulation at the right time. If such an improver is used it seems preferable to add it to the mix before pasteurization since the heat will destroy the enzyme and thus prevent too much coagulation and wheying-off. Unless the enzyme is destroyed by heat it will continue to work slowly even during the hardening period, and, as a result, the ice cream may shrink in the can or package. Ice creams containing improvers often have a curdled appearance when melted, due to a slight excess in the coagulation of the casein. The benefit of improvers is questionable except possibly in ice cream of low TS content.

Antioxidants. Antioxidants are substances that inhibit the development of "oxidized" flavor, often a troublesome defect in ice cream. They are successful only when added before the objectionable flavor develops. Several substances are known to have this effect: oat flour (a somewhat modified oat flour is being marketed under the trade name Avenex), an extract of oat flour, an extract of lettuce leaves, some vitamins, tannin, etc. The oat flour products are also credited with some merit as stabilizers. Although these products are frequently found in foods, their use in ice cream is illegal in some states.

The selection of a suitable stabilizer for use in the mix is influenced by many factors. One of the most important factors to consider is the adaptability of the product to the particular needs of the plant. Besides preference, availability, cost, and freedom from toxicity, other factors must be considered such as effect of the product on the properties of the mix, whether or not an aging period is necessary, kind of product being manufactured, method of processing, the effect on flavor, body and texture characteristics, and melting and storage properties of the ice cream.

The use of stabilizers changes the acidity of the mix slightly in some cases, produces a decided increase in mix viscosity, and increases the surface tension and whipping time slightly. In the finished ice cream, stabilizers have little effect on flavor, produce a smoother more resistant body and texture, may increase the rate of melting slightly, and improve storage qualities.

The amount of stabilizer used depends on the kind of stabilizer and the quality necessary to produce the desired stabilizing effect in the product being manufactured. There are four common ways of determining the amount of stabilizer to be used in the ice cream mix: the fat content of the mix, the TS content of the mix, the kind of freezer used, and the use of a constant percentage, which may range from 0.15 to 0.50%.

The maximum amount of stabilizer allowed in ice cream is 0.5%, while the maximum amount of mono- and diglycerides should be under 0.2% and the polyglycerides are limited to 0.1%. A guide to the amount of the basic stabilizers to use is given as in Table 6.1.

The method of incorporating stabilizers and emulsifiers in the mix is by mixing with 4–5 parts of sugar and adding before or during the heating process, dispersing by gently adding to the mix without special handling, or, in the case of algin stabilizers, suspending in cold water and adding to the mix when the mix temperature is 160°F, or using a hopper and a pump or other special arrangement.

When the batch method of pasteurization is employed, the stabilizer may be added to the cold or hot mix and there is more latitude for the selection of the stabilizer. In the HTST process of pasteurization, the stabilizer must be added to the cold mix ingredients and should disperse readily at a low temperature. The algin, guar, and CMC-type products are commonly used in this method of processing.

Table 6.1. A Guide to the Use of Stabilizers

	Percentage used	
Stabilizer	Ice cream	Sherbet, ice, and soft ice cream
Gelatin		
150 bloom	0.50	0.50
200 bloom	0.42	0.45
250 bloom	0.35	0.40
Sodium alginate (Dariloid)	0.27	0.33
CMC	0.16	0.20
Carageenan	0.10	0.25
Locust bean gum	0.25	0.25
Guar gum	0.25	0.25
Pectin	0.15	0.18

The ideal stabilizer for a presolution system should have the following properties: (1) should disperse readily in water without lumping; (2) should dissolve completely at room temperature; (3) should permit preparation of as concentrated a solution as possible (a 10–12% solution is about the maximum concentration that can be obtained with stabilizing materials now on the market); (4) should not develop viscosity on standing; and (5) must pump easily.

Proprietary stabilizers contain a combination of the various stabilizer and emulsifier materials with sugar as a carrier and salts. These combinations may be more effective in producing the characteristics desired than some of the stabilizing materials used alone.

Typical stabilizer combinations are CMC and gelatin; CMC and carrageenan; gelatin, CMC, and carrageenan; and CMC, locust bean gum, and carrageenan.

Figure 6.1 shows the effects of the use of stabilizers and emulsifiers on the internal structure of ice cream.

EMULSIFIERS

Emulsifiers are substances that tend to concentrate in the interface between the fat and the plasma and reduce the surface tension of the system.

The value of emulsifying agents in the manufacture of ice cream lies mainly with the improved whipping quality of the mix, the production of a drier ice cream with a smoother body and texture, superior drawing qualities at the freezer, and better control over various manufacturing processes.

Two types of emulsifiers are used in the manufacture of ice cream: (1) mono- and diglycerides derived by chemical reaction of naturally occurring glycerides, and (2) polyoxyethylene derivatives of hexahydric alcohols, glycol, and glycol esters.

The monoglycerides improve fat dispersion and whipping ability and have a moderate effect on stiffness and rate of melting. The polyderivatives are effective in producing dryness and stiffness, and increasing the melting time.

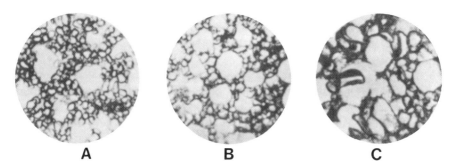

Fig. 6.1 Effect of stabilizers and emulsifiers on the internal structure of ice cream. (A) No stabilizer of emulsifier, (B) stabilizer, (C) stabilizer plus emulsifier.

Although emulsifiers such as mono- and diglycerides are more recently recognized products, milk contains certain natural emulsifying constituents, such as milk proteins, fat lecithin, phosphates, and citrates. Egg yolk products are high in lecithin and have long been used in ice cream. These products produce results similar to, but not as pronounced as, those produced by the commercial emulsifiers. Emulsifiers are available in liquid, semisolid, and powder forms and may include glycerides, lecithin, and fatty-acid esters. The mono- and diglyceride products have gained wide popular approval. In general, emulsifiers have little effect on the acidity (pH) or viscosity of the ice cream mix, but they tend to lower the surface tension and improve the whipping properties.

A noticeable reduction in whipping time is encountered when any emulsifier is used. The effect of emulsifiers on surface tension is most significant, and the determination of surface tension may be of value in estimating the effectiveness of an emulsifier product. The use of emulsifiers decreases the rate of melting in the finished ice cream. Structure measurements show that emulsifiers produce somewhat smaller ice crystals more evenly distributed and smaller air cells, which result in a smoother ice cream.

Many factors may affect the action of an emulsifier. Among these are the ingredients of the mix, procedure of processing, freezing, hardening, and the amount of emulsifier used. Emulsifiers must be used judiciously as regulated by prevailing plant conditions and practices.

Table 6.2 gives data typical of the effect of emulsifiers on the properties of the mix and the finished ice cream for a mix stabilized with gelatin and a heavily emulsified mix.

There are also disadvantages to the use of emulsifiers. Homogenization of the mix is essential to obtain best rsults. Some investigators think that they tend to favor the development of the defect called shrinkage. Excessive emulsification may cause a short body and texture characteristic, slow melting, and a curdy meltdown in the finished ice cream.

The use of emulsifiers in ice cream has been studied by many and it has been widely concluded that the value of emulsifying agents in the manufacture of ice cream is that they produce a mix that is more adaptable to general

Table 6.2. Physical Effects of Emulsifiers

Property	Mix stabilized with gelatin	Mix stabilized with gelatin and heavily emulsified
Surface tension (dynes)	51.9	48.3
Time to reach 90% overrun (min:sec)	8:30	4:45
Amount melted by weight when exposed at 85°F for 45 min (%)		
in batch freezer	23.7	5.2
in continuous freezer	31.4	13.8
Air cell size, diameter (μm)	204	146
Ice crystal size, length and width (μm)	44 ×32	40 ×30
Texture comments	Very slightly coarse	Smooth

processing procedures, enhance the whipping properties of the mix, and generally improve the body and texture of the finished ice cream.

Jensen *et al.* (1961) studied the composition of emulsifiers used in ice cream. The glyceride and fatty-acid composition of 20 commercial ice cream emulsifiers were determined: mono-, di-, and triglycerides were 20.6–93.5%, 6.5–51.3%, and 05–16.6%, respectively; most of the solid emulsifiers contained by weight 45.0–69.8% stearates, 23.8–48.8% palmitates, and smaller amounts of laurate, myristate, and oleate; the liquid emulsifiers contained 83% oleate or linoleate.

The two types of synthetic emulsifiers that are legal for use in ice cream, the polyoxyethylene sorbitan monooleate and polyoxyethylene sorbitan tristearate, known as polysorbate 80 and polysorbate 65, respectively, are known as the "monos."

7
Flavoring and Coloring Materials

Frozen desserts are valued mainly for their pleasing flavor and their cooling and refreshing effects. Since there are so many kinds of flavoring material and since they are sold under so many brands and grades, it is useful to understand their sources and to select and buy with great care. Among the flavoring substances that play an important part in frozen desserts are vanilla, chocolate and cocoa, fruits and fruit extracts, nuts, spices, and sugars. In the selection of flavoring materials it is important to consider the quality of the ice cream mix in which they are to be used, since slight off-flavors in it may obscure the delicate flavor of the flavoring material to be added.

American ice cream is noted for its wide range of flavors and various flavor combinations that use a variety of confections, bakery, liquors, and other materials. Some manufacturers have flavor lists consisting of as many as 500 or more different flavor recipes. Flavor preferences are undergoing some changes, and recent data (IAICM 1980) on sales according to flavor for ice cream, ice milk, and sherbet are shown in Table 7.1.

Vanilla and chocolate are still the dominant flavors, but there has been some shifting in rank of other flavors.

Of the many and varied flavoring materials available for vanilla, chocolate, fruit, and nut ice cream, only those that impart the delicate desired flavor to the finished product should be chosen.

Flavor is usually considered to have two important characteristics: type and intensity. Generally, the delicate, mild flavors are easily blended and tend not to become objectionable at high concentrations, while the harsh flavors are usually objectionable even in low concentrations. Therefore, delicate flavors are preferable to harsh flavors, but in any case a flavor should only be intense enough to be easily recognized and to present a delicate, pleasing taste.

The ice cream manufacturer has given considerable attention to standardizing the ingredients and composition of mixes, but problems of flavor standardization still exist for several reasons:

- There are so many flavoring products available that it is difficult to make the proper choice.
- The available flavoring material supply may vary from year to year.

Table 7.1. Flavor Preferences

	Ice cream			Ice milk			Sherbet	
Rank	Flavor	% of production	Rank	Flavor	% of production	Rank	Flavor	% of production
1	Vanilla	35.1	1	Vanilla	49.2	1	Orange	32.6
2	Chocolate	12.4	2	Chocolate	11.0	2	Rainbow	22.0
3	Neapolitan	7.4	3	Vanilla Fudge	7.2	3	Lime	13.4
4	Chocolate Chip	5.9	4	Neapolitan	6.1	4	Raspberry	11.5
5	Strawberry	5.6	5	Strawberry	4.0	5	Pineapple	10.7
6	Vanilla Fudge	4.2		Others	22.5		Others	9.8
7	Butter Pecan	2.7		Total	100.0		Total	100.0
8	Cherry	2.5						
9	Butter Almond	1.6						
10	French Vanilla	1.4						
	Others	21.2						
	Total	100.0						

Source: IAICM (1984).

Table 7.2. Market Classes of Ice Cream

Market group	Composition	Flavoring material
Economy brand	Meets minimum composition requirements only	Minimum rate of category II or III
Good average trade brand	Above minimum composition requirements	Minimum or above minimum rate of category II or I
Premium product	Higher fat and TS, lower overrun	Higher rate of category I
Superpremium product	Very high fat and TS, very low overrun	Highest rate of category I

- Serving conditions affect how pronounced a flavor will be and will thereby influence consumer acceptance.
- Since no two consumers have exactly the same sense of taste, opinions regarding choice of flavor are vastly different.

Because flavor is so important in influencing consumer acceptance, it is easy to lose sales because of a poorly flavored product.

The problems that can be caused in the addition of flavorings in the manufacturing processes are lack or excess of flavor; unnatural, wrong, imitation, or nontypical flavor; lack or excess of sweetness, and coarse flavor. In addition, added flavorings may affect appearance: lack or excess of flavor particles; poor distribution or uneven variegation patterns; particles too large or too small; wrong color or ingredient; ribbon that is too thick or too thin.

In accordance with the Federal Standards of Identity, flavoring materials and the labeling of finished frozen products are divided into three categories:

I   Pure extracts (10–20% of market)
II   Pure extracts with synthetic component (about 75% of market)
III Artificial flavors (about 10% of market)

Prevailing classes of ice cream are partly based on composition and partly on the flavoring materials used (see Table 7.2). Frozen-dessert flavoring practices indicate that the flavoring materials for premium and superpremium are not only of category I quality, but are of the highest usage level rate. Consumer reactions to the flavor intensity of these products are very favorable, as shown by increased sales.

There are a number of ways that flavoring materials can help ice cream manufacturers increase their sales:

- Developing improved processing methods for fruits and nuts.
- Upgrading overall quality by increasing flavor levels at slightly higher prices and greater profit margin.
- Adjusting the flavor level to avoid flavor defects in all lines.
- Using only flavors with good solvents to avoid solvent aftertaste.
- Using flavor extenders with caution.
- Conducting regular flavor evaluation product clinics and adjusting flavors to meet market demands.

Establishing favorable product acceptance by the consumer is a major objective in increasing product sales and the use of top-quality flavors has an important role in meeting this objective.

ICE CREAM FLAVOR SUBSTANCES

An abundant variety of flavoring substances has been provided by nature, and the chemist has attempted to duplicate this variety. Natural flavoring substances are sometimes limited in supply, but the chemically produced supplements have been made available in virtually unlimited quantities at low cost.

Flavor substances of natural and chemically produced origin are available mainly in mixtures for the proper flavoring of foods. Information occurring in the literature (Merory 1968) relative to food flavoring materials and the rise of these materials is limited, as there has been a degree of secrecy in flavor technology; but information is available covering the composition, manufacture, and use of food flavoring and there is information on natural and synthetic flavorings. Included among the natural flavorings are (1) noncitrus fruit; (2) citrus fruit; (3) tropical fruit; (4) sugar-free fruit; (5) natural flavors from botanicals; (6) spices; (7) cocoa and chocolate; (8) coffee; (9) natural flavorings from vanilla beans; and (10) nuts. The synthetic flavorings include aromatic chemicals and imitation flavors. Liqueur flavorings are also included: (1) alcohol; (2) whiskey and other distilled beverages; (3) fruit brandy distillate and brandy flavor essence: and (4) fruit liqueurs. All of the above-mentioned flavoring substances have an important part in flavoring the 50 or more major flavors as well as many of the less common flavors of ice cream.

There are many different flavoring materials available for flavoring vanilla, chocolate, and fruit and nut ice creams, but generally only those materials imparting a delicate, mild, natural flavor prove to be most satisfactory.

The delicate mild flavors imparted by natural flavoring materials only reach a level of intensity that produces a delicate pleasing taste, and there is little danger of overflavoring even at high concentrations. This is not true in the case of imitation flavoring materials, as these materials may result in harsh, pronounced, objectionable flavors even in low concentrations.

Investigations indicate that mix composition, processing methods, serving temperature, and color intensity (which affect the appearance, flavor, and sweetness of products) all influence consumer preference of ice cream.

A series of studies (Reid and Arbuckle, 1938) conducted with sherbets of different flavors and ice cream varying in fat content from 10 to 16%, MSNF from 9 to 15%, and sugar from 12 to 18% with serving temperatures ranging from 4° to 18°F showed that a majority of the consumers liked ice cream best when it was served at 8°F. As the serving temperature was increased from 6° to 18°F, the vanilla flavor was more pronounced. The ice cream was observed as being sweeter and the high-fat ice cream as less resistant to melting and more desirable as the serving temperature increased. Ice creams and sherbets of higher sugar content or of pronounced flavor were rated as best when served at temperatures lower than 8°F.

Studies (Cremers and Arbuckle, 1954) show there is a milk fat–air cell orientation in the freezing process that influences the smoothness and mellowness of ice cream. The fat concentrates on the surface in surrounding the air cell in the internal structure of ice cream and influences the smoothness of the product as well as imparting a full milkfat flavor when the optimum distribution prevails. This work indicates that careful overrun control in relation to product composition is important in gaining optimum flavor.

The MSNF contributes a slightly cooked and a slightly salty flavor due both to the heat-treatment and to the natural milk salts contained in the dairy products supplying this constituent.

In a series of articles reporting the influence of sugar in ice cream (Pangborn et al., 1957), a study of vanilla ice cream containing 11, 13, 15, 17, and 19% sugar showed that the three higher levels were liked equally well, but were preferred to a significant degree over the 11 and 13% levels.

Strawberry ice cream having sugar content of 15.9, 17.6, 19.2, and 20.8% was evaluated in a household survey. (Pangborn *et al.*, 1957). The ice cream containing 19.2% sugar was preferred over the other samples.

Results obtained with a professional panel in a study (Arbuckle *et al.* 1961) of the use of fruit concentrates and essences for flavoring ice cream indicated that a sugar level of 17% was most desirable for producing optimum fruit flavor. When the sugar content was over 17%, the mixes were rated as too sweet and lacking fruit flavor. The sweetness of a high sugar level may actually submerge the effect of some fruit flavorings.

The rates of 15% cane sugar equivalent for plain ice cream and 17–18% cane sugar equivalent for bulky flavors of ice cream have given good results for optimum acceptance.

VANILLA

Vanilla is without exception the most popular flavor for ice cream. Records show that about 75% of all ice cream contains vanilla flavoring. This flavoring material is usually obtained in extract form, but there is a rapidly growing demand for vanilla concentrates and paste, and for powdered vanilla and sugar preparations.

The finest vanilla has traditionally been obtained from the fruits of the orchid *Vanilla fragrans*, indigenous to Southeastern Mexico, where it was used by the Aztecs to season their chocolate.

The plant has been introduced into other tropical countries: islands in the Madagascar area (now providing 80% of the world's supply), Indonesia, certain islands in the West Indies, and other parts of Central America. The vanilla product of Tahiti is derived from *Vanilla tahitensis*, an inferior variety whose fruits impart a harsh flavor. The fruits of *Vanilla pompona* are known as vanillons and are similar to the Tahiti beans in flavor.

Vanillin ($C_8H_8O_3$) is the principal flavoring essential in vanilla. However, there is no free vanillin in the beans when they are harvested; it develops gradually during the curing period from glucosides, which break down during the fermentation and "sweating" of the beans. The sweating process consists of alternately drying the beans in the sun and wrapping them up at night so that they heat and ferment. This process, which is continued until the flavor and aroma are developed, takes 4 weeks to 4 months and reduces the beans to sufficient dryness so that they will not mold. Beans are sometimes artificially dried but this produces a product of inferior quality. At the end of the curing period the pods are carefully sorted into various grades based on their quality.

Vanilla flavoring is available in liquid or powder forms as pure vanilla, reinforced vanilla with vanillin, and imitation vanilla, and is classified as true, compound, and imitation.

True Vanilla Flavorings

True vanilla extract is prepared by the extraction of finely cut vanilla beans in a solution containing not less than 35% alcohol.

The present federal standard for vanilla extract calls for soluble matter from not less than 10 g of vanilla beans in 100 ml of alcohol, with or without added sugar, glycerine, or coloring matter. This amounts to 13.35 oz of beans to make 1 gal (128 fl oz) of extract. These true vanilla extracts are generally of such a strength that 5–6 oz of the extract are required to flavor 10 gal of ice cream mix.

Concentrated vanilla extract is made by distilling off a large part of the solvent, usually in vacuum, until the strength reaches the desired concentration which is then specified as fourfold, fivefold, etc. Each multiple must be derived from an original 13.35 oz of beans in the starting extract before concentration. The maximum strength of a direct extraction, without concentration, is 2 lb of vanilla beans in 1 gal of solvent. The amount of such products used should be slightly higher than the amount of a standard vanilla extract used divided by the multiple of the concentrate.

True vanilla powders are made by mixing finely ground vanilla beans with sugar, or by incorporating the vanilla extractives with a dry carrier, evaporating the solvent, and drying. The amount used would correspond by weight to the number of ounces of a standard strength extract.

Vanilla paste is made by mixing the concentrated extractives with a dry carrier to form a paste. The amount used would be the same as for powders.

True vanilla flavor conforms to the same standards as vanilla extract except that it contains less than 35% alcohol, propylene glycol, or other solvent as the carrier.

Compound Vanilla Flavorings

These flavorings consist of a combination of vanilla and vanillin. Not less than half of the flavor must be derived from the vanilla bean content. Not more than 1 oz of vanillin may be used in conjunction with 13.35 oz of vanilla beans. This type is available in various degrees of concentration.

Blends are true vanilla extract, flavor, or powder with added synthetics, where less than half of the flavor is derived from the vanilla beans.

Imitation Vanilla Flavorings

Artificial or synthetic vanillin is a product of slightly different flavor but the same general composition as that which occurs naturally in vanilla beans. Tests have shown that 1-1/8 oz of vanillin are equivalent in flavoring strength to 1 lb of vanilla beans. It has also been stated that a 0.7% solution of vanillin is equal in strength of flavor to single-strength vanilla extract.

Some preparations contain no vanilla bean extractives, and are made up entirely of combinations of substances such as synthetics and natural extractives other than from vanilla beans. These preparations may contain added water, alcohol, propylene glycol, vanillin, caramel color, etc.

For those who wish to economize on vanilla costs a suggested reinforcement for a vanilla extract is 2 oz of vanillin to 1 gal. A highly reinforced vanilla should not exceed 8 oz of vanillin per gallon.

An artificial flavoring extract strong enough so that 1/2 oz is sufficient to flavor 10 gal of ice cream usually contains 12–14 oz of vanillin to 1 gal. Fortunately, these imitations are seldom used exclusively in ice cream.

Other materials may be added to vanilla to produce a vanillalike flavor. These may include such substances as the synthetic vanilla like flavoring material, propenyl guaethol (0.0132–0.0166 g/10 gal mix), ethyl vanillin, anisyl aldehyde, and heliotropine (piperonal).

Vanilla Ice Cream

In the manufacture of vanilla ice cream the flavor materials should be used in sufficient amounts, and should be of the best quality. Careful selection of fine natural flavoring materials will do much to eliminate the "unnatural flavor" criticism so often directed at the finished product. In early experiments with vanilla ice cream, Pierce *et al.* (1924) showed that true vanilla flavors persist better than artificial flavors. All the various types and strengths of vanilla are available for use in ice cream.

The basic mix is processed and stored, and the cold mix is flavored with vanilla by thoroughly blending the flavoring material just previous to the freezing process.

The amount of vanilla used depends somewhat on mix composition: 4–6 oz of single-strength vanilla per 5 gal if the mix contains the normal 12% fat. The lower the butterfat content, the more vanilla is required, and as the MSNF is increased more vanilla is required. The sugar level also plays an important role. A low sugar level requires a higher vanilla level, but at a high sugar level the amount of vanilla makes little difference in consumer preference.

Tharp and Gould (1962) conducted a survey of 329 vanilla flavoring materials used by 34 companies in the ice cream industry. These materials were grouped as pure, fortified, and imitation and ranged in strength from single-fold to 22-fold. Approximately 75% of the products examined had concentrations of sixfold or less and about 35% were twofold. Costs varied from 0.2 to 7.2¢ per gallon of ice cream at 100% overrun. The cost per gallon for pure vanilla were 1.4 to 7.2¢ averaging 3.3¢; for fortified products, 0.2–4.2¢, averaging 1.7¢; and for imitation products, 0.2–3.5¢ averaging of 1.0¢. (These costs had increased eight- to tenfold by 1985.) They presented this usage level formula:

level of usage of n-fold vanilla = level of usage of singlefold vanilla/n

This survey showed that the wide range of vanilla flavoring materials available is reflected in cost, which is an important factor influencing flavor materials selection. Although it is sometimes contended that pure vanilla flavor becomes less intense during storage, Lucas (1929) concluded that it shows no tendency to disappear from ice cream during a storage period of 3 months at $-10°F$. However, flavors that may develop during storage will submerge the vanilla flavor.

CHOCOLATE AND COCOA

Chocolate and cocoa rank second only to vanilla as flavorings for ice cream. They are obtained from the cacao bean, the fruit of the tree *Theobroma cacao*, which grows in such tropical regions as Mexico, Central America, Ecuador, Venezuela, Brazil, West Indies, the African Gold Coast, and the East Indies.

The almond-sized cacao beans or seeds develop in a large pulpy pod, with 20–30 beans to the pod. The ripened pods, rich golden red in color, are cut from the trees, gathered in piles and left to ripen further for about 48 hr, after which they are slashed open, and the beans removed and placed in vats or bags to heat and ferment for about 10 days, or until the characteristic flavor and cinnamon-red color develop. The beans are then washed clean of the dried pulp, are dried slowly and sufficiently to prevent mold growth, and are then sorted and graded prior to shipment to manufacturers of chocolate and cocoa.

Processing the Cocoa Beans

At the factory the beans are first mechanically cleaned. Then they are roasted to drive off the moisture and to bring out the special chocolate flavor and aroma. The roasted beans are then cooled quickly by forced air, and are next run through a winnowing machine, which crushes them into small pieces and separates the shells from the nibs, the seed part, which is made into chocolate and cocoa. These nibs, containing approximately 50% of the fat of the bean, are then placed between heavy stone grinders or mills which reduce them to a liquid by the heat created through the friction of milling.

Chocolate liquor or pure bitter chocolate is the generic name for the liquid chocolate produced by these processes. This liquor may then be cooled in molds and put up in large slabs or in half-pound packages such as are sold in grocery stores as bitter cooking chocolate, or it may be further processed into cocoa.

Sweet milk chocolate is made from the chocolate liquor by adding the necessary proportions of sugar, milk, and cocoa butter, with or without vanilla flavoring. The blending of these ingredients requires a considerable amount of skill and special machinery.

Natural-process cocoa is made from chocolate liquor by subjecting it to high pressure in hydraulic presses. This process removes a large amount of the cocoa butter (fat), usually about 38–40% of the total, and leaves a hard, dry cake that normally contains about 22% fat, though some cocoas contain more and some less. It also contains nearly all the flavoring material from the cocoa bean (the fat is practically tasteless). This cocoa cake is then put through a number of processes known as milling, which result in the finely sifted cocoa.

Dutch process cocoa is made in the same way as the natural process cocoa, except for one thing: In the Dutch process the beans are treated with alkalis at the time of roasting to break up the cell structure. This alkali treatment makes the cocoa more soluble and helps give it the darker color that distinguishes Dutch process from natural cocoa. It also aids in bringing out the full, fine chocolate flavor when the cocoa is used in the finished product. Because the alkalis counteract the puckery acid taste found in natural cocoa, the Dutch process cocoa leaves no bitter taste when used as flavoring in ice cream.

A defect that sometimes appears in chocolate ice cream made with Dutch process cocoa is the formation of a greenish-black discoloration where the ice cream comes in contact with exposed iron on the inner surface of the packing cans, for example, if the cans are rusty or the tinning is scratched or worn off. In the "Dutching" process, the tannins the cocoas contain are made soluble by the added alkalis, and they react with the iron to form ferric tannate, which gives the discoloration to the ice cream. This can be avoided by using well-tinned cans, paper can liners, or paper containers.

Ramachandran *et al.* (1961) made a review of the literature covering the steps involved in changing the cocoa bean to edible cocoa or chocolate product with particular emphasis on factors affecting the flavor of ice cream.

Cocoa Characteristics

Cocoa is more concentrated for ice cream flavoring than chocolate liquor because it contains a higher percentage of the real chocolate flavor, and a lower percentage of the nearly tasteless fat. For example, 100 lb of cocoa contain 78 lb flavor plus 22 lb fat; and 100 lb of chocolate liquor contain 48 lb flavor plus 52 lb fat. It is evident, therefore, that in 100 lb of cocoa there is approximately 30 lb more real chocolate flavor than in 100 lb of chocolate liquor. Due to the prevailing high price of cocoa butter, it is more economical for the ice cream manufacturer to use cocoa rather than chocolate liquor.

The color of cocoa is the result of several factors: (1) the blend of beans, (2) the fat content, (3) treatment (Dutching), and (4) rate of chilling. The rate of chilling is an important factor and influences color by affecting the size of the fat globules in the cocoa. This influence is lost when the cocoa is used.

Cocoa is seldom adulterated. Sugar, starch, cocoa shells, ground wood fiber, and iron oxide at one time were often used as adulterants, but are seldom found in cocoas now. Some companies do, however, add to cocoa some aromatic substances such as cinnamon, oil of cloves, oil of bitter almond, or vanillin. Some of these substances in small quantities will give cocoa a higher, pleasant aroma.

Chocolate Ice Cream

Numerous early references occur in the literature on the manufacture of chocolate ice cream (Dahle 1927; Dahlberg and Hening 1928; Fabricius 1930; Martin 1931; Reid and Painter 1931; Tuckey *et al.* 1932). The results obtained by these workers provide the basis for many current manufacturing practices.

Chocolate products used in fiavoring ice cream are cocoa, chocolate liquor, cocoa and chocolate liquor blends, and chocolate syrups. The use of 3% cocoa, a 4% blend of cocoa (2.5%) and chocolate liquor (1.5%), or 5% chocolate liquor is very acceptable.

Decker (1950) concluded that a full chocolate flavor, but one without harshness or bitterness, is most desirable. A formula using 3% cocoa, 1.5% chocolate liquor, and 18% sugar met this requirement. He suggested that a variation of this formula could be made by replacing the chocolate liquor at the rate of

0.25% cocoa for each 0.5% chocolate liquor. Modified flavorings, such as vanillin or vanilla extract, were not recommended for use in ice cream.

Lindamood and Gould (1964a,b) stated that chocolate ice cream prepared with low-cocoa-fat products was generally superior to that prepared with fat liquors. The natural-processed product was preferred rather than the Dutch process chocolate flavoring material.

The amount of cocoa or chocolate liquor to use in ice cream depends upon several factors, such as consumer preference, color desired in ice cream, strength of flavor, and fat content of flavor. The usual recommendation is sometimes as much as 4 lb of cocoa or 6 lb of chocolate liquor to 100 lb of mix. Extra sugar should be added to compensate for the bitter flavor of the cocoa, the usual recommendation being the same weight of sugar as of cocoa or chocolate. The tendency seems to be to flavor chocolate ice cream too highly. It is apparent that a better product could be made by reducing the amount of flavor and using, instead, a finer grade of cocoa or chocolate liquor.

Preparing the Chocolate Syrup

The small ice cream manufacturer usually prefers to flavor chocolate ice cream by adding syrup at the freezer. Desirable results may be expected by using a formula of 20 lb cocoa, 20 lb sugar, and enough water to make 10 gal of finished syrup; 5–7 lb of this syrup may be used to 5 gal of mix. The syrup should be made up in a chocolate kettle or double boiler. Mix the sugar and cocoa or chocolate together and add enough water to make a heavy paste. Heat gradually and add water slowly as necessary. (The final syrup should contain enough water so that it will pour when cooled.) The syrup should be heated to the boiling point and cooled before using, so as not to prolong the freezing operation.

Preparing the Chocolate Ice Cream Mix

Whenever possible, an entire chocolate mix should be made by adding the cocoa (or chocolate) and extra sugar to the mix, along with the other dry ingredients, before pasteurization. The temperature of pasteurization is sufficient to incorporate the flavor properly. A chocolate mix made in this way whips more rapidly than plain mix plus syrup at the freezer. amd goves a better flavored, more uniform product, freer of dark specks.

The best chocolate ice cream is made when the chocolate mix is compounded and processed. A typical formula is fat, 10%; MSNF, 10%; sugar, 18%; cocoa, 2.5%; chocolate liquor, 1.5%; stabilizer, 0.2%; and TS, 42.2%.

Freezing Characteristics

Chocolate ice cream is one of the most difficult to freeze because it whips very slowly. This is due to the fact that chocolate mix is viscous. The viscosity may be reduced and whipping time improved by adding 1 lb of citrates or phosphates to 1000 lb of mix.

A comprehensive review of the literature with particular emphasis on the factors affecting the flavor of chocolate ice cream cites numerous references on the many chemical and physical alterations that occur during the production and manufacture of cocoa and chocolate. The information available does not reveal clearly the nature of chocolate flavor or the wide differences in flavor that prevail.

FRUITS IN ICE CREAM

The ice cream trade is one of the chief markets for fresh, frozen, and canned (pie grade) fruits, Strawberry ice cream ranks third among flavors, representing about 8% of the total amount of ice cream made. Other fruit flavors are popular in season and are consumed more or less throughout the year.

Fruit flavors are available as (1) extracts prepared from the fruit, (2) artificial compounds, and (3) true extracts fortified artificially. These flavors supplement the fruits in cases where it is necessary to avoid excessive amounts of fruit, but they are quite generally inferior to the flavor obtained from the fruit itself and do not supply the desired fruit pulp.

Defects in fruit ice cream may result from: (1) improperly handled fruit; (2) use of insufficient fruit; (3) poorly incorporated fruit; (4) use of poor quality fruit; (5) excessive fortified flavor and color resulting in unnatural flavor and color; and (6) use of poor quality base mix.

A special mix need not be used for fruit ice cream unless the basic mix contains more than 16% sugar. With a 16% sugar content a 3:1 fruit pack should be used. If the mix contains 15% sugar or less, the 2:1 pack is usually preferred.

If a special mix is prepared for use in the manufacture of fruit ice cream, such a mix may be of the following composition: fat, 13.5%; sucrose, 10.5%; MSNF, 12.5%; and stabilizer–emulsifier, 0.35%. Federal Standards of Identity allow a reduction of fat and total milk solids in fruit ice cream to 8% and 16%, respectively, and require the use of a factor of 1.4 in computing the allowed reduction.

Since fruit ice cream contains a higher percentage of sugar than plain ice cream it should be drawn from the freezer at about 1°F colder. A drawing temperature of 23°F for the batch freezer or 20°F for the continuous freezer is satisfactory under most condition.

Fresh Fruit

Fresh fruit must be considered the best source of flavor when available at sufficiently low prices. Fresh fruit ice creams also have a special sales appeal. The fruit should be washed and hulled or peeled and then mixed with sugar in the ratio of 2–7 lb fruit to 1 lb sugar (see Table 7.3) and held at about 40°F for 12–24 hr before using. During this aging period a large part of the juice and flavor of the fruit will combine with the sugar, by osmotic action, to form a

Table 7.3.　Amount and Preparation of Fruits and Nuts for Ice Cream

Flavor	Fruit–sugar ratio	Quantity of fruit in mix (%)	Kind of preparation	Added color
Apple	7:1	20–25	Sliced	Light yellow green
Apricot	3:1	20–25	Sliced, diced, or puree	Light orange yellow
Banana	—	18–20	Puree	[a]
Blackberry	3:1	20	Crushed or puree	Slight red
Blueberry	4:1	20	Crushed or puree	Light blue
Cherry	5:1	15–20	Whole or crushed	Light red
Fruit salad	3:1	15	Sliced or diced	[a]
Grape	—	25	Juice	Light purple
Peach	4:1	20–25	Sliced, diced, or puree	Light
Pineapple	4:1	12–15	Diced or crushed	[a]
Plum	4:1	25	Puree	Light red
Raspberry	2:1	10–12	Crushed or puree	Light purple
Strawberry	3:1–4:1	15–20	Sliced, crushed, or puree	Pink
Almond	[b]	3 lb:10 gal mix	Broken	[a]
Chocolate	[b]	2.7–3.5 lb cocoa		
		3.5–4.5 lb cocoa liquor blend	Syrup	[a]
		4.5–5.5 lb chocolate liquor per 10 gal mix		
Pecan	[b]	3 lb:10 gal mix	Broken	
Pistachio	[b]	4 lb:10 gal mix	Whole and broken	Light green
Walnut	[b]	4 lb:10 gal mix	Broken	[a]
Orange	5:1	14–18 oz:10 gal mix	Puree	Orange
Lemon	5:1	10–14 oz:10 gal mix	Puree	Yellow green
Lime	5:1	8–12 oz:10 gal mix	Puree	Green

[a]Natural, no color added.
[b]Sugar pack may range from 2:1 to 9:1.

fruit syrup. This syrup will impart to the ice cream the full flavor of the fruit much more effectively than would the fresh fruit if used immediately.

Strawberries need not be mashed or sliced. This is merely a waste of time and does not enhance their flavoring ability. Very seedy fruits such as raspberries should be puréed so that about 75% of the seeds are removed. Peaches should be sliced.

Fresh fruit and fresh frozen fruit are the most desirable flavoring materials. The aged fruit–sugar mixture used at the rate of 15–20% produces good results with many fruits. The fruit–sugar ratio may vary from 2:1 to as high as 9:1. Fruits may be used whole, sliced, crushed, diced, pureed (coarse, medium, or fine), or as juice. The use of whole or large slices of fruit sometimes results in coarse texture, which reduces consumer acceptance of the finished product. A greater amount of fruit is often required to obtain the desired flavor intensity when a puree is used (see Figs. 7.1–7.3).

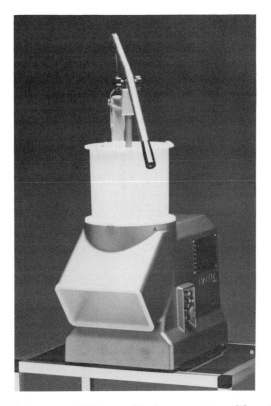

Fig. 7.1 Food disintegrator. This type of food processor is used for cutting, chopping, and pureeing fruits and other ingredients used in ice cream production and in toppings. (Courtesy Hallde Inc., Woodside, NJ.)

Good results from the standpoint of fruit distribution, appearance, and desirable texture and flavor characteristics result from the use of diced fruit or coarse pureed fruit. A combination of sliced fruit and fruit puree is sometimes used with success.

Kind of Pack to Use

Fresh or frozen packs are preferable for fruits such as strawberries, whose distinctive flavor is easily impaired by heating; while fruits like cherries or pineapple, whose flavors are relatively stable or improved by heating, are usually heat-preserved, that is, canned. For strawberries the 2:1 and 3:1 frozen packs are the most popular, with the tendency toward the latter. Peaches should also be frozen, the 3:1 pack being preferred. Raspberries are very satisfactory frozen, although they withstand heating much better than strawberries. Cherries are usually canned, although the frozen fruit is satisfactory. The 2:1 ratio pack should be used in both cases. Generally the

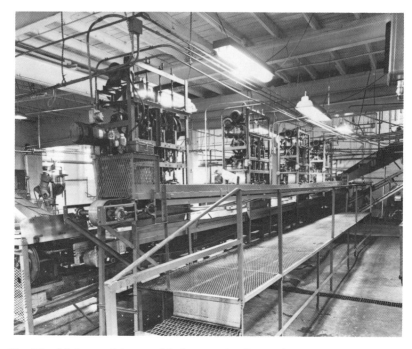

Fig. 7.2. Modern stainless steel fruit processing line produces processed fresh fruits for ice cream or sherbet mixes. (Courtesy Southern Packing Co., Baltimore, MD.)

maraschino process cherries are used. Frozen pineapples are used occasionally and have a very fine flavor but the canned fruit flavor is also very popular.

Amount to Use

The amount of fruit required to impart the desired flavor varies with the characteristic intensity of the flavor. This amount varies from 10 to 25% of the weight of the finished product. In every case, fruit ice cream should contain not less than 3% by weight of clean, mature, sound fruits or their juice. This minimum value is desirable and is already a legal requirement in some states. It is usually desirable also to have pieces of the fruit or pulp large enough so they can be easily recognized in the finished ice cream.

For strawberries the optimum amount seems to be about 15% of 2:1 or 3:1 pack. For cherry ice cream, as well as pincapple, 12–15% is satisfactory. When these fruits are high in price, less fruit is used, and enough true fruit extract is added to produce a flavor approximately the same as the natural fruit flavor. A little artificial color is added to give the delicate tints associated with these fruits. Raspberries are generally rather expensive, and so about 10% of fruit plus enough good raspberry extract to bring out the desired flavor should be used. For best results with peaches, about 20% of frozen pack fruit should be

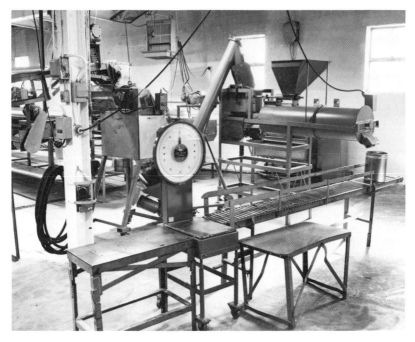

Fig. 7.3. For fruit purees, modern lines of stainless steel throughout produce the finest quality products. (Courtesy Southern Packing Co., Baltimore MD).

used along with a good peach brandy syrup. Of the mixed fruits and fruit combinations, about 15% seems to be the desirable amount to use.

Fruit Concentrates and Essences

Good results have been obtained using concentrated fruit juice and essences in ice cream and related frozen dairy foods. The most desirable use levels and best formulas have been established for peach, blueberry, grape, apple, red raspberry, and strawberry flavor concentrates. In most cases, the supplemental use of 3.5–10% fruit equivalent of concentrates improved flavor properties. The amount of flavoring material, the composition of the ice cream mix, and the sugar–acid ratio are factors that have been controlled in obtaining the most desirable flavor. Adjustment of the acidity and the sugar content of the mix produced desirable effects for the flavors studied except for apple products. Fruit concentrates and essences have been found to be valuable products in improving fruit ice cream and sherbet flavors, either when used to supplement the use of fruit or in some cases when used as the sole source of flavor.

The results indicate that the established flavors of ice cream can be improved by the addition of concentrated fruit juice, for example, peach or blueberry, and that the use of fruit concentrates or essences offers the possibility of the development of new flavors of ice cream, for example, grape or Montmorency cherry.

Arbuckle *et al.* (1961) used fruit concentrate and essence of seven different fruits including peach, apple, strawberry, blueberry, grape, red raspberry, and cherry to flavor ice cream, sherbets, ices, ice milk, and variegated ice cream. Many of the fruit concentrates and essences studied proved to be valuable and economical means of improving the flavor of fruit ice cream and related products, either when used to supplement the use of fruit, or in some cases, when used as the only source of fruit flavor.

Candied and Glaced Fruits

Candied or glaced fruits such as cherries, pineapple, and citron, and such candied fruit peels as orange, lemon, and grapefruit are very good flavoring materials. They are used chiefly in rich types of ice cream—puddings, aufaits, mousses—and as decorative material for fancy molded ice creams, sherbets, and ices.

Dried Fruits

Dried fruits such as apricots, figs, prunes, and raisins make tasty ice creams. Although of slightly different flavor than the corresponding fresh fruit, they usually are less expensive and often can be obtained at times when fresh fruit is very scarce or in places where it is practically unobtainable. Dates, figs, and raisins, particularly, have long been used in frozen puddings, but recently there has been a tendency to use these and other dried fruits as flavoring material for ice cream either separately or in combinations.

Freeze-Dried Fruits

Lazar (1970) studied the use of freeze-dried fruits in ice cream and found that an acceptable flavor was obtained only with the strawberries when freeze-dried peaches, strawberries, and bananas were studied. In all cases, the fruit remained leathery, and soaking in water or 25% sugar solution failed to eliminate the defect.

PROCEDURES AND RECIPES

Base Syrup

In making most fruit-flavored ice creams, the fruit is combined with a syrup base.

A base may be prepared for fruit-flavored syrup by using 55 lb sugar, 2.5 lb stabilizer (pectin gives very desirable results), and sufficient water to make 100 lb of base syrup. The syrup may then be prepared by using a 1:2 ratio of fruit puree to base syrup. The addition of 0.3 lb of citric acid per 100 lb of syrup may be used with good results for fruit flavors.

Strawberry Ice Cream

The adaptability of the cultivars of strawberries and the various methods of freezing them have been discussed by Tressler *et al.* (1968). Fabricius (1931) did a great deal of experimenting on the use of strawberries for ice cream manufacture. He found that variety was a deciding factor influencing the quality of flavor. Maturity was the second significant factor since berries picked when fully ripe gave a superior flavor over berries that had been picked for shipment. Fabricius' (1931) experiments also proved that cold-packed strawberries were superior to canned berries and that both gave products that were superior to those packed using strawberry extracts for flavoring. In the same test, Fabricius froze strawberries with and without sugar. Those frozen with sugar at $-20°F$ gave the best-flavored and best-textured ice cream. Hening and Dahlberg (1933) also found that ice creams in which sugar-packed berries were used gave the best products in flavor, appearance, and texture. They used sliced strawberries packed in 80% cane sugar syrup that had been stored at 0°F. The strawberries were mixed into the ice cream after it was drawn. The only objection to the product was the hardness of the sliced pieces of fruit. This was overcome by allowing the frozen berries to thaw and stand in their syrup overnight.

Strawberries frozen for use in ice cream should be packed in a fruit:sugar ratio of 2–3:1, or in a 40–50% sugar syrup; this was suggested by Mack and Fellers (1932), who also found that the percentage of fruit used affects the rate of freezing, the body and texture, and the flavor and appearance of ice cream. In making ice cream using 6–20% fruit, they noted that the product became progressively better flavored up to 15%. Higher percentages increased the fruit flavor only slightly and decreased the desirability of texture and body. These defects caused the product to deteriorate more rapidly in storage and so indirectly contributed to the factor of poorer flavor.

Hening and Dahlberg (1933) gave the following directions for making strawberry ice cream:

A strawberry variety that has been found to give good results in freezing tests should be used. The berries should be sliced. A ratio of berries to sugar of 2 to 1 or the use of a 75% sugar solution (2.5 lb of berries to 1.6 lb of syrup) will give good results. It is desirable to freeze the fruit quickly to 0°F ($-18°C$) and to hold it at 0°F ($-18°C$) or below to retain the maximum flavor. Small containers, such as the 30-lb tin single service container, can be more readily frozen and handled than barrels and proper proportions of berries to syrup can be secured more easily. Before using the berries they should be thawed at a temperature not exceeding 40°F (4°C) and soaked in their syrup for 12–24 hr to soften them.

It is desirable to make a special mix for fruit ice creams in which the fat content is about 2% higher and the serum solids 1.5% higher than in regular vanilla ice cream to make allowance for the diluting effect of the syrup. The sugar content of the mix should be about 2% below that of vanilla ice cream, as 5–6% sugar is added in the fruit juice. The use of 20% of fruit gives a very desirable, evident flavor and plenty of visible fruit. The syrup should be drained off the berries and the berries alone placed in the hardening room for about a 1/2 hr to chill well. The syrup and color should be added to the mix in the freezer. The berries can be readily mixed by hand with the frozen ice cream. A hopper is desirable, but a large can, such as a 10-gal. tin container, may be used for this purpose. It is essential to prechill the utensils and the berries to avoid increasing the temperature of the ice cream, thereby lessening the degree of smoothness and creaminess of the finished product.

It is perhaps regrettable that over the past 50 years, no investigator has made as comprehensive or as detailed a study on the use of frozen fruits in ice cream as did Mack and Fellers (1932) and Hening and Dahlberg (1933). Surely there is a need for such a study in view of the many new cultivars that have come into existence and are now being used in commercially frozen packs.

Arbuckle (1952) reported that a 3:1 berry–sugar ratio pack is the best for use in ice cream. If fruit particles in ice cream are icy the product will not have good consumer acceptance. For fruit to have the same consistency as the ice cream when served, he stated that the sugar content in the fruit should be at least 21%, which is possible 3:1 ratio. Arbuckle also advised that there seem to be two schools of thought in regard to the appearance of strawberry ice cream. one group believes that the berries should be completely broken up so that only the seeds show. The other group believes that the berries should appear in large pieces. He believed that both groups can be satisfied and suggests that half the berries be pulped and added to the flavor vat and that the remainder be added through the fruit feeder.

According to Struble (1951) the ice cream industry might use greater quantities of the frozen fruits (primarily strawberries) if the quality of the frozen fruit pack was improved. In reporting on an examination of a number of samples, Struble commented on the variation in the berry–sugar ratio. The lot in question was labeled 3:1, but in some containers, the contents anayzed as high as 12:1. Obviously, variation of that nature would make it next to impossible to prepare a high-quality ice cream, where the balanced ratio of butterfat to solids other than fat is so important. Another instance of poor quality noted in the above examination was the amount of undissolved sugar in the bottom of some containers in which the berries were packed; also too much extraneous matter was present, such as caps, weeds, and insects. In addition, Struble (1951) claimed that the use of frozen fruits in ice cream manufacture would materially increase if packers avoided varieties that do not have good berry flavor.

Struble (1952) repeated his suggestion to the packers that there be sufficient mixing of the sugar and berries so that there is never any trace of undissolved sugar in the tin. He recommended additional mixing beyond that necessary to dissolve the sugar. Struble also repeated his plea for better quality cold-packed fruit.

A report of Guadagni (1956) seems to minimize the importance of adding sugar to berries when packed for use in ice cream. He summarizes his report as follows:

It is increasingly apparent that the most important single factor affecting the flavor quality of strawberry ice cream is the selection of highly flavored varieties which are harvested at optimum maturity and promptly frozen. With high-quality berries, such factors as freezing rate, fruit-to-sugar ratio, "sugar curing," and stabilization seem to offer little or no advantage in the flavor quality of the finished ice cream.

This suggests that strawberry ice cream could be satisfactorily flavored by simply adding the proper amount of high-quality unsugared strawberry puree.

In part, the above summary is in agreement with Tressler (1946), who said: "For some unexplained reason, crushed and pureed fruits hold their flavor and color better than fruits which have not been crushed prior to freezing."

However, he did not recommend packing unsugared strawberry puree for use in ice cream: "For many purposes, the addition of sugar to the purée is desirable. The addition of sugar helps to hold the flavor and color and also retards oxidation."

Raspberry Ice Cream

The recipe quoted for strawberries is adaptable to raspberries and yields a good flavored, full-bodied ice cream.

Hening and Dahlberg (1933) found that a 20–25% quantity of raspberries produced an excellent flavor ice cream. The whole berry, which had been packed in 80% cane sugar syrup and stored at 0°F was mixed into the ice cream after it was drawn from the freezer. The syrup in which the berries was packed was added to the mix in the freezer. They noted that raspberry ice cream stored at 15°F for 6 months was of poorer flavor and texture than the same lot stored at 0°F for the same length of time.

Mack and Fellers (1932) reported that less fruit was necessary to make a desirable-flavored ice cream of raspberries than any other fruit flavor. They used 12–15% of raspberry purée from which 75% of the seeds had been removed. This gave a superior product in flavor, but still somewhat seedy in texture. After reducing the puree to 10% and combining with commercial extract, a product of equally good flavor and better texture was produced.

A marked difference in the desirability of different cultivars was found. Preferred in order were 'Cuthbert', 'Herbert', and 'St. Regis'. The varieties 'Newman', 'Latham', and 'Ontario' gave decidedly poorer products and deteriorated in storage more quickly. Raspberries of the first three cultivars yielded better-flavored ice creams when they had been packed in 3:1 ratios with cane sugar syrups. The ratio of 2:1 was also acceptable but not superior in flavor or texture.

Peach Ice Cream

The adaptability of different cultivars of peaches to freezing has been discussed by Tressler et al. (1968). 'Early Crawford' was the only cultivar used by Hening and Dahlberg (1933) in their studies. Mack and Fellers (1932) noted that good-flavored peach ice cream could be made with 'Hiley', 'J. H. Hale', 'Elberta', 'Champion', and 'Crawford'.

It was found that pulped peach skin would greatly increase the flavor of peach ice cream. Also in the same studies, Hening and Dahlberg found that peaches packed in 5:1 ratio of cane sugar and kept at 0°F produced a good-textured and flavored ice cream if 25–30% of fruit was used.

A slightly lower amount of fruit, 15–20%, was suggested by Mack and Fellers and a 3:1 ratio of fruit to sugar was considered by them to yield the best product.

They found that yellow-fleshed peaches gave a greater concentration of flavor than white, and since the fruit is firmer in texture, large shreds of the yellow peaches were evident in the ice cream. They did not find any variety to yield sufficient flavor unless a flavoring extract was added along with the fruit. By replacing 35% of the peaches with apricots, excellent results are claimed by some manufacturers. Pulped fruit was found to be easier to handle and yielded a more desirable flavor and appearance since shreds of the peaches were visible.

The following directions for making peach ice cream are given by Haning and Dahlberg (1933):

> Fresh, ripe peaches of a standard variety with a fairly pronounced flavor should be dipped in boiling water, skinned, and ground or very finely sliced. The pulp should be mixed with sugar at the rate of 5 to 1 and immediately frozen to and held at 0°F (−18°C) or below.
>
> A day before using, the frozen peaches should be held at 40°F (4°C) to thaw. The color and the peaches may be added to the ice cream mix in the freezer as there is little advantage in endeavoring to retain pieces of peach in the ice cream due to the blending of color with the ice cream and to lack of a pronounced flavor. About 25% of peaches gave a recognizable, mild peach flavor. Peaches do not increase the moisture and sugar content of the ice cream as much as strawberries or raspberries, so they may be advantageously added to the regular vanilla mix, but the flavor will be best if the mix is rather rich.
>
> As previously mentioned, approximately 20–30% of the fresh, ripe peaches may be skinned like an apple and, after grinding the skins finely and adding 20% of sugar, cooked for 5 min just below the boiling point. The cooked skins with pulp may then be frozen and used to increase the intensity of the peach flavor by replacing 5–10% of the peaches in the ice cream. The skins must be fine enough to avoid detection in the ice cream.
>
> One percent of apricot added to peach ice cream increased the intensity of the flavor noticeably. Although the flavor was characteristic of apricots, few persons recognized their presence.

Cherry Ice Cream

Sour cultivars of cherries were found to be superior to other kinds of cherries in the production of ice cream. Mack and Fellers (1932) list in the order of preference 'Montmorency', 'Early Richmond', and 'May Duke'. The 'Morello' variety is less desirable and none of these varieties gives as good a flavor as processed maraschino cherries. The addition of a good commercial cherry extract, or the use of a small amount of oil of bitter almonds, added to the thawed frozen fruit of any of the above varieties, will give a flavor of ice cream comparable to that made from maraschino cherries. For 10 gal of fruit it is necessary to add only 1–2 ml of oil of bitter almonds or benzaldehyde. This must be thoroughly mixed through the fruit before adding to the ice cream mix.

The following recipe for cherry ice cream was developed by Hening (1935):

> Eleven pounds of Montmorency cherries packed in the ratio of 4 to 1 plus 2-1/2 lb of sugar were thawed and allowed to soak in their syrup for 20 hr prior to their use in ice cream. It took the greater part of this time to dissolve the additional sugar. This total of 13-1/2 lb of cherries and syrup was added in the early part of the freezing period to the 31-1/2 lb of mix in the freezer. This mix contained 14% fat, 11% MSNF, 14% sugar, and 0.5% of a medium grade gelatin. The scraper and dasher broke up the cherries and after the ice cream was hardened, small pieces of cherry were attractively distributed through the ice cream. These pieces were not hard or icy and they increased the cherry flavor in the ice cream.

Thirty percent of cherries and syrup may seem like an excessive amount, but since the cherry flavor is mild, this amount can be used to very good advantage. Cherry ice cream is very refreshing and was pronounced very good by everyone tasting it. The addition of a small amount of almond flavor or bitter almond oil produced an unusual and pleasing flavor. Experiments with cherries to which cherry extract had been added before freezing the cherries indicated that excellent flavor could be secured with a little less fruit, but the proportion of fruit in the ice cream needed to be high.

Pineapple Ice Cream

Mack and Fellers (1932) showed that 12–15% fruit gave the most desirable flavor and texture to pineapple ice cream. In a comparison of pineapples packed in Hawaii and Puerto Rico by crushing and canning, the flavor imparted by the Hawaiian packs was noticeably stronger and better. They also had the advantages of firmer flesh, less syrup, and better color.

Frozen pineapple was not available for the work done by Mack and Fellers but it is believed that considering the excellent product that can be obtained by freezing pineapple, they could have produced equally satisfactory results with frozen pineapple in place of the heat-preserved fruit they used.

Other Fruit Ice Creams

Mack and Fellers (1932) also made studies of fruit ice creams and fruit ices using less common flavors. In such fruits as wild and Evergreen blackberries, cranberries, Damson plums, red currants, rhubarb, and nectarines, they attained surprising results.

In using blackberries of both wild and Evergreen varieties, the products were only of fair quality since the good natural flavor was offset by a decidedly inferior appearance. This was also true when red currants, Damson plums, and rhubarb were added to the ice cream mix. These same fruits gave good quality products when made into frozen ices.

Nectarines imparted a flavor not unlike peaches when used in ice cream, but the frozen product was unattractive in appearance after storage.

In ice cream, cranberries lost their characteristic flavor, but in frozen ices, the pulped fruit gave a product superior to the fruit packed whole or sliced. Cranberry pulp or sliced cranberries were rated the best packs in appearance and flavor when they were frozen with sugar in a 1:1 ratio. Regardless of the method of freezing, the fruit kept perfectly in storage.

Apricot ice cream was produced by Hening and Dahlberg (1933) using a 4:1 fruit:sugar ratio. The pulp was preheated to 180°–190°F (82°–88°C) and held for 5 min before freezing. When the fruit was stirred into the ice cream after it was drawn from the freezer, the skins of the apricot were much less noticeable than when they were added to the mix in the freezer. The flavor was satisfactory and the color and texture acceptable.

Hening (1949), in developing a new method of producing apple juice, found that the resulting product could be used to add apple flavor to ices and ice cream. In making juice he found it advantageous to add ascorbic acid in apple juice solution during or immediately after milling and before pressing. Thirty-five percent of this apple juice was blended with an ice cream mix that contained 14% milkfat, 10% MSNF, and 15% sugar. While this ice cream was a delicious product, the mix appeared diluted. Later experiments indicated that 20% of the 37% soluble solids apple juice concentrate resulted in an excellent product, when an additional 5% sugar was added to the apple juice concentrate.

NUTS

Nutmeats and nut extracts are quite extensively used as flavorings in ice cream. Pecans, walnuts, almonds, pistachios, filberts, and peanuts are among the most popular. Nutmeats should be sound and clean and free from rancid flavors. They should be stored in tight containers in a cool place until used. Considerable care should be used in preparing them for the ice cream mix, to make certain that no foreign material, such as pieces of shell or pieces of wood and nails from containers, get into the mix. Nuts such as almonds, filberts, and pistachios should be blanched to remove their dark outer skin.

Since nutmeats are often high in bacteria count and sometimes are not hygienically handled, they can contaminate the mix and be the source of high count and sometimes pathogenic bacteria count in the ice cream unless they receive special heat-treatment. Some manufacturers dry-heat the nuts to pasteurizing temperatures or above, while others have found that they can greatly reduce bacterial count and improve the flavor of some nutmeats by dipping them in a boiling, slightly salted sugar solution for a few seconds. To prevent sogginess, the meats are afterwards dried for 3–4 min at 250°–300°F. All nutmeats should be chopped into very small pieces before they are added to the mix.

SPICES AND SALT

Spices such as cinnamon, cloves, nutmeg, allspice, and ginger are used to a limited extent as flavorings in ice cream, sherbets, and ices. Ginger ice cream is a favorite in some localities. Cinnamon, nutmeg, and cloves are often used to enhance or vary the flavor of chocolate ice cream, and they are used in combination with fruits or fruit extracts in such frozen products as puddings, eggnog, and punch.

Spices may be purchased either in dried and finely ground form or as extracts. Their flavors are very pungent and therefore only small amounts are required to produce the desired flavoring effect.

Salt, although not a spice, is often used in very small quantities to enhance the flavor of ice creams, especially in mixes containing eggs—custards and rich puddings—and in nut ice cream.

VARIEGATED OR RIPPLED ICE CREAM

Variegated ice cream is becoming increasingly popular. This product is produced by injecting approximately 10% of a prepared base into the ice cream.

Most popular flavors of variegated ice cream are chocolate, butterscotch, marshmallow, fudge, strawberry, pineapple, raspberry, and caramel. This type of ice cream provides almost unlimited possibilities for flavor combinations. The methods for the manufacture of variegated ice cream as given by Dahle (1941b) are as follows:

> Many types of pumps, fillers, etc., are available for use with the continuous freezers which give a nice "waviness" of flavor to the ice cream, and more uniformity than with some of the apparatus used for batch freezers. Some of the equipment used for incorporating the flavor with the batch freezer is far from sanitary, but it works fairly well. The pressure tank apparatus requires two operations for best results.
>
> Some small manufacturers using batch freezers have done a good job by pouring in the flavor from the measuring can as the ice cream is coming from the freezer. This takes two operators, one to pour and the other to throttle the gate of the freezer. The one who pours has the pouring lip of a 2-qt container against the stream of ice cream coming from the batch freezer. Brick ice cream can be made from batch ice cream by merely pouring the flavor on layers of vanilla ice cream in the tray. This is a clumsy way to operate, but it is being practiced by many small manufacturers using batch freezers.

Today, variegated ice cream is an important product, believed to rank fourth behind vanilla, chocolate, and strawberry in sales across the country. Variegator machines are available that make possible precise control of the amount of the variegating desired in packages ranging from pints to half-gallons.

COLOR IN ICE CREAM

Ice cream should have a delicate, attractive color that suggests or is readily associated with its flavor. Only colors certified by the FDA should be used.

Almost all flavors of ice cream should be slightly colored. Enough yellow color is generally added to vanilla ice cream to give it the shade of natural ceram produced in the summer months. Fruit ice creams need to be colored because about 15% fruit, the maximum commonly used, produces only a slight effect on color. Chocolate ice cream is one of the exceptions. It rarely needs to be colored, for the required amount of a Dutch process cocoa will produce sufficient color.

Most colors are of synthetic origin. A weak alkaline solution of annatto color is about the only vegetable color used in ice cream. However, instead of a good egg-shade yellow, this produces a pinkish tinge. Most ice cream makers purchase the desired colors in liquid or paste form.

Preparation of Coloring Solutions

It is more economical to purchase food colors in powder form and dissolve them in boiling water as needed. Blending of these "primary colors" to give desired shades requires some artistic ability and experience. Such coloring solutions, if contaminated, will become very high in bacteria count. In this way the bacteria content of the ice cream is increased and the growth of the organisms partially destroys the color pigment. Therefore color solutions should not be prepared in large amounts, should be boiled, and should be stored in a cool place. A good practice is to add 0.1% of sodium benzoate to the solution to keep it sterile.

FD&C Approved Food Colors

The colors approved by the Federal Food, Drug and Cosmetic Act can be obtained by writing to the FDA. Color solutions of a strength commonly used may be prepared by dissolving 4 oz of a primary or basic color per gallon of water, or 0.5 oz pt to make a liquid solution of about 3%. Use 1 oz of this liquid solution to 5 gal of mix.

8
Calculation of Ice Cream Mixes

THE IMPORTANCE OF CALCULATIONS

Since the palatability, quality, body and texture, and cost of the ice cream hinge upon our ability to select and use, in the right proportion, the various ingredients from those that are available, it becomes essential for us to learn to calculate accurately the amount of each ingredient that goes into the mix we desire to make. In other words, as ice cream makers, we need to know how much it costs to make a gallon of ice cream; how much ice cream can be made from a gallon of mix; how much cream, sugar, etc., are needed to make 100 lb (or any other number of pounds) of mix. Answers to such questions can be obtained only if we know how to make at least simple, although time-consuming, calcuations.

A knowledge of calculations is also helpful in properly balancing a mix, especially in establishing and maintaining uniform quality, and in producing ice cream that conforms to the necessary legal standards. Some authorities think that an ice cream maker's knowledge of making ice cream is in direct proportion to the ability to make the necessary calculations.

The method and procedure of making calculations are demonstrated by a few typical problems, which are presented in detail for the benefit of the reader who might be confused by figures alone, i.e., without explanation of the processes involved. However, the presentation here attempts to focus attention on *the method* and *the procedure* with a minimum of effort in performing the necessary arithmetic. It is assumed that the reader is most interested in learning a quick and easy way to arrive at the correct answer and therefore little explanation is given of the mathematics involved in deriving the formulas or the logic in setting up the equations.

Much practice is usually necessary to develop speed and accuracy in making calculations. This practice can be obtained by using the demonstrated problems as a pattern for setting up and solving many similar problems.

Ice cream mixes may be divided into two groups: simple and complex. Simple mixes require the least calculations and are made of ingredients each of which supplies one constituent. Complex mixes are more difficult to calculate. They include mixes where at least one constituent is obtained from two or more products. Simple mixes may be figured by multiplication, addition, subtraction, or division while complex mixes require the use of the Pearson square method, the serum point method, or algebra.

MATHEMATICAL PROCESSES MOST FREQUENTLY USED

The discussion in this chapter on calculating ice cream mixes assumes a knowledge of arithmetic, especially decimals and percentages. Even so, it may be helpful to state the following mathematical facts that will be used frequently:

1. A fraction indicates the process of division. Thus

$$\frac{2.25}{5} \text{ or } 2.25/5$$

means that 2.25 is divided by 5 to give 0.45, or

$$\frac{2.25}{5} = 2.25 \div 5 = 0.45$$

2. When a percentage figure is used in division or multiplication, the percent sign is dropped and the decimal point is moved two places to the left. Thus 94% = 0.94 and 2.25/94% indicates that 2.25 is divided by 0.94, or

$$\frac{2.25}{94\%} = 2.25 \div 0.94 = 2.39$$

Similarly, 63/100% indicates that 63 is divided by 1.00, or

$$\frac{63}{100\%} = 63 \div 1.00 = 63$$

3. When the amount of milk (pounds) and the test (percentage of fat in the milk) are given, the amount of fat (pounds) is obtained by multiplication:

$$50 \text{ lb milk} \times 4\% = 50 \times 0.04 = 2.00 \text{ lb fat}$$

4. When the amount of fat and the test are given, the amount of milk (or cream) is obtained by division:

$$\frac{2.00 \text{ lb fat}}{4\%} = \frac{2.00}{0.04} = 50 \text{ lb milk}$$

5. When the amount of milk and fat are given, the test is obtained by division:

$$\frac{2.00 \text{ lb fat}}{50 \text{ lb milk}} = 0.04 = 4\%$$

METHODS OF CALCULATING MIXES

Several methods of calculating mixes are available, but some are too tedious, too complicated, or unsatisfactory for calculating the more complex mixes. The Pearson square, algebraic, serum point, formula tables, tabulations, or graphic methods and, more recently, computer-developed formulations have all been used.

The Pearson square method is successful when the calculation is limited to the proportion of milk and cream needed, but it will not readily calculate the amount of MSNF needed. The algebraic method is equally accurate and applicable to the most complex problems, but it involves rather lengthy calculations and a thorough knowledge of setting up and solving simultaneous equations. It is definitely cumbersome and slow. The serum point method and various arithmetic methods are basically identical with the formulas presented in these chapters. However, the use of the formulas simplifies the procedure and thus makes it easier to learn.

The use of recipe tables or tabulations that indicate the amount of each ingredient has the advantage of eliminating errors in calculation and saving valuable time. However, a new table must be prepared for every slight change in the desired composition of the mix, and for changes in the source of the constituents. For example, if the mix is prepared using sugar and sweetened condensed skim milk, the table must allow for all variations in the test of the sweetened condensed skim milk in regard to both sugar composition and MSNF. Such a table would be practically useless when liquid sugar is substituted for sugar. This indicates the large number of tables necessary to provide for all possible variations in composition and ingredients. Such a compilation in one volume would be too cumbersome for convenient reference. A final advantage of the formulas given in these chapters is that they make possible the calculation of all the tables required by the particular conditions of any manufacturer whenever the tables justify the effort of preparation.

STANDARDIZING MILK AND CREAM

Sometimes it is desirable to use a simple and easy method for standardizing milk and cream so that stocks on hand are always of the same tests, a convenience in calculating mixes.

There are several methods of standardizing which are very satisfactory. To find the proportions of milk and cream to use, either of the following methods may be employed.

Pearson Square Method

Draw a rectangle with two diagonals. At the upper left-hand corner, write the test of the cream to be standardized. At the lower left-hand corner write the test of the milk to be used in standardizing. In the center of the rectangle, place the desired test. At the right-hand corners write the differences between the numbers at the left-hand corner and the number in the center. The number at the upper right-hand corner represents the number of pounds of cream of the richness indicated by the number at the upper left-hand corner. The number at the lower right-hand corner indicates the number of pounds of milk of the richness indicated by the number at the lower left-hand corner. By mixing milk and cream in these proportions the desired test will be obtained.

For example, say 35% cream is to be standardized to 20% using 4% milk, as shown in Fig. 8.1. The difference 20 − 4 = 16 represents the amount of 35% cream that must be mixed with 15 lb of 4% milk to make 31 lb of 20% cream. When the proportions of milk and cream have been found, any amount of 35% cream may be standardized to 20% by mixing with 4% milk in the proportions of 16/31 of cream to 15/31 of milk. For example, if 310 lb of 20% cream is wanted, then 16/31 × 310 = 160 lb, the amount of 35% cream needed, and 15/31 × 310 = 150 lb, the amount of 4% milk needed.

If skim milk is used instead of whole milk the figures would be as shown in Fig. 8.2. In this case a mixture composed of 20/35 cream and 15/35 skim milk will test 20%.

Arithmetical Method

Another method of standardizing that is quite simple and accurate and involves little calculating is as follows: Multiply the amount of cream by the

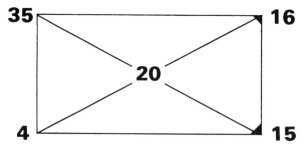

Fig. 8.1. Pearson square method for standardizing a 35% cream to 20% using 4% milk. The number in the lower right-hand corner is the difference of the number in the upper-left-hand corner and the number in the center. The number in the upper right-hand corner is the difference of the number in the lower left-hand corner and the number in the center.

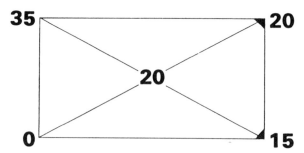

Fig. 8.2. Pearson square method for standardizing a 35% cream to 20% using skim milk (0% fat).

difference between its test and the required test, and divide the product by the difference between the required test and the test of the milk to be added.

Problem 1. Standardize 120 lb of 30% cream to 20%, using 4.2% milk.

Solution. The difference between the test of cream and the required test is $30 - 20 = 10$. The difference between the required test and the test of the milk is $20 - 4.2 = 15.8$.

Using these figures we have $120 \times 10 \div 15.8 = 75.95$ lb. Therefore, 75.95 lb of 4.2% milk are required to reduce the test of 120 lb of 30% cream to 20%. The accuracy of this method is shown by the following calculations. The amount of fat in 75.95 lb of 4.2% milk is

$$75.95 \times 4.2\% = 3.1899 \ \text{lb}$$

The amount of fat in 120 lb of 30% cream is

$$120 \times 30\% = 36 \ \text{lb}$$

Thus we have a total of 195.95 lb of milk and cream, containing a total of 39.1899 lb of fat. The same amount of 20% cream contains

$$195.95 \times 20\% = 39.19 \ \text{lb}$$

Problem 2. Calculate the quantities of the ingredients needed for a 100-lb mix containing 12% fat, 15% sugar, and 0.5% stabilizer, using 40% cream and 4% milk.

Solution

Step 1. First prepare a proof sheet, which is useful in calculating the mix and in checking the accuracy of the calculations (see Fig. 8.3). Enter the amount of sugar and stabilizer required—15 and 0.5 lb, respectively—for a total of 15.5 lb. This leaves 84.5 lb to be supplied by milk and cream.

Step 2. Calculate to the nearest 0.1% the percentage of fat needed in the 84.5 mixture of milk and cream to provide 12% fat in the total 100 lb mix:

$$\frac{12}{84.5} \times 100 = 14.2\%$$

Step 3. Use the Pearson square method first to determine the proportions of milk and cream (see Fig. 8.4). Then calculate the amounts needed to produce 84.5 lb:

$$25.8 \times 10.2 = 36.0 \ \text{parts}$$
$$84.5/36.0 = 2.347 \ \text{lb/part}$$

	Ingredient weight (lb)	Calculated constituents				
Ingredients		Fat (lb)	MSNF (lb)	Sugar (lb)	Stabilizer (lb)	TS (lb)	Cost ($)
	—	—	—	—	—	—	—
Total						
Calculated %						
Check with desired wt. desired %						

Fig. 8.3. Sample proof sheet.

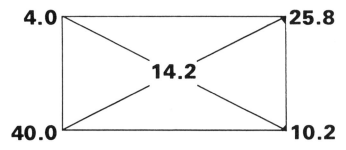

Fig. 8.4. Application of Pearson square method to Problem 2.

Then

$$25.8 \times 2.347 = 60.5 \quad \text{lb 4\% milk}$$
$$10.2 \times 2.347 = 24.0 \quad \text{lb 40\% cream}$$

The completed proof sheet is shown in Fig. 8.5.

CALCULATING MIXES WITH THE
SERUM POINT METHOD

1. List the amount and composition of the desired mix.

2. Determine the amount (pounds) of fat, serum solids (MSNF), stabilizer, emulsifier, etc., by using the formula

amount of ingredient = (amount of mix) × (proportion of ingredient)

3. Calculate the amount (pounds) of the serum of the mix (recall that serum is water and serum solids), by subtracting all of the other ingredients from the total mix:

serum = mix − (fat + sugar + stab. + emul.)

4. To calculate the amount of condensed milk needed, it is necessary to know the amount of serum solids and the amount of serum in 1 lb of the condensed milk, and the amount of serum solids and serum (calculated in steps 2 and 3, respectively) in the mix. The formula for the amount of condensed milk (in pounds) is then given by[1]

$$\text{cond.} = \frac{(\text{serum solids needed}) - (\text{serum of mix} \times 0.09)}{(\text{serum solids/lb of cond. milk}) - (\text{serum/lb of cond. milk} \times 0.09)}$$

---

[1]The figure 0.09 represents the percentage of total solids in 1 lb of skim milk, in this case 9%. However, if skim milk tests 8.8% TS, then the figure 0.088 must be used.

| Ingredients | Ingredient weight (lb) | Calculated constituents | | | | | |
		Fat (lb)	MSNF (lb)	Sugar (lb)	Stabilizer (lb)	TS (lb)	Cost ($)
Sugar	15.0			15.0		15.0	
Stabilizer	0.5				0.5	0.5	
Cream, 40%	24.0	9.6	1.3			10.9	
Milk, 4%	60.5	2.4	5.3			7.7	
Total	100.00	12.0	6.8	15.0	0.5	34.1	—
Calculated %		12.0	6.8	15.0	0.5	34.1	
Check with desired wt. desired %		12.0	6.8	15.0	0.5		

Fig. 8.5. Completed proof sheet for Problem 2.

5. If there is any fat or sugar in the condensed milk, it must be calculated:

$$\text{fat} = (\text{cond. milk}) \times (\text{decimal proportion of fat})$$
$$\text{sugar} = (\text{cond. milk}) \times (\text{decimal proportion of sugar})$$

6. Calculate the amount of fat needed from the milk and cream by subtracting the amount of fat in the condensed milk from the total amount of fat needed in the mix:

$$\text{fat (milk/cream)} = \text{fat (mix)} - \text{fat (cond.)}$$

7. Calculate the amount of sugar that must be added to the mix by subtracting the amount of sugar in the condensed milk from the total amount needed in the mix:

$$\text{sugar (needed)} = \text{sugar (total)} - \text{sugar (cond. milk)}$$

8. If there is no fat or sugar in the condensed milk, omit steps 6 and 7.
9. Calculate the amount of milk and cream needed by subtracting the total of all ingredients from the amount of the total mix:

$$\text{milk/cream} = (\text{total mix}) - (\text{total other ingredients})$$

10. The amount of cream needed can be calculated as follows:

$$\text{cream} = \frac{(\text{fat needed}) - [(\text{milk and cream needed}) \times (\text{fat \% in milk})]}{(\text{amount of fat/lb of cream}) - (\text{amount of fat/lb of milk})}$$

11. Calculate the amount of milk needed by subtracting the amount of cream from the amount of milk and cream.
12. The total weight of all ingredients will now equal the amount of mix required.
13. Verify the calculations.

For example, to calculate the ingredients needed for 100 lb of a mix containing 12% fat, 11% serum solids, 15% sugar, 0.3% stabilizer if we have the following ingredients on hand: 40% cream, 4% milk, condensed milk (27% serum solids), sugar, and stabilizer, we apply the serum point method.

1. The amounts and composition are given in the initial conditions.
2. Step 2 is easily calculated from the desired mix proportions as 12 lb fat, 11 lb serum solids, 15 lb sugar, and 0.3 lb stabilizer.
3. The total serum amount is $100 - (15 + 12 + 0.3) = 72.7$ lb.
4. The amount of condensed milk is given by the serum point formula as

$$\frac{11 - (72.7 \times 0.09)}{0.27 - (1 \times 0.09)} = 24.76 \quad \text{lb}$$

5. There is no fat or sugar in the condensed milk, and so we go on to step 9.

9. The amount of milk and cream are calculated as $100 - (24.76 + 15 + 0.3) = 59.94$ lb.

10. The amount of cream needed is

$$\frac{12 - (59.94 \times 0.04)}{0.40 - 0.04} = 26.67 \quad \text{lb.}$$

11. The amount of milk needed is then $59.94 - 26.67 = 33.27$ lb.

12. A check of the weights of the ingredients will show that they add up to 100 lb of mix.

13. All of the calculations should then be verified by using a proof sheet.

MIX DECISIONS

Before a mix can be calculated, a number of key decisions have to be made by the ice cream manufacturer:

1. Composition of mix: the proportionate amount of each of the constituents must first be specified (e.g., percentage fat).
2. Size of batch: the size of the batch is usually constant within a factory; it is most frequently calculated on a 100-lb basis and then the figures are increased for larger batches.
3. Choice of ingredients: from the available ingredients, a decision must be made on the basis of quality, characteristics, and cost.
4. Composition of ingredients: the composition of ingredients can be determined from a table, but the best results are obtained when they are based on the exact analysis of the actual ingredients.
5. Classification of the mix; when the above information has been obtained, the mix can be classified as either simple or complex, and calculations can be made accordingly.

After these decisions have been made, the following steps are taken to calculate the mix:

1. Prepare a proof sheet and record each subsequent calculation.
2. Calculate the amount of each ingredient that supplies only one constituent to the mix (usually sugar and stabilizer).
3. Calculate the amount of each product that supplies concentrated serum solids or fat. Record the amounts of the constituents supplied.
4. Calculate the amount of each remaining dairy product. Record the amounts of the constituents supplied.
5. Total each constituent column in the proof sheet and compare the "needed" and "total" columns.

SIMPLE MIXES

Simple mixes require the least calculation and include such mixes as one made of stabilizer, sugar, and cream, and condensed skim milk or non-fat dry milk solids; or one made from ingredients each of which supply only one constituent. Mixes having two sources of one constituent are more complex, but sometimes the calculation may be reduced to the same simple procedure that is used for the simplest mixes.

Problem 3. How much 30% cream, nonfat dry milk solids testing 97% MSNF, cane sugar, dried egg yolk, stabilizer, and water will be needed to make 450 lb of mix testing 10% fat, 11% MSNF, 14% sugar, 0.5% egg yolk solids, and 0.5% stabilizer?

Solution

Step 1. List the available ingredients and the number of pounds of each constituent in the desired mix, as in Table 8.1.

Step 2. Make a proof sheet and enter the weight and percentage of each constituent of the desired mix in the desired wt and % columns. Enter the information obtained in each succeeding step. (See complete proof sheet, Fig. 8.6.)

Step 3. Compute the amount of each ingredient that supplies only one constituent. In this problem these will be the stabilizer product, supplying all of the stabilizer, and the cane sugar, supplying all of the sugar.

The stabilizer containe 90% TS. Therefore, 90% of the weight stabilizer needed must equal 2.25 lb, the desired amount of stabilizer (the moisture-free part of the stabilizer). From this it follows that

$$2.25/0.90 = 2.50 \quad \text{lb}$$

Enter 2.50 in weight column of proof sheet and enter 2.25 in the stab, and the total solids columns. Cane sugar is 100% sugar and so 63 lb of cane sugar is needed. Enter this figure in the weight, sugar, and TS columns of the proof sheet.

Step 4. Compute the amount of those ingredients that supply more than one constituent of the mix but are the only remaining source of some one

Table 8.1. Available Ingredients/Desired Composition Table for Problem 3

Available ingredients		Desired mix composition		
Ingredient	Constituent (%)[a]	Constituent	Proportion (%)	Weight (lb)
Stabilizer	TS (90%)	Fat	10	45.0
Dried egg yolks[b]	Fat (62.5%)	MSNF	11	49.5
	TS (94%)			
Cane sugar	Sugar (100%)	Sugar	14	49.5
Nonfat dry milk	TS (97%)	Egg yolk solids[b]	0.5	2.25
	MSNF (97%)	Stabilizer[c]	0.5	2.25
Cream	Fat (30%)			
	MSNF (6.24%)			
Water				

[a]The figures are approximate, and are taken from Table 5.7.
[b]Although egg products are not widely used in ice cream manufacture, they are included here for illustrative purposes.
[c]Stabilizer in these calculations means the moisture-free part only. It also includes the emulsifier.

constituent—in this problem, the dried egg yolk, which is the only source of egg solids.

$$2.25/0.94 = 2.39 \quad \text{lb}$$

Enter this in the weight column, and enter 2.25 lb in the egg solids and TS columns of proof sheet.

Also calculate the amount of other constituents supplied by the dried egg yolk, namely, fat:

$$2.39 \times 0.625 = 1.49 \quad \text{lb}$$

Enter in proof sheet. This 1.49 lb of fat is part of the 2.25 lb of egg solids or TS. Frequently the fat supplied by the eggs is disregarded, but sometimes, as in this problem, it is considered as a part of the fat that is desired in the mix. Thus the 45 lb of fat desired less the 1.49 lb of fat supplied by the dried egg yolk leaves 43.51 lb of fat to be supplied by other ingredients, in this case, the cream. Hence the weight of the 30% cream needed is

$$43.51/0.30 = 145.03 \quad \text{lb}$$

Enter in proof sheet. This cream furnishes not only fat but also MSNF, which is computed as follows:

$$145.03 \times 0.624 = 9.05 \quad \text{lb}$$

Enter in proof sheet. The total 49.5 lb of MSNF desired less the 9.05 lb MSNF supplied by the cream leaves 40.45 lb lf MSNF to be obtained from the remaining ingredients, namely, the nonfat dry milk. Therefore, it follows that the weight of the nonfat dry milk solids needed is

$$40.45/0.97 = 41.70 \quad \text{lb}$$

Enter in proof sheet. Enter 40.45 lb in MSNF and TS columns of proof sheet.

Finally, the above calculated amounts of each ingredient are totaled, and this sum is subtracted from the total 450 lb of mix desired. The difference represents the amount of water needed:

$$450.00 - (2.50 + 2.39 + 63.00 + 145.03 + 41.70 =$$
$$450.00 - 254.62 = 195.38 \quad \text{lb}$$

Enter in proof sheet.

Step 5. At this time it may also be desirable to compute the cost of the mix by entering in the proof sheet the actual cost of the ingredients used. (See Chapter 10; cost figures are assumed, not actual.)

Step 6. To find the percentage (test) of each constituent in the mix, each column should now be totaled. The calculated test for any constituent is obtained by dividing the total of that column by the total weight of the ingredients. For example, the calculated MSNF test is obtained by dividing 49.50 lb MSNF by 450 lb, the total weight of the ingredients, giving 11.0%. Similarly 160.51 lb, the total weight of TS, is divided by 450 lb to give 35.67% TS. In similar manner find the percentage of each of the remaining constituents, and enter the figures in their respective columns in proof sheet.

Step 7. Determine the correctness of the calculation from the proof sheet by comparing the calculated percentage for each constituent with the corresponding desired test. When the difference between these two percentages is less than one-tenth, the mix is assumed to be correctly calculated (see Fig. 8.6).

COMPLEX MIXES

Complex mixes, according to our classification, include all mixes, except those classed as simple mixes, and mixes made in a vacuum pan. They can usually be identified by the fact that at least one constituent is obtained from two or more ingredients. These complex mixes are most rapidly calculated by using formulas in the following steps:

1. List the available ingredients and the number of pounds of each constituent in the desired mix (see Table 8.1).

2. Make a proof sheet and enter the weight and percentage of each constituent of the desired mix. Enter the information obtained in each succeeding step.

3. Compute the amount of each ingredient that supplies only one constituent. (This usually includes the stabilizer, egg products, and sugar substitutes.)

4. Calculate the amount of condensed or powdered dairy products needed, using one of the following formulas:

(I) Amount of nonfat dry milk solids or condensed skim milk (when using fresh whole or skim milk):[2]

$$\frac{(\text{MSNF needed}) - (\text{serum of mix} \times 0.09)}{\text{MSNF per pound nonfat dry milk solids}} \qquad \text{(I)}$$

(II) Amount of condensed whole or condensed skim milk (when using fresh whole or skim milk):

$$\frac{(\text{MSNF needed}) - (\text{serum of mix} \times 0.09)}{\text{MSNF/lb cond. milk} - (\text{serum/lb cond. milk} \times 0.09)} \qquad \text{(II)}$$

5. Calculate the amount of sugar needed.

---

[2]Although not absolutely accurate, this formula can be used for practical operation when butter is the source of fat.

| Ingredients | Ingredient weight (lb) | Calculated constituents | | | | | | |
		Fat (lb)	MSNF (lb)	Sugar (lb)	Egg solids (lb)	Stabilizer (lb)	TS (lb)	Cost ($)
Stabilizer	2.50					2.25	2.25	
Dried egg yolk	2.39	1.49			2.25		2.25	
Cane sugar	63.00			63.00			63.00	
Cream (30%)	145.03	43.51	9.05				52.56	
Nonfat dry milk solids	41.70		40.45				40.45	
Water	195.38							
Total	450.00	45.00	49.50	63.00	2.25	2.25	160.51	—
Calculated %		10.00	11.00	14.00	0.50	0.50	35.67	
Check with desired wt.	450.00	45.00	49.50	63.00	2.25	2.25	162.00	
desired %		10.00	11.00	14.00	0.50	0.50	36.00	

Fig. 8.6. Completed proof sheet for problem 3.

6. Calculate the amount of cream (or butter) needed by using the following:
(III) Amount of cream or butter needed when using fresh whole milk:

$$\frac{(\text{fat needed}) - (\text{milk and cream needed} \times \text{proportion of fat milk})}{(\text{fat per pound of cream}) - (\text{fat per pound of milk})} \qquad (\text{III})$$

7. Calculate the amount of sweetened whole or skim milk needed.
8. Add up each column in the proof sheet and compute the percentages.
9. Examine your figures for accuracy by checking them against the desired amounts and percentages.
10. Compute the cost of the mix.

Problem 4. MSNF from Three Sources. Calculate the amount of ingredients needed to make 200 lb of mix testing 14% fat, 9% MSNF, 13% sugar, and 0.5% stabilizer. The available ingredients are 40% cream, 4% milk, condensed skim milk (27% MSNF, 27% TS), cane sugar, and stabilizer.

Solution. This is a complex mix since the MSNF will be obtained from three sources (condensed skim milk, cream, and milk).

Step 1. Make a list of available ingredients and the constituents desired (Table 8.2).
Step 2. Make a proof sheet and enter the information from step 1.
Step 3. In this problem, there is only one source of stabilizer, and it contains 90% TS, the balance being water. Therefore 90% of the number of pounds of stabilizer needed must equal 1.0 lb, the desired amount of stabilizer in the mix, and so 1.0/0.90 = 1.11 lb, the amount of stabilizer needed. This figure is entered in the weight column of the proof sheet.
The 1.1 lb of stabilizer product supplies 1.0 lb of dry stabilizer, which also counts as 1 lb TS. Enter these figures in the stabilizer and TS columns, respectively.
In this problem, no egg products are used and no sugar substitutes are used; therefore, these require no calculation. Also, cane sugar is the only source of sugar, and so 26 lb is needed.
Step 4. To find the amount of condensed skim milk needed, we use formula (I). The figures we need for the formula are obtained as follows:
From step 1, the amount of MSNF needed is 18 lb. To obtain the amount of serum of the mix, first find the sum of the fat (28 lb, from step 1), the stabilizer (1.11 lb, from step 3), and the sugar (26 lb, from step 3), which is 55.11 lb. Then subtract this from the desired total weight of the mix, 200.00 lb, leaving 144.89 lb, the amount of serum of the mix. We obtain the amount of MSNF in 1 lb of condensed skim milk by multiplying the 1 lb by 27% which gives 0.27.
We substitute these figures in formula (I):

$$\frac{18 \text{ lb} - (144.89 \text{ lb} \times 0.09)}{0.27 - 0.09} = \frac{18 - 13.04}{0.27 - 0.09} = \frac{4.96}{0.18} = 27.56 \quad \text{lb}$$

Table 8.2. Available Ingredients/Desired Composition Table for Problem 4

Available ingredients		Desired mix composition		
Ingredient	Constituent (%)	Constituent	Proportion (%)	Weight (lb)
Stabilizer	TS (90%)	Fat	14	28
Cane sugar	Sugar (100%)	MSNF	9	18
Condensed skim milk	TS (27%)	Sugar	13	26
	MSNF (27%)	Stabilizer	0.5	1
Cream	Fat (40%)			
	MSNF (5.35%)			
Whole milk	Fat (4%)			
	MSNF (8.79%)			

the amount of sweetened condensed skim milk needed. This figure is entered in the weight column of the proof sheet.

We also enter in their respective columns the amount of MSNF and TS supplied by the 27.56 lb condensed skim milk. We obtained these by multiplying the 27.56 lb by the respective percentages of MSNF and TS:

$$27.56 \times 27\% \text{ MSNF} = 7.44 \text{ lb MSNF}$$
$$27.56 \times 27\% \text{ TS} = 7.44 \text{ lb TS}$$

Step 5. The amount of sugar needed has been calculated in step 3.

Step 6. The amount of cream needed is calculated with the aid of formula (III), using the following figures:

From step 1, the amount of fat needed is 28 lb. To calculate the amount of milk and cream needed, we first find the sum of the stabilizer (1.11 lb, from step 3), the condensed skim milk (27.56 lb, from step 4), and the sugar (26 lb, from step 3), which is 54.67 lb. Then subtract this from the desired total weight of the mix, 200 lb, which leaves 145.33 lb, the amount of milk and cream needed. We obtain the amount of fat in 1 lb of 40% cream by multiplying the 1 lb by 0.40, which gives 0.40 lb; and the amount of fat in 1 lb of 4% milk by multiplying the 1 lb by 0.04, which gives 0.04 lb. We substitute these figures in formula (III):

$$\frac{28 \text{ lb} - (145.33 \text{ lb} \times 0.04)}{0.40 - 0.04} = \frac{28 \text{ lb} - 5.813 \text{ lb}}{0.36} = \frac{22.187}{0.36} = 61.63 \text{ lb}$$

the amount of 40% cream needed.

This figure is entered in the weight column of the proof sheet.

We also enter in their respective columns the amounts of fat, MSNF, and TS contained in the 61.63 lb of cream. We obtain these by multiplying the 61.63 lb by the respective percentages of fat, MSNF, and TS:

$$61.63 \text{ lb} \times 40\% = 24.65 \text{ lb fat}$$
$$61.63 \text{ lb} \times 5.35\% = 3.30 \text{ lb MSNF}$$

and adding:

$$24.65 \text{ lb} + 3.30 \text{ lb} = 27.95 \text{ lb TS}$$

Step 7. The amount of milk needed is computed by subtracting the amount of cream (61.63 lb, from step 6) from the amount of milk and cream needed (145.33 lb, from Step 6), to obtain 83.70 lb. This is entered in the weight column. We calculate the amounts of fat, MSNF, and TS contained in the milk by multiplying 83.70 lb by the respective percentages:

$$83.70 \times 0.04 = 3.35 \text{ lb fat}$$
$$83.70 \times 0.0879 = 7.36 \text{ lb MSNF}$$

and adding:

$$3.35 + 7.36 = 10.71 \quad \text{lb TS}$$

and these are entered in their respective columns.

Step 8. Each column of the proof sheet is now totaled. These totals should agree with the corresponding figures of the desired mix (see Fig. 8.7). (The calculations in this book were done using four decimal places, although in most cases only two are recorded. One unit in the second decimal place is equivalent to only about one-sixth of an ounce.)

The percentage of TS is calculated as follows:

$$\frac{73.10 \text{ lb TS}}{200 \text{ lb mix}} = 0.3655 = 36.55\% \quad \text{TS}$$

Similar computations will yield the calculated percentage for each of the constituents.

Step 9. The correctness of the calculations may be determined by comparing the calculated percentage for each constituent with the corresponding test of the desired mix. For example, in this problem, the calculated percentage of MSNF is 9.05% (18.10 lb MSNF/200 lb mix), compared with 9.0% MSNF of the desired mix. Since the difference between these two percentages is less than 0.1, it is not significant. Similar comparisons for each constituent show no significant differences, and therefore the calculations are correct.

Step 10. The actual cost depends upon many factors, and so the figures are not included in this problem, but the methods of calculating an assumed cost are demonstrated in problem 9, Chap. 10.

Problem 5. More Than One Source of Sugar, MSNF, and Fat. Calculate the amount of ingredients needed to make 900 lb of mix testing 12% fat, 10% MSNF, 14% sugar, and 0.4% stabilizer. The available ingredients are 40% cream, 4.0% milk, dehydrated corn syrup solids to supply 25% of the sugar, sweetened condensed skim milk (42% sugar, 30% MSNF), cane sugar, and stabilizer.

Solution. This complex mix has three sources of sugar, three sources of MSNF, and two sources of fat.

Step 1. List the available ingredients and desired constituents (Table 8.3).

Step 2. Make a proof sheet and enter the information from step 1.

Step 3. In this problem there is only one source of stabilizer, and it contains 90% TS. Therefore, 90% of the number of pounds needed equals 3.6 lb, the desired amount of stabilizer (from Step 1), and so 3.6/0.90 = 4.0 lb of stabilizer is needed. This figure is entered in the weight column of the proof sheet. Enter 3.6 lb in the stabilizer and TS columns.

Dehydrated corn syrup solids are used to supply 25% of the desired sugar. Therefore, 126 × 0.25 = 31.50 lb of sugar to be obtained from the dehydrated corn syrup solids, which contain only 47% sucrose equivalent. It follows that

Ingredients	Ingredient weight (lb)	Calculated constituents					
		Fat (lb)	MSNF (lb)	Sugar (lb)	Stabilizer (lb)	TS (lb)	Cost ($)
Stabilizer	1.11				1.00	1.00	
Cane sugar	26.00			26.00		26.00	
Cond. skim milk	27.56		7.44			7.44	
Cream, 40%	62.63	24.65	3.30			27.95	
Milk, 4%	83.70	3.35	7.36			10.71	
Total	200.00	28.00	18.10	26.00	1.00	73.10	—
Calculated %		14.00	9.05	13.00	0.50	36.55	
Check with desired wt.	200.00	28.00	18.00	26.00	1.00	73.00	
desired %		14.00	9.00	13.00	0.50	36.50	

Fig. 8.7. Completed proof sheet for problem 4.

Table 8.3. Available Ingredients/Desired Composition Table for Problem 5

Available ingredients		Desired mix composition		
Ingredient	Constituent (%)	Constituent	Proportion (%)	Weight (lb)
Stabilizer	TS (90%)	Fat	12	108
Dehydrated corn syrup solids	Sugar (47%)	MSNF	10	90
	TS (96.5%)	Sugar	14	126
Sweetened condensed skim milk	Sugar (42%)	Stabilizer	0.4	3.6
	MSNF (30%)			
Cane sugar	Sugar (100%)			
Cream	Fat (40%)			
Milk	Fat (4%)			

the amount of dehydrated corn syrup solids needed is 31.5 = 67.02 lb. This figure is entered in the weight column of the proof sheet.

We also enter the 31.5 lb of sugar in the sugar column. To obtain the TS in the corn syrup solids, we multiply the amount (67.02 lb) by the percentage of TS (96.5%) to obtain 64.67 TS, which we enter in the TS column.

Step 4. To find the amount of sweetened condensed skim milk needed, we use formula (II). The figures we need for the formula are obtained as follows:

From step 1, the amount of MSNF needed is 90 lb. To obtain the amount of serum of the mix, first find the sum of the fat (108.0 lb, from step 1 or 2), the stabilizer (4.0 lb, from step 3), the dehydrated corn syrup solids (67.02 lb, step 3), and the sugar not supplied by the corn syrup solids (126 − 31.5 = 94.50), which is 273.52 lb. Then subtract this from the desired total weight of the mix: 900.00 − 273.52 = 626.48 lb serum of the mix.

We obtain the amount of MSNF in 1 lb of sweetened condensed milk by multiplying the 1 lb by 30%, which gives 0.30. To obtain the amount of serum in 1 lb of sweetened condensed milk we multiply 1 lb sweetened condensed skim milk by 42% sugar to get 0.42 lb sugar. Then subtract the 0.42 lb from the 1 lb sweetened condensed skim milk, which leaves 0.58 lb serum, only the water and MSNF.

We substitute these figures in formula (II):

$$\frac{90.00 \text{ lb} - (626.48 \text{ lb} \times 0.09)}{0.30 - (0.58 \times 0.09)} = \frac{90 - 56.38}{0.30 - 0.052} = \frac{33.62}{0.248} = 135.56 \text{ lb}$$

the amount of sweetened condensed skim milk needed.

This figure is entered in the weight column of the proof sheet.

We also enter in their respective columns the amount of MSNF, sugar, and TS contained in the 135.66 lb sweetened condensed skim milk. We obtain these by multiplying the 135.66 lb by the respective percentages of MSNF, sugar, and TS:

$$135.56 \times 0.3 = 40.67 \text{ lb MSNF}$$
$$135.56 \times 0.42 = 56.94 \text{ lb sugar}$$
$$135.56 \times 0.72 = 97.60 \text{ lb TS}$$

Step 5. To calculate the amount of cane sugar needed, we add the amounts provided by the corn syrup solids (31.5 lb) and by the sweetened condensed skim milk (56.94 lb). Since the total amount of sugar desired is 126 lb and 88.44 lb has been supplied by other ingredients, then 126 − 88.44 = 37.56 lb of sugar remains to be supplied by the cane sugar. Since cane sugar is 100% sugar, then 37.56 lb of cane sugar is needed. This amount can be entered in the weight, sugar, and TS columns on the proof sheet.

Step 6. The amount of cream is calculated with the aid of formula (III), using the following figures:

From step 1, the amount of fat needed is 108 lb. To calculate the amount of milk and cream needed, we first find the sum of the stabilizer (4 lb, from step 3), the dehydrated corn syrup solids (67.02 lb, from step 3), the sweetened condensed skim milk (135.56 lb, from step 4), and the cane sugar (37.56, from step 5), which is 244.14 lb. Then subtract this from the desired total weight of the mix, 900 lb, which leaves 655.86 lb, the amount of milk and cream needed. We obtain the amount of fat in 1 lb of cream by multiplying the 1 lb by 0.40, which gives 0.40 lb, and the amount of fat in 1 lb of milk, by multiplying the 1 lb by 0.04, which gives 0.04 lb. We substitute these figures in formula (III):

$$\frac{108.00\ lb\ -\ (665.86\ lb\ \times\ 0.04)}{0.40\ -\ 0.04} = \frac{108.00\ lb\ -\ 26.23\ lb}{0.36} = \frac{81.77}{0.36} = 227.13\ lb$$

the amount of 40% cream needed. This number is entered in the weight column of the proof sheet.

We also enter in their respective columns the amounts of fat, MSNF, and TS contained in the cream. We obtain these by multiplying the 227.13 lb by the respective percentages:

$$227.13\ lb\ \times\ 0.40\ fat\ =\ 90.85\quad lb\ fat$$
$$227.13\ lb\ \times 0.0535\ MSNF\ =\ 12.15\quad lb\ MSNF$$

and adding:

$$90.85\ +\ 12.15\ =\ 103.00\quad lb\ TS$$

Step 7. The amount of milk needed is obtained by subtracting the amount of cream (277.13 lb) from the amount of milk and cream (655.86 lb, Step 6), which leaves 428.73 lb. This is entered in the weight column. We calculate the amounts of fat, MSNF, and TS contained in the milk by multiplying 428.73 lb by the respective percentages:

$$428.73\ lb\ \times\ 0.04\ =\ 17.15\quad lb\ fat$$
$$428.73\ lb\ \times\ 0.0879\ =\ 37.68\quad lb\ MSNF$$

and adding:

$$17.15\ +\ 37.68\ =\ 54.83\quad lb\ TS$$

Step 8. Each column of the proof sheet is now totaled. These totals should agree with the corresponding figures of the desired mix (see Fig. 8.8).

The percentage of TS is computed as follows:

$$\frac{361.28\ lb\ TS}{900\ lb\ mix} = 0.4014 = 40.14\%\quad TS$$

Similarly we compute the percentages of the remaining constituents.

Step 9. The correctness of the calculations is determined by comparing the calculated percentages for each constituent with the corresponding test of the desired mix.

Step 10. If desired, we compute the cost of the mix.

Ingredients	Ingredient weight (lb)	Calculated constituents					
		Fat (lb)	MSNF (lb)	Sugar (lb)	Stabilizer (lb)	TS (lb)	Cost ($)
Stabilizer	4.00				3.60	3.60	
Dehydrated corn syrup solids	67.02			31.50		64.68	
Sweetened condensed skim milk	135.56		40.67	56.94		97.61	
Cane sugar	37.56			37.56		37.56	
Cream, 40%	227.13	90.85	12.15			103.00	
Milk, 4%	428.73	17.15	37.68			54.83	
Total	900.00	108.00	90.50	126.00	3.60	361.28	—
Calculated %		12.00	10.06	14.00	0.40	40.14	
Check with desired wt.	900.00	108.00	90.00	126.00	3.60	327.60	
desired %		12.00	10.00	14.00	0.40	36.40	

Fig. 8.8. Completed proof sheet for problem 5.

There are times when it is necessary to use up odd lots of products that result from variation from the planned production schedule. These may include ice cream mixes of different composition cream, condensed milk, whole milk, or skim milk. These products can be utilized in making a mix of a desired composition.

The use of odd lots or leftovers does not imply in any way the use of inferior quality products. It should be understood that the odd lots of products used in ice cream mixes should be of the highest quality. Accurate information of the composition of such products must be available if these small lots are to be used to the best advantage. Problem 6 illustrates such a case.

Problem 6.   Using Leftovers.   This problem shows how to make use of leftovers, or relatively small amounts of several ingredients. The procedure can also be used when there are several lots of cream, none large enough to make the entire batch of mix.

A 900-lb mix testing 12% fat, 10% MSNF, 14% sugar, 0.5% egg solids, and 0.3% stabilizer is desired. The following materials are leftovers to be used to avoid loss: 40 lb frozen 50% cream, 90 lb 30% cream, 25 lb sweetened condensed skim milk (42% sugar, 28% MSNF), 100 lb 3% milk, and 30 lb corn syrup. The following ingredients are also available: stabilizer, cane sugar, frozen egg yolk (33% fat, 50% TS), condensed skim milk (32% TS), 40% cream, and 4% milk.

Solution

Step 1.   List the available ingredients and desired constituents (Table 8.4).

Step 2.   Make a proofsheet and enter the information from step 1.

Step 3.   Since there are several ingredients to be completely used, enter the amount of each of these immediately in the weight column of the proof sheet. Then compute the amount of each constituent contained in each ingredient and enter these amounts in their respective columns. For instance, 40 lb frozen cream multiplied by its fat test (50%) gives 20 lb fat, multiplied by its MSNF test (4.45%) gives 1.78 lb MSNF, and multiplied by its TS test (54.45%) gives 21.78 lb TS. Similar multiplications are made for the 30% cream, sweetened condensed skim milk, 3% milk, and corn syrup.

When these data have been entered in the proof sheet it is apparent that no stabilizer has been obtained, and that 2.7 lb is needed. In this problem there is only one source of stabilizer, and it contains 90% TS. Thus 2.7/0.90 = 3.0 lb of stabilizer product is needed. This figure is entered in the weight column of the proof sheet. The 2.7 lb of stabilizer is entered in the stabilizer and TS columns.

Again referring to the partially completed proof sheet, it is apparent that 4.50 lb of egg solids must be obtained from the frozen egg yolk, which is 50% TS and therefore 50% egg solids. Thus 4.50/0.50 = 9.0 lb of frozen egg yolk is needed. This figure is entered in the weight column of the proof sheet. We obtain the amount of each constituent furnished by the frozen egg yolk by multiplying the 9 lb by the respective percentages of fat, egg solids, and TS:

$$9 \times 0.33 = 2.97 \text{ lb fat}$$
$$9 \times 0.50 = 4.50 \text{ lb egg solids}$$
$$9 \times 0.50 = 4.50 \text{ lb TS}$$

Table 8.4. Available Ingredients/Desired Composition Table for Problem 6

Available ingredients		Desired mix composition		
Ingredient	Composition (%)	Constituent	Proportion (%)	Weight (lb)
Frozen cream	Fat (50%)	Fat	12	108
	MSNF (4.45%)	MSNF	10	90
Cream	Fat (30%)	Sugar	14	126
	MSNF (6.24%)	Egg solids	0.5	4.5
Sweetened		Stabilizer	0.3	2.7
condensed				
skim milk	MSNF (28%)			
	Sugar (42%)			
Milk	Fat (3%)			
	MSNF (8.33%)			
Corn syrup	Sugar (67%)			
	TS (83%)			
Stabilizer	TS (90%)			
Frozen egg yolk	Fat (33%)			
	TS (50%)			
Cane sugar	Sugar (100%)			
Condensed skim				
milk	MSNF (32%)			
	TS (32%)			
Cream	Fat (40%)			
	MSNF (5.35%)			
Milk	Fat (4%)			
	MSNF (8.79%)			

These amounts are entered in their respective columns.

Once again, refer to the partially completed proof sheet. It now appears that all of the stabilizer and all of the egg solids have been provided for. Also, it appears that the sweetened condensed skim milk and the corn syrup will furnish 30.60 lb of sugar, leaving some to come from the cane sugar, which is the only remaining source of sugar. Subtracting the 30.60 lb from the desired 126 lb leaves 95.40 lb of sugar to be obtained from cane sugar, which is 100% sugar. Thus 95.40 lb, is the amount of cane sugar needed. This figure is entered in the weight, the sugar, and TS columns of the proof sheet.

By adding each column as it now stands, it appears that provision has been made for 392.4 lb total weight, 52.97 lb of fat, 22.73 lb of MSNF, 126 lb of sugar, 4.50 lb of egg solids, and 2.7 lb of stabilizer. Subtracting each of these from its corresponding figures in the desired mix leaves 507.60 lb total weight, 55.03 lb of fat, and 67.27 lb of MSNF. These figures will be used in the following steps:

Step 4. To find the amount of condensed skim milk needed, it will be necessary to use formula (I). The figures to substitute in the formula are obtained as follows:

From step 3, the amount of MSNF needed is 67.27 lb. We obtain the amount of serum by subtracting the amount of fat (step 3) from the total weight (step 3): 507.60 − 55.03 = 452.57 lb of serum. Finally, the amount of MSNF in 1 lb of condensed skim milk is 0.32 lb (obtained by multiplying 1 lb × 32%, which is the MSNF test). We substitute these figures in formula (I):

$$\frac{67.27 \text{ lb} - (452.57 \text{ lb} \times 0.09)}{0.32 - 0.09)} = \frac{67.27 - 40.73}{0.23} = \frac{26.45}{0.23} = 115.39 \quad \text{lb}$$

the amount of condensed skim milk needed. This figure is entered in the weight column of the proof sheet.

We also enter in their respective columns the amount of MSNF and TS in the condensed skim milk. We obtain these by multiplying the 115.39 lb by the respective percentages of MSNF and TS:

$$115.39 \times 0.32 = 36.92 \quad \text{lb MSNF}$$
$$115.39 \times 0.32 = 36.92 \quad \text{lb TS}$$

Step 5.   The amount of sugar was calculated as part of step 3.

Step 6.   The amount of cream is calculated by using formula (III), with the following figures:

From step 3, the amount of fat needed is 55.03 lb. To calculate the amount of milk and cream needed, we subtract the amount of condensed skim milk (115.39, step 4) from the total weight (507.60 lb, step 3), which is 392.21 lb. The amount of fat in 1 lb of 40% cream is 0.40 lb, and the amount of fat in 4% milk is 0.04 lb. These figures are then substituted into formula (III):

$$\frac{55.03 - (392.21 \times 0.04)}{0.40 - 0.04} = \frac{55.03 - 15.69}{0.40 - 0.04} = \frac{39.34}{0.36} = 109.28 \quad \text{lb}$$

which is the amount of cream needed. This figure is entered in the weight column of the proof sheet.

We also enter in their respective columns the amount of fat, MSNF, and TS contained in the cream. We obtain these by multiplying the 109.28 lb by the respective percentages:

$$109.28 \times 0.40 = 43.71 \quad \text{lb fat}$$
$$109.28 \times 0.0535 = 5.85 \quad \text{lb MSNF}$$
$$109.28 \times 0.4535 = 49.56 \quad \text{lb TS}$$

Step 7.   The amount of milk needed is computed by subtracting the amount of cream (109.28 lb, step 6) from the amount of milk and cream (392.21 lb, step 6), which is 282.93 lb. This is entered in the weight column. We calculate the amount of fat, MSNF, and TS contained in the milk by multiplying the 282.93 lb by the respective percentages:

$$282.93 \times 0.04 = 11.32 \quad \text{lb fat}$$
$$282.93 \times 0.0879 = 24.87 \quad \text{lb MSNF}$$
$$282.93 \times 0.1279 = 36.19 \quad \text{lb TS}$$

Step 8.   Each column of the proof sheet is now totaled. These totals should agree with the corresponding figures of the desired mix (see Fig. 8.9).

The TS test is computed as follows:

$$\frac{333.40 \text{ lb TS}}{900 \text{ lb mix}} = 0.3704 = 37.04\% \text{ TS}$$

Similarly, we calculate the percentages of the remaining constituents.

Step 9.   The correctness of the calculations is determined by comparing the calculated percentage for each constituent with the corresponding test of the desired mix.

Step 10.   If desired, we compute the cost of the mix.

PLAIN MIX FORMULAS

The ice cream maker who prefers not to calculate mixes will find that the following formulas (adapted from Leighton 1945) give quite satisfactory results. Tables 8.5–8.14 present a number of mix formulas for ice cream ranging in fat content from 10 to 18%. Tables 8.5 and 8.6 first list the proportions of constituents for ice creams that do not and that do use some form of concentrated milk, for various fat contents. Tables 8.7–8.14 then give different combinations of milk products that can be used to produce the ice creams.

The formulas are all figured on a 100-lb basis, which is easily converted to other amounts. For example, if the desired amount of a mix is expressed as 500 gal, the gallons must first be converted to pounds by multiplying by the average weight per gallon of mix, 9.2 lb, which gives 4600 lb. This represents a 46-fold increase in the amounts in the tables, and so the ingredients in the tables must be multiplied by 46 to obtain the amount required for the batch.

These mixes are complete, except for color and flavor materials, which do not add significantly to weight. (Refer to Chapter 7 for information on adding flavorings to mixes.)

Table 8.5.   Proportions of the Constituents of Different Types of Ice Cream That Do Not Use Concentrated Milk[a]

	Type				
Constituent	14	15	16	17	18
Fat	14.00	15.00	16.00	17.00	18.00
MSNF	6.36	6.27	6.18	6.09	6.00
Sugar	15.00	15.00	15.00	15.00	15.00
Stabilizer	0.30	0.30	0.30	0.30	0.30
TS	35.66	36.57	37.48	38.39	39.30
Water	64.34	63.43	62.52	61.61	60.70

[a]Type refers to the percentage of butterfat in the ice cream.

Ingredients	Ingredient weight (lb)	Calculated constituents						
		Fat (lb)	MSNF (lb)	Sugar (lb)	Egg solids (lb)	Stabilizer (lb)	TS (lb)	Cost ($)
Cream, frozen, 50%	40.00	20.00	1.78				21.78	
30%	90.00	27.00	5.62				32.62	
Sweetened condensed skim milk	25.00		7.00	10.50			17.50	
Milk, 3%	100.00	3.00	8.33				11.33	
Corn syrup	30.00			20.10			24.90[a]	
Stabilizer	3.00					2.70	2.70	
Egg yolk, frozen	9.00	2.97			4.50		4.50[a]	
Cane sugar	95.40			95.40			95.40	
Condensed skim milk	115.39		36.92				36.92	
Cream, 40%	101.28	43.71	5.85				49.62	
Milk, 4%	282.93	11.32	24.87				36.19	
Total	900.00	108.00	90.37	126.00	4.50	2.70	333.40	
Calculated %		12.00	10.04	14.00	0.50	0.30	37.04	
Check with desired wt.	900.00	108.00	90.00	126.00	4.50	2.70	331.20	
desired %		12.00	10.00	14.00	0.50	0.30	36.80	

Fig. 8.9. Completed proof sheet for problem 6.

Table 8.6. Proportions of the Constituents of Different Types of Ice Cream That Use Some Form of Concentrated Milk

Constituent	Type								
	10	11	12	13	14	15	16	17	18
Fat	10.00	11.00	12.00	13.00	14.00	15.00	16.00	17.00	18.00
MSNF	11.00	10.50	10.00	9.50	9.00	8.50	8.00	7.50	7.00
Sugar	15.00	15.00	15.00	15.00	15.00	15.00	15.00	15.00	15.00
Stabilizer	0.30	0.30	0.30	0.30	0.30	0.30	0.30	0.30	0.30
TS	36.30	36.80	37.30	37.80	38.30	38.80	39.30	39.80	40.30
Water	63.70	63.20	62.70	62.20	61.70	61.20	60.70	60.20	59.70

Table 8.7. Different Proportions of Ingredients for Ice Cream —No Concentrated Milk

		Type				
		14	15	16	17	18
(1)	Cream (50% fat)	28.00	30.00	32.00	34.00	36.00
	Skim milk	56.70	54.70	52.70	50.70	48.70
(2)	Cream (40% fat)	35.00	37.50	40.00	42.50	45.00
	Skim milk	49.70	47.20	44.70	42.20	39.70
(3)	Cream (30% fat)	46.66	50.00	53.33	56.66	60.00
	Skim milk	38.04	34.70	31.37	28.04	24.70
(4)	Cream (20% fat)	70.00	75.00	80.00	—	—
	Skim milk	14.70	9.70	4.70	—	—
(5)	Cream (50% fat)	23.46	25.64	27.80	29.91	32.10
	Whole milk (3.7% fat)	61.24	59.06	56.90	54.79	52.60
(6)	Cream (40% fat)	29.92	32.69	35.45	38.18	40.94
	Whole milk (3.7% fat)	54.78	52.01	49.25	46.52	43.76
(7)	Cream (30% fat)	41.29	45.10	48.91	52.67	56.48
	Whole milk (3.7% fat)	43.41	39.60	35.79	32.03	28.22
(8)	Cream (20% fat)	66.61	72.76	78.91	—	—
	Whole milk (3.7% fat)	18.09	11.94	5.79	—	—
Add to any above combination:						
	Sugar	15.00	15.00	15.00	15.00	15.00
	Stabilizer	0.30	0.30	0.30	0.30	0.30
	Total	100.00	100.00	100.00	100.00	100.00

Table 8.8. Different Proportions of Ingredients for Ice Cream—With Dry Skim Milk[a]

		10	11	12	13	14	15	16	17	18
						Type				
(1)	Cream (50% fat)	20.00	22.00	24.00	26.00	28.00	30.00	32.00	34.00	36.00
	Skim milk	59.70	58.20	56.70	55.20	53.70	52.20	50.70	49.20	47.70
(2)	Cream (40% fat)	25.00	27.50	30.00	32.50	35.00	37.50	40.00	42.50	45.00
	Skim milk	54.70	52.70	50.70	48.70	46.70	44.70	42.70	40.70	38.70
(3)	Cream (30% fat)	33.33	36.66	40.00	43.33	46.66	50.00	53.33	56.66	60.00
	Skim milk	46.37	43.54	40.70	37.87	35.04	32.20	29.37	26.54	23.70
(4)	Cream (20% fat)	50.00	55.00	60.00	65.00	70.00	75.00	80.00	—	—
	Skim milk	29.70	25.20	20.70	16.20	11.70	7.20	2.70	—	—
(5)	Cream (50% fat)	15.21	17.33	19.45	21.57	23.70	25.83	27.96	30.08	32.20
	Whole milk (3.7% fat)	64.49	62.87	61.25	59.63	58.00	56.37	54.74	53.12	51.50
(6)	Cream (40% fat)	19.40	22.10	24.80	27.51	30.22	32.92	35.63	38.34	41.05
	Whole milk (3.7% fat)	60.30	58.10	55.90	53.69	51.48	49.28	47.07	44.86	42.65
(7)	Cream (30% fat)	26.76	30.50	34.25	37.98	41.70	45.43	49.17	52.90	56.63
	Whole milk (3.7% fat)	52.94	49.70	46.45	43.22	40.00	36.77	33.53	30.30	27.07
(8)	Cream (20% fat)	43.17	49.20	55.22	61.25	67.27	73.30	79.32	—	—
	Whole milk (3.7% fat)	36.53	31.00	25.48	19.95	14.43	8.90	3.38	—	—
	Add to any above combination:									
	Dry skim milk	5.00	4.50	4.00	3.50	3.00	2.50	2.00	1.50	1.00
	Sugar	15.00	15.00	15.00	15.00	15.00	15.00	15.00	15.00	15.00
	Stabilizer	0.30	0.30	0.30	0.30	0.30	0.30	0.30	0.30	0.30
	Total	100.00	100.00	100.00	100.00	100.00	100.00	100.00	100.00	100.00

[a]95% solids.

Table 8.9. Different Proportions of Ingredients for Ice Cream
—With Unsweetened Condensed Milk[a]

		Type								
		10	11	12	13	14	15	16	17	18
(1)	Cream (50% fat)	20.00	22.00	24.00	26.00	28.00	30.00	32.00	34.00	36.00
	Skim milk	41.00	41.25	41.50	41.80	42.10	42.40	42.70	42.95	43.19
(2)	Cream (40% fat)	25.00	27.50	30.00	32.50	35.00	37.50	40.00	42.50	45.00
	Skim milk	36.00	35.75	35.50	35.30	35.10	34.90	34.70	34.45	34.19
(3)	Cream (30% fat)	33.33	36.66	40.00	43.33	46.66	49.99	53.33	56.66	60.00
	Skim milk	27.67	26.59	25.50	24.47	23.44	22.41	21.37	20.29	19.19
(4)	Cream (20% fat)	50.00	55.00	60.00	65.00	70.00	—	—	—	—
	Skim milk	11.00	8.25	5.50	2.80	0.10	—	—	—	—
(5)	Cream (50% fat)	16.73	18.70	20.68	22.66	24.63	26.61	28.59	30.57	32.53
	Whole milk (3.7% fat)	44.27	44.55	44.82	45.14	45.47	45.79	46.11	46.38	46.66
(6)	Cream (40% fat)	21.33	23.85	26.37	28.89	31.41	33.93	36.45	38.97	41.50
	Whole milk (3.7% fat)	39.67	39.40	39.13	38.91	38.69	38.47	38.25	37.98	37.69
(7)	Cream (30% fat)	29.44	32.92	36.40	39.82	43.35	46.82	50.30	53.77	57.25
	Whole milk (3.7% fat)	31.56	30.33	29.10	27.98	26.75	25.58	24.40	23.18	21.94
(8)	Cream (20% fat)	47.49	53.10	58.72	64.32	69.92	—	—	—	—
	Whole milk (3.7% fat)	13.51	10.15	6.78	3.48	0.18	—	—	—	—
	Add to any above combination:									
	Unsweetened condensed skim milk	23.70	21.45	19.20	16.90	14.60	12.30	10.00	7.75	5.51
	Sugar	15.00	15.00	15.00	15.00	15.00	15.00	15.00	15.00	15.00
	Stabilizer	0.30	0.30	0.30	0.30	0.30	0.30	0.30	0.30	0.30
	Total	100.00	100.00	100.00	100.00	100.00	100.00	100.00	100.00	100.00

[a]Concentration 3:1; contains 27% MSNF.

Table 8.10. Different Proportions of Ingredients for Ice Cream
—With Sweetened Condensed Skim Milk[a]

		Type								
		10	11	12	13	14	15	16	17	18
(1)	Cream (50% fat)	20.00	22.00	24.00	26.00	28.00	30.00	32.00	34.00	36.00
	Skim milk	54.74	53.63	52.68	51.59	50.56	49.53	48.49	47.45	46.40
(2)	Cream (40% fat)	25.00	27.50	30.00	32.50	35.00	37.50	40.00	42.50	45.00
	Skim milk	49.74	48.18	46.63	45.09	43.56	42.03	40.49	38.95	37.40
(3)	Cream (30% fat)	33.33	36.66	40.00	43.33	46.66	49.99	53.33	56.66	60.00
	Skim milk	41.41	39.02	36.63	34.26	31.90	29.54	27.16	24.79	22.40
(4)	Cream (20% fat)	50.00	55.00	60.00	65.00	70.00	—	—	—	—
	Skim milk	24.74	20.68	16.63	12.59	8.56	—	—	—	—
(5)	Cream (50% fat)	15.63	17.71	19.79	21.87	23.96	26.04	28.13	30.21	32.30
	Whole milk (3.7% fat)	59.11	57.97	56.84	55.72	54.60	53.49	52.36	51.24	50.10
(6)	Cream (40% fat)	19.93	22.58	25.24	27.89	30.55	33.20	35.86	38.53	41.20
	Whole milk (3.7% fat)	54.81	53.10	51.39	49.70	48.01	46.33	44.63	42.92	41.20
(7)	Cream (30% fat)	27.51	31.17	34.83	38.49	42.16	45.82	49.49	53.13	56.80
	Whole milk (3.7% fat)	47.23	44.51	41.80	39.10	36.40	33.71	31.00	28.32	25.60
(8)	Cream (20% fat)	44.69	50.44	56.19	62.10	68.00	73.91	79.83	—	—
	Whole milk (3.7% fat)	30.05	25.24	20.44	15.49	10.56	5.62	0.66	—	—
Add to any above combination:										
	Sweetened condensed skim milk[a]	17.22	15.57	13.92	12.27	10.61	8.96	7.31	5.65	4.00
	Sugar	7.74	8.45	9.15	9.84	10.53	11.21	11.90	12.60	13.30
	Stabilizer	0.30	0.30	0.30	0.30	0.30	0.30	0.30	0.30	0.30
	Total	100.00	100.00	100.00	100.00	100.00	100.00	100.00	100.00	100.00

[a]Contains 30.0% MSNF, 42% sugar, 28% water.

Table 8.11. Different Proportions of Ingredients for Ice Cream —With Unsweetened Condensed Skim Milk[a] and Liquid Sugar[b]

			Type								
			10	11	12	13	14	15	16	17	18
(1)	Cream (50% fat)		20.00	22.00	24.00	26.00	28.00	30.00	32.00	34.00	36.00
	Skim milk		30.42	30.70	30.99	31.29	31.59	31.86	32.14	32.39	32.65
(2)	Cream (40% fat)		25.00	27.50	30.00	32.50	35.00	37.50	40.00	42.50	45.00
	Skim milk		25.42	25.20	24.99	24.79	24.59	24.36	24.14	25.89	23.65
(3)	Cream (30% fat)		33.33	36.66	40.00	43.33	46.66	49.99	53.33	56.66	60.00
	Skim milk		17.09	16.04	14.99	13.96	12.93	11.87	10.81	9.73	8.65
(4)	Cream (20% fat)		—	—	—	—	—	—	—	—	—
	Skim milk		—	—	—	—	—	—	—	—	—
(5)	Cream (50% fat)		17.61	19.57	21.54	23.51	25.48	27.47	29.46	31.43	33.40
	Whole milk (3.7% fat)		32.81	33.13	33.45	33.78	34.11	34.39	34.68	34.96	35.25
(6)	Cream (40% fat)		22.42	24.95	27.49	30.03	32.57	35.08	37.59	40.16	42.74
	Whole milk (3.7% fat)		28.00	27.75	27.50	27.26	27.02	26.78	26.55	26.23	25.91
(7)	Cream (30% fat)		30.90	34.39	37.88	41.25	44.62	48.20	51.78	55.34	58.90
	Whole milk (3.7% fat)		19.52	18.31	17.11	16.04	14.97	13.66	12.36	11.05	9.75
(8)	Cream (20% fat)		—	—	—	—	—	—	—	—	—
	Whole milk (3.7% fat)		—	—	—	—	—	—	—	—	—
	Add to any above combination:										
	Unsweetened condensed skim milk[a]		27.28	25.00	22.71	20.41	18.11	15.84	13.56	11.31	9.05
	Liquid sugar[b]		22.00	22.00	22.00	22.00	22.00	22.00	22.00	22.00	22.00
	Stabilizer		0.30	0.30	0.30	0.30	0.30	0.30	0.30	0.30	0.30
	Total		100.00	100.00	100.00	100.00	100.00	100.00	100.00	100.00	100.00

[a]Concentration 3:1; contains 27% MSNF.
[b]Concentration 68:1; i.e., 1 gal = 11 lb, containing 7.5 lb sugar.

Table 8.12 Different Proportions of Ingredients for Ice Cream—With Sweetened Condensed Skim Milk and Liquid Sugar

		Type								
		10	11	12	13	14	15	16	17	18
(1)	Cream (50% fat)	20.00	22.00	24.00	26.00	28.00	30.00	32.00	34.00	36.00
	Skim milk	50.65	49.25	47.86	46.44	45.02	43.59	42.16	40.82	39.48
(2)	Cream (40% fat)	25.00	27.50	30.00	32.50	35.00	37.50	40.00	42.50	45.00
	Skim milk	45.65	43.75	41.86	39.94	38.02	36.09	34.16	32.32	30.48
(3)	Cream (30% fat)	33.33	36.66	40.00	43.33	46.66	50.00	53.33	56.66	60.00
	Skim milk	37.32	34.59	31.86	29.11	26.36	23.59	20.83	18.16	15.48
(4)	Cream (20% fat)	50.00	55.00	60.00	65.00	70.00	—	—	—	—
	Skim milk	20.65	16.25	11.86	7.44	3.02	—	—	—	—
(5)	Cream (50% fat)	15.95	18.07	20.19	22.28	24.37	26.49	28.62	30.75	32.89
	Whole milk (3.7% fat)	54.70	53.18	51.67	50.16	48.65	47.10	45.54	44.07	42.59
(6)	Cream (40% fat)	20.32	23.01	25.70	28.39	31.09	33.79	36.50	39.17	41.84
	Whole milk (3.7% fat)	50.33	48.24	46.16	44.05	41.93	39.80	37.66	35.65	33.64
(7)	Cream (30% fat)	28.11	31.81	35.51	39.19	42.87	46.63	50.39	54.10	57.81
	Whole milk (3.7% fat)	42.54	39.44	36.35	33.25	30.15	26.96	23.77	20.72	17.67
(8)	Cream (20% fat)	46.24	51.81	57.38	63.25	69.13	—	—	—	—
	Whole milk (3.7% fat)	24.41	19.44	14.48	9.19	3.89	—	—	—	—
	Add to any above combination:									
	Sweetened condensed skim milk	18.43	16.88	15.32	13.76	12.21	10.67	9.14	7.53	5.93
	Liquid sugar	10.62	11.57	12.52	13.50	14.47	15.44	16.40	17.35	18.29
	Stabilizer	0.30	0.30	0.30	0.30	0.30	0.30	0.30	0.30	0.30
	Total	100.00	100.00	100.00	100.00	100.00	100.00	100.00	100.00	100.00

USE OF COMPUTERS IN ICE CREAM PRODUCTION

Computer controls for ice cream production have been described by Kreider and Snyder (1964) and Byars (1969). Bohn (1971) reviewed the use of computers in ice cream manufacture and stated that in addition to providing the basic quantitative specifications for ice cream mixing, computers can be programmed to perform a minimum cost analysis on the basis of availale data. It is possible to have the computer indicate the exact amounts of each available ingredient to prepare a particular mix at a minimum cost. Also, the computer will specify the cost range within which it is feasible to use each ingredient. Further, a detailed cost analysis can be generated relative to quality regulations.

This is accomplished through a technique known as linear programming. The computer is given the quantities of ingredients available to the manufacturer together with a composition breakdown for each of the ingredients and its unit cost. It is also supplied with the acceptable composition range for each element (butterfat, etc.) of the finished product. These parameters are then automatically inserted into linear programming equations, which the computer uses to calculate the exact amount of each ingredient to comprise the ice cream mix. In addition to specifying the amount of each ingredient used to make up a fixed amount of mix, the computer will indicate the amount of each ingredient that will minimize the cost of the mix within the specified quality and composition restrictions. It also will establish a cost ceiling for each ingredient above which it would be economically advantageous to exclude it from the mix in favor of another one.

This information is made available in a minimum amount of time, and computer accuracy eliminates the risk of human error through manual calculations.

Byars (1969) gave an example of using the computer to minimize the cost of the mix. He used the following method:

(1) Establish the desired mix formula and amount desired with minimum, maximum, or exact equal limitations for each ingredient.

(2) Establish the ingredients available, costs per pound, and analyses of the ingredients.

(3) Specify maximum amount of each product available.

(4) Establish abbreviations used for ingredients for computer analysis.

(5) Develop linear programming equations with the objective of minimizing costs and the constraint equations involved.

It was concluded that computerized linear programming performed blending demands at minimum cost and supplied other valuable information.

Use of Computers in Least-Cost Formulation
of Ice Cream Mixes

Bell (1983) developed the material that follows on p. 157 on the use of computers in the formulation of ice cream mixes.

Table 8.13. Different Proportions of Ingredients for Ice Cream—With 50% of Fat Added in the Form of Butter,[a] Unsweetened Condensed or Dry Skim Milk, and Water or Whole Milk

		Type								
		10	11	12	13	14	15	16	17	18
(1)	Cream (40% fat)	12.50	13.75	15.00	16.25	17.50	18.75	20.00	20.25	22.50
	Unsweetened condensed skim milk	24.40	22.30	20.20	17.90	15.60	13.40	11.20	8.97	6.75
	Water	41.70	41.95	42.20	42.65	43.10	43.42	43.75	44.10	44.45
(2)	Cream (40% fat)	12.50	13.75	15.00	16.25	17.50	18.75	20.00	21.25	22.50
	Dry skim milk	5.00	4.55	4.10	3.65	3.20	2.75	2.30	1.85	1.40
	Water	61.10	59.70	58.30	56.90	55.50	54.07	52.65	51.22	49.80
(3)	Cream (20% fat)	25.00	27.50	30.00	32.50	35.00	37.50	40.00	42.50	45.00
	Unsweetened condensed skim milk	24.40	22.30	20.20	17.90	15.60	13.40	11.20	8.97	6.75
	Water	29.20	28.20	27.20	26.40	25.60	24.67	23.75	22.85	21.95
(4)	Cream (20% fat)	25.00	27.50	30.00	32.50	35.00	37.50	40.00	42.50	45.00
	Dry skim milk	5.00	4.55	4.10	3.65	3.20	2.75	2.30	1.85	1.40
	Water	48.60	45.95	43.30	40.65	38.00	35.32	32.65	29.97	27.30

	8.25	9.47	10.70	11.85	13.00	14.30	15.60	16.90	18.20
(5) Cream (40% fat)	24.40	22.30	20.20	17.90	15.60	13.40	11.20	8.97	6.75
Unsweetened condensed skim milk	45.95	46.23	46.50	47.05	47.60	47.87	48.15	48.45	45.75
Whole milk (3.7% fat)	6.23	7.65	9.08	10.44	11.80	13.15	14.50	15.80	17.10
(6) Cream (40% fat)	5.00	4.55	4.10	3.65	3.20	2.75	2.30	1.85	1.40
Dry skim milk	67.37	65.80	64.22	62.71	61.20	59.67	58.15	56.67	55.20
Whole milk (3.7% fat)	18.50	21.20	23.90	26.55	29.20	32.00	34.80	37.40	40.00
(7) Cream (20% fat)	24.40	22.30	20.20	17.90	15.60	13.40	11.20	8.97	6.75
Unsweetened condensed skim milk	35.70	34.50	33.30	32.35	31.40	30.17	28.95	27.95	26.95
Whole milk (3.7% fat)	14.10	17.10	20.10	23.10	26.10	29.10	32.10	35.15	38.20
(8) Cream (20% fat)	5.00	4.55	4.10	3.65	3.20	2.75	2.30	1.85	1.40
Dry skim milk	59.50	53.35	53.20	50.05	46.90	43.72	40.55	37.32	34.10
Whole milk (3.7% fat)									
Add to any above combination:									
Butter	6.10	6.70	7.30	7.90	8.50	9.13	9.75	10.38	11.00
Sugar	15.00	15.00	15.00	15.00	15.00	15.00	15.00	15.00	15.00
Stabilizer	0.30	0.30	0.30	0.30	0.30	0.30	0.30	0.30	0.30
Total	100.00	100.00	100.00	100.00	100.00	100.00	100.00	100.00	100.00

[a] 82% butterfat.

Table 8.14. Different Proportions of Ingredients for Ice Cream—With Half the Normal Sucrose Replaced by Corn Syrup, Maintaining a Sweetness of 13.5[a,b]

			10	11	12	13	14	15	16	17	18
							Type				
(1)	Cream (50% fat)		20.00	22.00	24.00	26.00	28.00	30.00	32.00	34.00	36.00
	Skim milk		33.42	33.71	34.00	34.27	34.55	34.83	35.11	35.41	35.70
(2)	Cream (40% fat)		25.00	27.50	30.00	32.00	35.00	37.50	40.00	42.50	45.00
	Skim milk		28.42	28.21	28.00	27.77	27.55	27.33	27.11	26.91	26.70
(3)	Cream (30% fat)		33.33	36.66	40.00	43.33	46.66	49.99	53.33	56.66	60.00
	Skim milk		20.09	19.05	18.00	16.94	15.89	14.84	13.78	12.75	11.70
(4)	Cream (20% fat)		50.00	—	—	—	—	—	—	—	—
	Skim milk		3.42	—	—	—	—	—	—	—	—
(5)	Cream (50% fat)		17.28	19.26	21.24	23.21	25.19	27.17	29.15	31.13	33.11
	Whole milk (3.7% fat)		36.14	36.45	36.76	37.06	37.36	37.66	37.96	38.28	38.59
(6)	Cream (40% fat)		22.11	24.63	27.16	29.68	32.20	34.71	37.22	39.74	42.26
	Whole milk (3.7% fat)		31.31	31.08	30.84	30.59	30.35	30.12	29.89	29.67	29.44
(7)	Cream (30% fat)		30.50	34.03	37.56	40.99	44.43	47.90	51.37	54.84	58.31
	Whole milk (3.7% fat)		22.92	21.68	20.44	19.28	18.12	16.93	15.74	14.57	13.39
(8)	Cream (20% fat)		49.21	—	—	—	—	—	—	—	—
	Whole milk (3.7% fat)		4.21	—	—	—	—	—	—	—	—
Add to any above combination:												
Unsweetened condensed skim milk			26.28	23.99	21.70	19.43	17.15	14.87	12.59	10.29	8.00
Sucrose			7.50	7.50	7.50	7.50	7.50	7.50	7.50	7.50	7.50
Corn syrup			12.50	12.50	12.50	12.50	12.50	12.50	12.50	12.50	12.50
Stabilizer			0.30	0.30	0.30	0.30	0.30	0.30	0.30	0.30	0.30
Total			100.00	100.00	100.00	100.00	100.00	100.00	100.00	100.00	100.00

[a]The amount of sugar used is calculated to be that amount which will make the finished mix as sweet as one containing 13.5 per cent sucrose.
[b]Corn syrup containing 80.3% solids. High equivalent syrup of 82% solids of greater sweetness can be used in compounding these mixes by adding from 3 to 6 lb of water to 100 lb of syrup.

The applications for computer formulation of ice cream mixes have been realized for several years; however, the techniques are still somewhat new to many people in the industry. Traditional methods of calculations are not outdated; simply, computers greatly minimize the amount of time required to perform calculations and eliminate occurrences of human error.

Computers used for formulation of ice cream products use a technique known as linear programming. The linear program takes into account all variables and factors that have an impact on each formula and on all ingredients in those formulas. Quantitative analyses of raw materials are used in solving formulas within set boundaries.

With an increased product line due to increased production capacities, greater variations of consumer preferences, and expanded availability of raw materials, the number of variables that must be considered is no longer merely percentages of butterfat and MSNF. Combined with the ever-increasing need to minimize costs and maximize profits, calculations require more attention and thus more time.

Hand calculation methods of formulation become more and more cumbersome with this increased complexity of product line. With each finished product, there is also an accompanying set of government regulations. Further, there are limitations on availability of raw materials, limitations on amounts which can be physically kept on hand, limitations based on shipping schedules, and limitations imposed by seasonal supply of raw dairy products. When coupled with government regulations, these factors leave little room for control of costs using typical methods of formulation.

However, despite limitations on raw materials, materials still account for 60–80% of the product cost. Armed with this fact, it then is essential to use these items in the most cost-effective manner possible and still meet the quality restrictions imposed—both by plant standards and government regulations. Consideration of all variables for each raw material based on numeric values for test analyses is extremely time consuming and laborious when calculations must be done by typical methods. Using specially designed computer software this can be handled quickly and efficiently.

While this method of formulation is a great time saver, the computer merely serves as a tool for the process. Therefore, information fed into the system must be accurate and up to date, or else solution values from the linear program will not be useful.

In the same manner as with hand calculations, a determination must be made as to which products will be formulated. Each product formula (recipe) should contain applicable limitations on the proportions of butterfat, MSNF, sugars, stabilizers and emulsifiers, artificial sweeteners, coloring and flavoring, and so forth. These quality restrictions are called constraints in the examples that follow. Constraints may be imposed by government regulations or by quality parameters defined by the producer.

Each raw dairy item can be defined in terms of its butterfat, MSNF, and TS. Sweeteners can be expressed as a percentage of cane solids, corn syrup solids, or other sweeteners specific to the plant situation. Each of these quantitative definitions is called a characteristic. As the computer can only review each ingredient in terms of the characteristic values given it, the analysis should be as accurate as possible. Each of these ingredient characteristics references a formula constraint. The linear program reviews each raw material in terms of its possible contribution to the formula. This contribution is its characteristic value.

Using a linear program to solve formulations could yield several solutions for each formula. If there are a number of ingredients with similar characteristics, these could be combined in a variety of ways to meet the quality restrictions placed on each product, but only one solution will be the least-cost solution. Therefore, the program looks at all the possible combinations of raw materials, and then gives the one combination that satisfies the cost limitation as well.

In the examples that follow (Fig. 8.10), five general mixes have been set up for use in computer formulation runs. Among the five formulas there are some ingredients common to all. These are shown in the available ingredients file (Fig. 8.11). As shown, these ingredients are defined in terms of characteristic values. (Ingredients can be defined in terms of more characteristics than those shown here.)

Each formula has been established with constraint values that must be met (see Table 8.15). With seven dairy ingredients in the available ingredients file, there are several combinations that will satisfy each formula's constraints, but there is only one least-cost solution. All five formulas are submitted to the computer at the same time in what is called a multiproduct run. Taking

SEQUENCE NUMBER	FORMULA NAME	FINISHED WEIGHT	PERCENT SHRINK	BATCH NUMBER / NUMBER OF BATCHES
1	5 10% WHITE MIX	9200.00	0.00000	1.0
2	14 3% WHITE MIX	4600.00	0.00000	1.0
3	17 10% CHOC MIX	4600.00	0.00000	1.0
4	20 SHERBET	4600.00	0.00000	1.0
5	24 14% WHITE MIX	4600.00	0.00000	1.0

Fig. 8.10. Production run. Copyright 1983, Computer Concepts Corporation. All rights reserved.

INGREDIENT	COST/UNIT	% FAT	%MOISTURE	% MILK SOLIDS N/F	% TOTAL SOLIDS	% DAIRY	MINIMUM	MAXIMUM
1 WHOLE MILK	0.13014*	3.25000	88.0500	8.70000	11.9500	100.000		
5 CREAM	0.72087*	38.3500*	56.2500	5.40000*	43.7500	100.000		
10 SKIM MILK	0.07275*	0.00000*	91.0000*	9.00000*	9.00000*	100.000		
12 CONDENSED	0.30455	0.00000	66.1000	33.9000	33.9000	100.000		
13 BUTTER MILK COND	0.28000	4.00000	0.00000	30.0000	34.0000	100.000		
14 SKIM MLK PWDR	0.96750*	0.00000*	3.00000	97.0000*	97.0000	100.000		
16 WHEY POWDER	0.14500*	1.40000*	6.13500	92.4650*	93.8650	100.000		
40 CORN SYRUP	0.08867*	0.00000	19.3000*	0.00000	80.7000*	0.00000		
43 LIQUID CANE SUGAR	0.30000*	0.00000	33.7000*	0.00000	69.8600	0.00000		
71 EMUL/STAB	1.20000	0.00000*	0.00000*	0.00000*	100.000*	0.00000		
74 FRODEX	0.25430	0.00000	0.00000	0.00000	100.000	0.00000		
134 COCOA	0.62000	0.00000*	0.00000	0.00000	100.000	0.00000		
300 WATER	0.00001	0.00000	100.000	0.00000	0.00000	0.00000		

Fig. 8.11. Available ingredients file listing. Copyright 1983, Computer Concepts Corporation. All rights reserved.

ingredients from the available ingredients file, the program satisfies the constraints for each formula.

The examples show all five formulas after being solved by the linear program. In the first example (Figs. 8.12–8.16) all ingredients were considered to have been available in unlimited quantities; therefore the program could pick which materials would solve the formula constraints and do so at the lowest cost. This low cost does not mean that quality was sacrifieced, for the quality restrictions were met by incorporating them as constraints.

Because not all ingredients are available at all times or some ingredients must be forced into usage, the program can easily solve the same formulas based on new restrictions. In the available ingredients file that follows (Fig. 8.17), whole milk needed to be used up. Therefore, a minimum on that ingredient was forced in. The amount of cream that could be used was limited to 5000 lb, which was given as a maximum. When the same five formulas were recalculated by computer, the constraints were all met, the minimum and maximums on these two ingredients were met, but the costs as compared with

Table 8.15. Composition Constraints (%) on Seven Dairy Product Ingredients

	Type of mix (fat content)				
Ingredient	White	White	Chocolate	Sherbet	White
Fat	10.1	3.1	9.4	0.5	14.0
MSNF	10.0	12.0	9.5	3.0	10.0
Cane solids	9.1	11.0	12.4	18.0	16.0
Corn syrup solids	9.5		4.8	6.0	
Stabilizer/emulsifier	0.5	0.4	0.6		0.5
Cocoa			2.6		
Frodex	3.0				
Whey solids		3.0	2.375		
Finished weight (lb)	9200	4600	4600	4600	4600

```
INGREDIENT          TOTAL      BATCH    GALLONS  PERCENT  MINIMUM  MAXIMUM  -------------COST/UNIT-------------
                    WEIGHT     WEIGHT            BATCH    PERCENT  PERCENT    LOW     ACTUAL   HIGH    PENALTY
   1 WHOLE MILK                                                            0.11844  0.13014          0.01170
   5 CREAM          2143.33    2143.33  258.86 23.30 FW                    0.40341  0.72087  0.93143
  10 SKIM MILK                                                            0.06263  0.07275          0.01012
  12 CONDENSED                                                             0.23587  0.30455
  13 BUTTER MILK COND 2680.87  2680.87         29.14 FW                    0.07520  0.28000  0.31311
  14 SKIM MLK PWDR                                                         0.67488  0.96750          0.29262
  40 CORN SYRUP      1083.02   1083.02   97.22 11.77 FW                             0.08867
  43 LIQUID CANE SUGAR 1196.00 1196.00  107.36 13.00 FW                             0.30000
  71 EMUL/STAB       46.00     46.00     4.60  0.50 FW                              1.20000
 300 WATER          2050.78    2050.78  246.19 22.29 FW           -0.14994  0.00001  0.01395
-----------------------------------------------------------------------------------------------------------
FINISHED WEIGHT     9200.00    9200.00  714.23 100.00 FW                   0.30497 TOTAL COST=     2805.74
-----------------------------------------------------------------------------------------------------------

CONSTRAINT          SOLUTION   MINIMUM  MAXIMUM  PENALTY
                    VALUE      VALUE    VALUE    COST
   2 % FAT (TOTAL)  10.10      10.10        FW   0.01782
  54 %MSNF (INC WHEY) 10.00    10.00        FW   0.00696
  35 % EMUL & % STAB  0.50      0.50    0.50 FW  -0.01200
  29 % CANE SOLIDS   9.10       9.10    9.10 FW  -0.00429
  30 % CORN SYRUP SLDS 9.50     9.50    9.50 FW  -0.00110
  55 % TOTAL SOLIDS  39.18                   FW
  98 FINISHED WEIGHT 9200.00    9200.00 9200.00 FW  0.30497
```

Fig. 8.12. Multiproduct run (white mix, 10%) with no ingredient minimums or maximums. Copyright© Computer Concepts Corp., 1983.

INGREDIENT	TOTAL WEIGHT	BATCH WEIGHT	GALLONS	PERCENT BATCH	MINIMUM PERCENT	MAXIMUM PERCENT	COST/UNIT LOW	ACTUAL	HIGH	PENALTY
1 WHOLE MILK							0.11844	0.13014		0.01170
5 CREAM	223.44	223.44	26.99	4.86 FW			0.40341	0.72087	0.93143	
10 SKIM MILK							0.06263	0.07275		0.01012
12 CONDENSED							0.23587	0.30455		0.06868
13 BUTTER MILK COND	1374.44	1374.44		29.88 FW			0.1133?	0.28000	0.31311	
14 SKIM MLK PWDR							0.67488	0.96750		0.29262
16 WHEY POWDER	138.00	138.00	15.13	3.00 FW				0.14500	0.66827	
43 LIQUID CANE SUGAR	722.86	722.86	64.89	15.71 FW				0.30000		
71 EMUL/STAB	18.40	18.40	1.84	0.40 FW				1.20000		
74 FRODEX	138.00	138.00	15.13	3.00 FW				0.25430		
300 WATER	1984.86	1984.86	238.28	43.15 FW			-0.14994	0.00001	0.01395	
FINISHED WEIGHT	4600.00	4600.00	362.26	100.00 FW				0.18260 TOTAL COST=		839.98

CONSTRAINT	SOLUTION VALUE	MINIMUM VALUE	MAXIMUM VALUE	PENALTY COST
2 % FAT (TOTAL)	3.10	3.10	FW	0.01782
54 %MSNF (INC WHEY)	12.00	12.00	FW	0.00696
17 % WHEY SOLIDS	3.00		3.00 FW	0.00523
29 % CANE SOLIDS	11.00	11.00	11.00 FW	-0.00429
32 % FRODEX	3.00	3.00	3.00 FW	-0.00254
35 % EMUL & % STAB	0.40	0.40	0.40 FW	-0.01200
98 FINISHED WEIGHT	4600.00	4600.00	4600.00 FW	0.18260

Fig. 8.13. Multiproduct run (white mix, 3%) with no ingredient minimums or maximums. Copyright © Computer Concepts Corp., 1983.

INGREDIENT	TOTAL WEIGHT	BATCH WEIGHT	GALLONS	PERCENT BATCH	MINIMUM PERCENT	MAXIMUM PERCENT	COST/UNIT LOW	ACTUAL	HIGH	PENALTY
1 WHOLE MILK							0.12772	0.13014		0.00242
5 CREAM	1123.52	1123.52	135.69	24.42 FW			0.03924	0.72087	0.74939	
10 SKIM MILK	1796.34	1796.34	196.97	39.05 FW			0.04294	0.07275	0.07539	
12 CONDENSED	335.22	335.22	35.85	7.29 FW			0.27400	0.30455	0.32592	
14 SKIM MLK PWDR							0.89196	0.96750		0.07554
16 WHEY POWDER	109.25	109.25	11.98	2.37 FW				0.14500	0.87463	
40 CORN SYRUP	273.61	273.61	24.56	5.95 FW				0.08867		
43 LIQUID CANE SUGAR	814.86	814.86	73.15	17.71 FW				0.30000		
71 EMUL/STAB	27.60	27.60	2.76	0.60 FW				1.20000		
134 COCOA	119.60	119.60	13.11	2.60 FW				0.62000		
300 WATER							-0.01103	0.00001	0.01104	
FINISHED WEIGHT	4600.00	4600.00	494.07	100.00 FW				0.31185 TOTAL COST=		1434.51

CONSTRAINT	SOLUTION VALUE	MINIMUM VALUE	MAXIMUM VALUE	PENALTY COST
1 COST/UNIT ($/LB.)	0.00		FW	
2 % FAT (TOTAL)	9.40	9.40	FW	0.01777
54 %MSNF (INC WHEY)	9.50	9.50	FW	0.00931
55 % TOTAL SOLIDS	39.28		FW	
17 % WHEY SOLIDS	2.37		2.37 FW	0.00730
27 % COCO FLAVORING	2.60	2.60	2.60 FW	-0.00631
29 % CANE SOLIDS	12.40	12.40	12.40 FW	-0.00444
30 % CORN SYRUP SLDS	4.80	4.80	4.80 FW	-0.00124
35 % EMUL & % STAB	0.60	0.60	0.60 FW	-0.01211
98 FINISHED WEIGHT	4600.00	4600.00	4600.00 FW	0.31185

Fig. 8.14. Multiproduct run (chocolate mix, 10%) with no ingredient minimums or maximums. Copyright © Computer Concepts Corp., 1983.

INGREDIENT	TOTAL WEIGHT	BATCH WEIGHT	GALLONS	PERCENT BATCH	MINIMUM PERCENT	MAXIMUM PERCENT	LOW	ACTUAL	HIGH	PENALTY
								----------COST/UNIT----------		
1 WHOLE MILK							0.12772	0.13014		0.00242
5 CREAM	59.97	59.97	7.24	1.30 FW			0.04365	0.72087	0.74947	
10 SKIM MILK	1497.35	1497.35	164.18	32.55 FW			0.00001	0.07275	0.07540	
12 CONDENSED							0.27400	0.30455		0.03055
14 SKIM MLK PWDR							0.78399	0.96750		0.18351
40 CORN SYRUP	342.01	342.01	30.70	7.43 FW				0.08867		
43 LIQUID CANE SUGAR	1182.86	1182.86	106.18	25.71 FW				0.30000		
300 WATER	1517.81	1517.81	182.21	33.00 FW			-0.01103	0.00001	0.07275	
FINISHED WEIGHT	4600.00	4600.00	490.52	100.00 FW				0.11682	TOTAL COST=	537.36

CONSTRAINT	SOLUTION VALUE	MINIMUM VALUE	MAXIMUM VALUE	PENALTY COST
1 COST/UNIT ($/LB.)	0.00		FW	
2 % FAT (TOTAL)	0.50	0.50	FW	0.01766
29 % CANE SOLIDS	18.00	18.00	18.00 FW	-0.00429
30 % CORN SYRUP SLDS	6.00	6.00	6.00 FW	-0.00110
54 %MSNF (INC WHEY)	3.00	3.00	FW	0.00808
55 % TOTAL SOLIDS	27.46		FW	
98 FINISHED WEIGHT	4600.00	4600.00	4600.00 FW	0.11682

Fig. 8.15. Multiproduct run (sherbet) with no ingredient minimums or maximums. Copyright © Computer Concepts Corp., 1983.

INGREDIENT	TOTAL WEIGHT	BATCH WEIGHT	GALLONS	PERCENT BATCH	MINIMUM PERCENT	MAXIMUM PERCENT	LOW	ACTUAL	HIGH	PENALTY
								----------COST/UNIT----------		
1 WHOLE MILK							0.12771	0.13014		0.00243
5 CREAM	1580.14	1580.14	190.84	34.35 FW			0.15195	0.72087	0.74957	
10 SKIM MILK	995.03	995.03	109.10	21.63 FW			-1.52050	0.07275	0.07541	
12 CONDENSED							0.23543	0.30455		0.06912
13 BUTTER MILK COND	950.40	950.40		20.66 FW			0.14035	0.28000	0.33934	
43 LIQUID CANE SUGAR	1051.43	1051.43	94.38	22.86 FW				0.30000		
71 EMUL/STAB	23.00	23.00	2.30	0.50 FW				1.20000		
FINISHED WEIGHT	4600.00	4600.00	396.63	100.00 FW				0.39578	TOTAL COST=	1820.60

CONSTRAINT	SOLUTION VALUE	MINIMUM VALUE	MAXIMUM VALUE	PENALTY COST
1 COST/UNIT ($/LB.)	0.00		FW	
2 % FAT (TOTAL)	14.00	14.00	FW	0.01751
29 % CANE SOLIDS	16.00	16.00	16.00 FW	-0.00409
35 % EMUL & % STAB	0.50	0.50	0.50 FW	-0.01186
54 %MSNF (INC WHEY)	10.00	10.00	FW	0.00653
55 % TOTAL SOLIDS	40.47		FW	
98 FINISHED WEIGHT	4600.00	4600.00	4600.00 FW	0.39578

Fig. 8.16. Multiproduct run (white mix, 14%) with no ingredient minimums or maximums. Copyright © Computer Concepts Corp., 1983.

INGREDIENT	COST/UNIT	% FAT	%MOISTURE	% MILK SOLIDS N/F	% DAIRY	MINIMUM	MAXIMUM
				% TOTAL SOLIDS			
1 WHOLE MILK	0.13014*	3.25000	88.0500	8.70000	11.9500	100.000	2500.00
5 CREAM	0.72087*	38.3500*	56.2500	5.40000*	43.7500	100.000	5000.00
10 SKIM MILK	0.07275*	0.00000*	91.0000	9.00000*	9.00000*	100.000	
12 CONDENSED	0.30455	0.00000	66.1000	33.9000	33.9000	100.000	
13 BUTTER MILK COND	0.28000	4.00000	0.00000	30.0000	34.0000	100.000	
14 SKIM MLK PWDR	0.96750*	0.00000*	3.00000	97.0000*	97.0000	100.000	
16 WHEY POWDER	0.14500*	1.40000*	6.13500	92.4650*	93.8650	100.000	
40 CORN SYRUP	0.08867*	0.00000	19.3000*	0.00000	80.7000*	0.00000	
43 LIQUID CANE SUGAR	0.30000*	0.00000	33.0000*	0.00000	69.8600	0.00000	
71 EMUL/STAB	1.20000	0.00000*	0.00000*	0.00000*	100.000*	0.00000	
74 FRODEX	0.25430	0.00000	0.00000	0.00000	100.000	0.00000	
134 COCOA	0.62000	0.00000*	0.00000	0.00000	100.000	0.00000	
300 WATER	0.00001	0.00000	100.000	0.00000	0.00000	0.00000	

Fig. 8.17. Available ingredients file listing for example in Figs. 8.18–8.22.

the unlimited-supply run had increased. However, the solutions were still least-cost based on the new limitations. (The same five formulas with the new minimums and maximums are shown in Figs. 8.18–8.22. A comparison between the two multiproduct runs is shown in Table 8.16.

INGREDIENT	TOTAL WEIGHT	BATCH WEIGHT	GALLONS	PERCENT BATCH	MINIMUM PERCENT	MAXIMUM PERCENT	LOW	ACTUAL	HIGH	PENALTY
1 WHOLE MILK							0.12087	0.13014		0.00927
5 CREAM	2143.33	2143.33	258.86	23.30 FW			0.40341	0.72087	0.88779	
10 SKIM MILK							0.06263	0.07275		0.01012
12 CONDENSED							0.23587	0.30455		0.06868
13 BUTTER MILK COND	2680.87	2680.87		29.14 FW			0.07520	0.28000	0.31311	
14 SKIM MLK PWDR							0.67488	0.96750		0.29262
40 CORN SYRUP	1083.02	1083.02	97.22	11.77 FW				0.08867		
43 LIQUID CANE SUGAR	1196.00	1196.00	107.36	13.00 FW				0.30000		
71 EMUL/STAB	46.00	46.00	4.60	0.50 FW				1.20000		
300 WATER	2050.78	2050.78	246.19	22.29 FW			-0.14994	0.00001	0.01395	
FINISHED WEIGHT	9200.00	9200.00	714.23	100.00 FW				0.30497 TOTAL COST=		2805.74

CONSTRAINT	SOLUTION VALUE	MINIMUM VALUE	MAXIMUM VALUE	PENALTY COST
2 % FAT (TOTAL)	10.10	10.10	FW	0.01782
54 %MSNF (INC WHEY)	10.00	10.00	FW	0.00696
35 % EMUL & % STAB	0.50	0.50	0.50 FW	-0.01200
29 % CANE SOLIDS	9.10	9.10	9.10 FW	-0.00429
30 % CORN SYRUP SLDS	9.50	9.50	9.50 FW	-0.00110
55 % TOTAL SOLIDS	39.18		FW	
98 FINISHED WEIGHT	9200.00	9200.00	9200.00 FW	0.30497

Fig. 8.18. Multiproduct run (white mix, 10%) with restrictions on whole milk and cream. Copyright© Computer Concepts Corp., 1983.

INGREDIENT	TOTAL WEIGHT	BATCH WEIGHT	GALLONS	PERCENT BATCH	MINIMUM PERCENT	MAXIMUM PERCENT	LOW	ACTUAL	HIGH	PENALTY
1 WHOLE MILK							0.12087	0.13014		0.00927
5 CREAM	223.44	223.44	26.99	4.86 FW			0.40341	0.72087	0.88779	
10 SKIM MILK							0.06263	0.07275		0.01012
12 CONDENSED							0.23587	0.30455		0.06868
13 BUTTER MILK COND	1374.44	1374.44		29.88 FW			0.11306	0.28000	0.31311	
14 SKIM MLK PWDR							0.67488	0.96750		0.29262
16 WHEY POWDER	138.00	138.00	15.13	3.00 FW				0.14500	0.66827	
43 LIQUID CANE SUGAR	722.86	722.86	64.89	15.71 FW				0.30000		
71 EMUL/STAB	18.40	18.40	1.84	0.40 FW				1.20000		
74 FRODEX	138.00	138.00	15.13	3.00 FW				0.25430		
300 WATER	1984.86	1984.86	238.28	43.15 FW			-0.14994	0.00001	0.01395	
FINISHED WEIGHT	4600.00	4600.00	362.26	100.00 FW				0.18260 TOTAL COST=		839.98

CONSTRAINT	SOLUTION VALUE	MINIMUM VALUE	MAXIMUM VALUE	PENALTY COST
2 % FAT (TOTAL)	3.10	3.10	FW	0.01782
54 %MSNF (INC WHEY)	12.00	12.00	FW	0.00696
17 % WHEY SOLIDS	3.00		3.00 FW	0.00523
29 % CANE SOLIDS	11.00	11.00	11.00 FW	-0.00429
32 % FRODEX	3.00	3.00	3.00 FW	-0.00254
35 % EMUL & % STAB	0.40	0.40	0.40 FW	-0.01200
98 FINISHED WEIGHT	4600.00	4600.00	4600.00 FW	0.18260

Fig. 8.19. Multiproduct run (white mix, 3%) with restrictions on whole milk and cream. Copyright© Computer Concepts Corp., 1983.

INGREDIENT	TOTAL WEIGHT	BATCH WEIGHT	GALLONS	PERCENT BATCH	MINIMUM PERCENT	MAXIMUM PERCENT	LOW	ACTUAL	HIGH	PENALTY
1 WHOLE MILK	1963.11	1963.11	228.53	42.68 FW			0.10287	0.13014	0.13015	
5 CREAM	957.16	957.16	115.60	20.81 FW			0.72079	0.72087	1.04264	
10 SKIM MILK							0.07274	0.07275		0.00001
12 CONDENSED	334.82	334.82	35.81	7.28 FW			0.27400	0.30455	0.32592	
14 SKIM MLK PWDR							0.89198	0.96750		0.07552
16 WHEY POWDER	109.25	109.25	11.98	2.37 FW				0.14500	0.87465	
40 CORN SYRUP	273.61	273.61	24.56	5.95 FW				0.08867		
43 LIQUID CANE SUGAR	814.86	814.86	73.15	17.71 FW				0.30000		
71 EMUL/STAB	27.60	27.60	2.76	0.60 FW				1.20000		
134 COCOA	119.60	119.60	13.11	2.60 FW				0.62000		
300 WATER							-0.01104	0.00001		0.01105
FINISHED WEIGHT	4600.00	4600.00	505.50	100.00 FW				0.31288	TOTAL COST=	1439.26

CONSTRAINT	SOLUTION VALUE	MINIMUM VALUE	MAXIMUM VALUE	PENALTY COST
1 COST/UNIT ($/LB.)	0.00		FW	
2 % FAT (TOTAL)	9.40	9.40	FW	0.01777
54 %MSNF (INC WHEY)	9.50	9.50	FW	0.00931
55 % TOTAL SOLIDS	39.28		FW	
17 % WHEY SOLIDS	2.37		2.37 FW	0.00730
27 % COCO FLAVORING	2.60	2.60	2.60 FW	-0.00631
29 % CANE SOLIDS	12.40	12.40	12.40 FW	-0.00444
30 % CORN SYRUP SLDS	4.80	4.80	4.80 FW	-0.00124
35 % EMUL & % STAB	0.60	0.60	0.60 FW	-0.01211
98 FINISHED WEIGHT	4600.00	4600.00	4600.00 FW	0.31185

Fig. 8.20. Multiproduct run (chocolate mix, 10%) with restrictions on whole milk and cream. Copyright© Computer Concepts Corp., 1983.

INGREDIENT	TOTAL WEIGHT	BATCH WEIGHT	GALLONS	PERCENT BATCH	MINIMUM PERCENT	MAXIMUM PERCENT	LOW	ACTUAL	HIGH	PENALTY
1 WHOLE MILK	536.89	536.89	62.50	11.67 FW			0.13013	0.13014	0.13015	
5 CREAM	14.47	14.47	1.75	0.31 FW			0.72077	0.72087	0.72094	
10 SKIM MILK	1005.65	1005.65	110.27	21.86 FW			0.07274	0.07275	0.07276	
12 CONDENSED							0.27400	0.30455		0.03055
14 SKIM MLK PWDR							0.78399	0.96750		0.18351
40 CORN SYRUP	342.01	342.01	30.70	7.43 FW				0.08867		
43 LIQUID CANE SUGAR	1182.86	1182.86	106.18	25.71 FW				0.30000		
300 WATER	1518.12	1518.12	182.25	33.00 FW			-0.01103	0.00001	0.01395	
FINISHED WEIGHT	4600.00	4600.00	493.65	100.00 FW				0.11710	TOTAL COST=	538.66

CONSTRAINT	SOLUTION VALUE	MINIMUM VALUE	MAXIMUM VALUE	PENALTY COST
1 COST/UNIT ($/LB.)	0.00		FW	
2 % FAT (TOTAL)	0.50	0.50	FW	0.01766
29 % CANE SOLIDS	18.00	18.00	18.00 FW	-0.00429
30 % CORN SYRUP SLDS	6.00	6.00	6.00 FW	-0.00110
54 %MSNF (INC WHEY)	3.00	3.00	FW	0.00808
55 % TOTAL SOLIDS	27.46		FW	
98 FINISHED WEIGHT	4600.00	4600.00	4600.00 FW	0.11682

Fig. 8.21. Multiproduct run (sherbet) with restrictions on whole milk and cream. Copyright© Computer Concepts Corp., 1983.

Table 8.16. Multiple Formulations—Ingredient Usage Comparisons

		Ingredient	No minimums or maximums		Restrictions on milk and cream		Difference	
			Usage	Cost	Usage	Cost	Usage	Cost
1		Whole milk			2500.00	325.35	-2500.00	-325.3500
5		Cream	5130.40	3698.33	4918.54	3545.60	211.86	152.7526
10		Skim milk	4288.72	312.00	2000.68	145.55	2288.04	166.4548
12		Condensed	335.22	102.09	334.82	101.97	0.40	0.1221
13		Buttermilk, condensed	5005.71	1401.60	5005.71	1401.60	0.00	0.0000
16		Whey powder	247.25	35.85	247.00	35.85	0.00	0.0000
40		Corn syrup	1698.64	150.62	1698.64	150.62	-0.00	-0.0000
43		Liquid cane sugar	4968.00	1490.40	4968.00	1490.40	-0.00	-0.0001
71		Emulsifier/ Stabilizer	115.00	138.00	115.00	138.00	-0.00	-0.0000
74		Frodex	138.00	35.09	138.00	35.09	0.00	0.0000
134		Cocoa	119.60	74.15	119.60	74.15	0.00	0.0000
300		Water	5553.45	0.06	5553.76	0.06	-0.30	-0.0000
		Totals	27,600.00	7438.19	27,600.00	7444.24	0.00	-6.0479
		Cost/unit		0.26950		0.26972		-0.00022

INGREDIENT	TOTAL WEIGHT	BATCH WEIGHT	GALLONS	PERCENT BATCH	MINIMUM PERCENT	MAXIMUM PERCENT	----------COST/UNIT----------			
							LOW	ACTUAL	HIGH	PENALTY
1 WHOLE MILK							0.13013	0.13014		0.00001
5 CREAM	1580.14	1580.14	190.84	34.35 FW			0.15195	0.72087	0.72096	
10 SKIM MILK	995.03	995.03	109.10	21.63 FW			-1.52050	0.07275	0.07276	
12 CONDENSED							0.23543	0.30455		0.06912
13 BUTTER MILK COND	950.40	950.40		20.66 FW			0.14035	0.28000	0.31311	
43 LIQUID CANE SUGAR	1051.43	1051.43	94.38	22.86 FW				0.30000		
71 EMUL/STAB	23.00	23.00	2.30	0.50 FW				1.20000		
FINISHED WEIGHT	4600.00	4600.00	396.63	100.00 FW				0.39578 TOTAL COST=		1820.60

CONSTRAINT	SOLUTION VALUE	MINIMUM VALUE	MAXIMUM VALUE	PENALTY COST
1 COST/UNIT ($/LB.)	0.00		FW	
2 % FAT (TOTAL)	14.00	14.00	FW	0.01751
29 % CANE SOLIDS	16.00	16.00	16.00 FW	-0.00409
35 % EMUL & % STAB	0.50	0.50	0.50 FW	-0.01186
54 %MSNF (INC WHEY)	10.00	10.00	FW	0.00653
55 % TOTAL SOLIDS	40.47		FW	
98 FINISHED WEIGHT	4600.00	4600.00	4600.00 FW	0.39578

Fig. 8.22. Multiproduct run (white mix, 14%) with restrictions on milk and cream. Copyright © Computer Concepts Corp., 1983.

In real plant situations the use of a computer for formulation of ice cream mixes can mean a significant time savings for personnel involved. Further, the use of this system makes optimal use of raw materials by considering ingredients that must be forced into usage or items that are limited in availability. Computers maintain product quality standards by use of restrictions that are set by the plant. Formulation using a linear program not only meets ingredient availability limitations and quality restrictions, but does so on a least-cost basis.

Restandardizing and Calculating
Some Unusual Mixes

RESTANDARDIZING A MIX OR CORRECTING MIXES
HAVING AN UNDESIRED COMPOSITION

Sometimes when a mix has been made it is found by analysis to have a composition different from that which is desired. This incorrect mix can easily be corrected by restandardizing, i.e., by adding sufficient quantities of one or several ingredients to give the desired composition. This obviously increases the total amount of the mix and requires a vat large enough to hold the added ingredients plus the incorrect mix, so that they may be properly blended. Usually the total weight of all the added ingredients will not be more than one-third the weight of the incorrect mix.

If vat space is limited, it may be convenient to store a part (usually half) of the incorrect mix while the other part is used as one ingredient of the next batch of mix, thus distributing the incorrect mix between the next two batches. If vat space is available, the entire incorrect mix may be used as one ingredient of a batch having a total weight approximately one-third larger than the weight of the incorrect mix. In this manner the calculations will be similar to those of Problem 7, and a smaller amount of added ingredients will be used.

Problem 7. Restandardizing an Incorrect Mix. Calculate the amount of ingredients required to make 1800 lb of mix testing 14% fat, 10% MSNF, 14% sugar, and 0.3% stablizer. We want to use 900 lb (half of a batch incorrectly made) of mix testing 10% fat, 11% MSNF, 14% sugar, 0.5% stabilizer, and 35.5% TS. In addition to this mix, 40% cream, 4% milk, sweetened condensed skim milk (42% sugar, 30% MSNF), cane sugar, and stabilizer are available.

Solution. This problem is solved by using the same formulas and procedure steps that are used for other complex mixes (see Chapter 8, Problem 6).

Step 1. List the available ingredients and the desired mix composition constituents (Table 9.1).

Step 2. Make a proof sheet and enter the information from step 1.

Step 3. Since 900 lb of incorrect mix is all going to be used, it may be entered in the proof sheet immediately. The amount of each constituent in the

Table 9.1. Available Ingredients/Desired Composition Table for Problem 7

Available ingredients		Desired mix composition		
Ingredient	Constituent (%)	Constituent	Proportion (%)	Weight (lb)
Incorrect mix	Fat (10%)	Fat	14	252.0
	MSNF (11%)	MSNF	10	180.0
	Sugar (14%)	Sugar	14	252.0
	Stabilizer (0.5%)	Stabilizer	0.3	5.4
	TS (35.5%)			
Stabilizer	TS (90%)			
Sweetened				
condensed				
skim milk	MSNF (30%)			
	Sugar (42%)			
Cane sugar	Sugar (100%)			
Cream	Fat (40%)			
	MSNF (5.35%)			
Milk	Fat (4%)			
	MSNF (8.79%)			

incorrect mix is obtained by multiplying the proportion of the constituent times the 900 lb:

$$900 \times 0.10 = 90.00 \text{ lb fat}$$
$$900 \times 0.11 = 99.00 \text{ lb MSNF}$$
$$900 \times 0.14 = 126.00 \text{ lb sugar}$$
$$900 \times 0.005 = 4.50 \text{ lb stabilizer}$$
$$900 \times 0.355 = 319.50 \text{ lb TS}$$

Subtracting each of these amounts from the corresponding figure for the desired mix leaves 900 lb mix, 162 lb fat, 81 lb MSNF, 126 lb sugar, and 0.9 lb stabilizer still needed.

There is only one source of stabilizer and it contains 90% TS. Therefore, the 0.9 lb of needed stabilizer will require 1.0 lb stabilizer (0.9/0.90 = 1.0 lb), which is entered in the weight column. We also enter 0.9 lb in both the stabilizer and TS columns.

Step 4. To find the amount of sweetened condensed skim milk needed, it will be necessary to use formula (II). The figures to substitute in the formula are obtained as follows:

From step 3, the amount of MSNF needed is 81 lb. We obtain the amount of serum by subtracting the amount of fat (162 lb), sugar (126 lb), and stabilizer (1 lb) from the remaining total weight: 900 − 289 = 611 lb. Next we obtain the amount of MSNF in 1 lb of sweetened condensed skim milk by multiplying the MSNF test (30%) by 1 lb: 0.30 × 1 = 0.30 lb.

To find the amount of serum in 1 lb of sweetened condensed skim milk, we subtract the amount of sugar (0.42 × 1 = 0.42 lb) from the 1 lb: 1 − 0.42 = 0.58 lb serum. We finally substitute these figures into formula (II):

$$\frac{81 - (611 \times 0.09)}{0.30 - (0.58 \times 0.09)} = \frac{81 - 54.99}{0.30 - 0.052} = \frac{26.01}{0.248} = 104.88 \text{ lb}$$

the amount of sweetened condensed skim milk needed. We enter this figure in the weight column.

We also enter the amounts of MSNF, sugar, and TS in their respective columns. We obtain these by multiplying the 104.88 lb by the respective percentages of MSNF, sugar, and TS:

$$104.88 \times 0.30 = 31.46 \quad \text{lb MSNF}$$
$$104.88 \times 0.42 = 44.05 \quad \text{lb sugar}$$
$$104.88 \times 0.72 = 75.51 \quad \text{lb TS}$$

Step 5. To calculate the amount of sugar needed, first subtract the 44.05 lb sugar supplied by sweetened condensed skim milk from the 126 lb sugar needed. This leaves 81.95 lb sugar to be obtained from cane sugar which is 100% sugar. This means that 81.95 lb of cane sugar is needed and that figure can be entered in the proof sheet under weight, sugar, and TS.

Step 6. The amount of cream needed is calculated by using formula (III) with the following figures:

From step 3, the amount of fat needed is 162 lb. To calculate the amount of milk and cream needed, we subtract the amount of stabilizer (1 lb, step 3), sweetened condensed skim milk (104.88 lb, step 4), and cane sugar (81.95 lb, step 5) from the remaining total weight (900 lb, step 3): $900 - 187.83 = 712.17$ lb, the amount of milk and cream needed. The amount of fat in 1 lb of 40% cream is 0.40 lb, and the amount of fat in 1 lb of 4% milk is 0.04 lb. These figures are then substituted into formula (III):

$$\frac{162 - (712.17 \times 0.04)}{0.40 - 0.04} = \frac{162 - 28.49}{0.36} = 370.86 \quad \text{lb}$$

the amount of cream needed. This figure is entered in the weight column of the proof sheet.

We also enter in their respective columns the amount of fat, MSNF, and TS contained in the cream. We obtain these by multiplying the weight of the cream (370.86 lb) by the respective percentages:

$$370.86 \times 0.40 = 148.34 \quad \text{lb fat}$$
$$370.86 \times 0.0535 = 19.84 \quad \text{lb MSNF}$$
$$370.86 \times 0.4535 = 168.19 \quad \text{lb TS}$$

Step 7. The amount of milk needed is obtained by subtracting the amount of cream (370.86 lb, step 6) from the amount of milk and cream (712.17 lb, step 6), which is 341.31 lb. This figure is entered in the weight column. We calculate the amount of fat, MSNF, and TS contained in the milk by multiplying the 341.31 lb by the respective percentages:

$$341.31 \times 0.04 = 13.65 \quad \text{lb fat}$$
$$341.31 \times 0.0879 = 30.00 \quad \text{lb MSNF}$$
$$341.31 \times 0.1279 = 43.65 \quad \text{lb TS}$$

Step 8. Each column of the proof sheet is now totaled. These totals should agree with the corresponding figures of the desired mix (see Fig. 9.1). The TS test is computed as follows:

$$\frac{689.80 \text{ lb TS}}{1800 \text{ lb mix}} = 0.3832 = 38.32\% \quad \text{TS}$$

Likewise, we compute the percentages of all the remaining constituents.

Step 9. The correctness of the calculations is determined by comparing the calculated percentage for each constituent with the corresponding test of the desired mix.

Step 10. Calculate the actual cost if desired and enter in proof sheet.

UNUSUAL COMPLEX MIXES

On rare occasions, an unusual combination of ingredients for an ice cream mix will be selected for reasons of economy. These unusual combinations make the calculations somewhat longer and slightly more complicated. They can be grouped in two general types, illustrated by Problems 8 and 9.

The first unusual mix is when no dry source of sucrose is available and there are three sources of MSNF, one of which is a sweetened condensed milk product.

Problem 8. Calculate the amount of ingredients needed to make 900 lb mix testing 12% fat, 10% MSNF, 14% sugar, and 0.4% stabilizer. The available ingredients are 40% cream, 4% milk, corn syrup (47% sucrose equivalent, 64.68% TS) to supply 25% of the sugar, sweetened condensed whole milk (8% fat, 42% sugar, 23% MSNF), liquid sugar (67% sugar, 67% TS), and stabilizer.

Solution. This complex mix has three sources of sugar, three sources of MSNF, and three sources of fat. Therefore, the calculations will be made using formulas (II) and (III).

Steps 1–3. These steps are completed as in problem 3, and yield the partially completed proof sheet shown in Fig. 9.2.

Step 4. To find the amount of sweetened condensed whole milk needed, we use formula (II), with the following figures:

The amount of MSNF needed is 90 lb (from step 2). To obtain the serum of the mix, we subtract the amount of stabilizer (4.00 lb), fat, (108.00 lb), corn syrup (67.02 lb), sugar (94.50 lb, from liquid sugar and sweetened condensed whole milk—this represents 75% of the 126.00 lb of sugar needed), and estimated water in the liquid sugar (21.48 lb)[1] from the total weight: 900 − 295.00 = 605 lb.

---

[1]Since it is necessary in formula (II) to use the amount of sugar source and in this case some of the 94.50 lb of sugar will come from liquid sugar, then the amount of sugar source must be greater than 94.50. However, we cannot at this point tell how much greater it will be. We thus make an estimate of 21.48 lb, but any other estimate would do, since the revision process we shall go through in step 4a will always provide us with an accurate estimate.

Ingredients	Ingredient weight (lb)	Calculated constituents					
		Fat (lb)	MSNF (lb)	Sugar (lb)	Stabilizer (lb)	TS (lb)	Cost ($)
Incorrect mix	900.00	90.00	99.00	126.00	4.50	319.50	
Stabilizer	1.00				0.90	0.90	
Sweetened condensed skim milk	104.88		31.46	44.05		75.51	
Cane sugar	81.95			81.95		81.95	
Cream, 40%	370.86	148.35	19.84			168.19	
Milk, 4%	341.31	13.65	30.00			43.65	
Total	1800.00	252.00	180.30	252.00	5.40	689.80	—
Calculated %		14.00	10.01	14.00	0.30	38.32	
Check with desired wt.	1800.00	252.00	180.00	252.00	5.40	689.40	
desired %		14.00	10.00	14.00	0.30	38.30	

Fig. 9.1. Completed proof sheet for Problem 7.

| | | Calculated constituents | | | | | |
Ingredients	Ingredient weight (lb)	Fat (lb)	MSNF (lb)	Sugar (lb)	Stabilizer (lb)	TS (lb)	Cost ($)
Stabilizer	4.00				3.60	3.60	
Corn syrup	67.02			31.50		64.68	
Sweetened condensed whole milk							
Liquid sugar							
Cream, 40%							
Milk, 4%							
Total	—	—	—	—	—	—	—
Calculated %							
Check with desired wt.	900.00	108.00	90.00	126.00	3.60	327.60	
desired %		12.00	10.00	14.00	0.40	36.40	

Fig. 9.2. Partially completed proof sheet for Problem 8.

To obtain the amount of serum in 1 lb of sweetened condensed whole milk, we subtract the amount of MSNF (0.23 lb), sugar (0.42 lb), and fat (0.08 lb): $1 - 0.50 = 0.50$ lb, and substitute these figures into formula (II):

$$\frac{90 - (605 \times 0.09)}{0.23 - (0.50 \times 0.09)} = \frac{90 - 54.45}{0.23 - 0.045} = \frac{35.55}{0.185} = 192.16 \quad \text{lb}$$

the amount of sweetened condensed milk needed.

Since the calculation involved an estimate (of the water in the liquid sugar), this figure may be incorrect. Therefore, we must test its accuracy before proceeding with other calculations.

Step 4a. The 192.16 lb of milk will supply $192.16 \times 0.42 = 80.707$ lb of sugar. To obtain the amount of sugar supplied by the liquid sugar, we subtract this figure from the total amount of sugar supplied by the liquid sugar and the condensed milk: $94.50 - 80.707 = 13.793$ lb. Since the liquid sugar contains 67% sugar, then the amount of liquid sugar needed is given by

$$13.793/0.67 = 20.59 \quad \text{lb}$$

The total amount of sugar plus water is then obtained by adding $80.707 + 20.59 = 101.297$. However, the amount of sugar supplied by the two ingredients added to the amount of water that we estimated in step 4, $94.50 + 21.48 = 115.98$, which differs by more than 1 lb, and so our original estimate was incorrect. Therefore, we must repeat steps 4 and 4a, using a revised estimate. The revised estimate must be such as to make the total somewhere between the two figures calculated above. This time we estimate the amount of water in the liquid sugar as 8.0 lb, which gives a total of $94.50 + 8.0 = 102.50$ lb.

In repeating step 4, this reduces the amount of serum from 295.00 to 281.52 lb, which gives a serum total of $900 - 281.52 = 618.48$ lb. Substituting into formula (II):

$$\frac{90 - (618.48 \times 0.09)}{0.23 - (0.50 \times 0.09)} = \frac{34.34}{0.185} = 185.60 \quad \text{lb}$$

the amount of serum in the mix. Repeating step 4a to test the accuracy of our new estimate, the amount of sugar is then $185.60 \times 0.42 = 77.952$ lb from the milk. The amount of liquid sugar needed is then

$$\frac{94.50 - 77.952}{0.67} = \frac{16.548}{0.67} = 24.70 \quad \text{lb}$$

Adding, the amount of sugar plus water is then $77.95 + 24.70 = 102.65$ lb. The amount of sugar supplied by the two ingredients plus the estimated water is $94.50 + 8.0 = 102.50$ lb. Since the difference between the calculated and estimated amounts is less than 1 lb, our calculation of 185.60 lb of sweetened condensed whole milk is correct. (Sometimes it is necessary to make several revised estimates.)

We can now calculate the amounts of sugar, fat, MSNF, and TS contributed by the milk by multiplying the 185.60 lb by the respective percentages:

$$185.60 \times 0.42 = 77.954 \quad \text{lb sugar}$$
$$185.60 \times 0.08 = 14.848 \quad \text{lb fat}$$
$$185.60 \times 0.23 = 42.689 \quad \text{lb MSNF}$$
$$185.60 \times 0.73 = 135.491 \quad \text{lb TS}$$

Step 5. The amount of liquid sugar needed as determined in step 4a is 24.70 lb, which contain 67% sugar or $24.70 \times 0.67 = 16.55$ lb sugar. This figure can be entered in the sugar and the TS columns of the proof sheet.

Step 6. To find the amount of cream needed, we use formula (III). The total amount of fat needed is obtained by subtracting the amount of fat supplied by the milk ($18.5.60 \times 0.08 = 14.85$ lb) from the amount of fat desired: $108.00 - 14.85 = 93.15$ lb.

To obtain the amount of milk and cream needed, we subtract the amount of stabilizer (4.0 lb, step 2), corn syrup (67.02 lb, step 1), sweetened condensed whole milk (185.60 lb, step 4), and liquid sugar (24.70 lb, step 4a) from the total mix: $900 - 281.32 = 618.68$ lb.

The amount of cream is obtained by substituting into formula (III):

$$\frac{93.15 - (618.68 \times 0.04)}{0.40 - 0.04} = \frac{68.405}{0.36} = 190.01 \quad \text{lb}$$

This amount of cream supplies 76.00 lb of fat, 10.165 lb of MSNF, and 86.165 lb of TS, which can all be entered into their respective columns (see Fig. 9.3).

The rest of the steps are the same as for previous problems.

The second type of unusual combination of ingredients occurs when sweet cream and a condensed whole milk product (such as sweetened condensed whole milk, whole milk powder, or sweet cream buttermilk powder) are used as the only sources of milk solids.

This type of problem usually involves many ingredients, and there may be four or more sources of fat or milk MSNF. Such mixes are usually made to the desired volume by adding water. The calculation procedure involves determining the amounts of constituents supplied by products of which amounts are specified, and then the amounts of products supplying the remaining required stabilizer, fats, MSNF, sugar, and the amount of water needed.

Problem 9. A 700-lb mix testing 14% fat, 9% MSNF, 15% sugar, and 0.3% stabilizer is desired. The following materials are leftovers to be used up to avoid loss: 50 lb cream (30% fat, 6.24% MSNF) and 100 lb milk (3% fat, 8.33% MSNF). The following ingredients are also available: stabilizer, cane sugar, 40% cream, sweetened condensed whole milk (8% fat, 23% MSNF, 42% sugar), and water.

Solution. Steps 1–3 completed as in problem 6 will produce the partially completed proof sheet in Fig. 9.4.

It now appears that 547.67 lb total weight containing 80 lb fat, 51.55 lb

Ingredients	Ingredient weight (lb)	Calculated constituents					
		Fat (lb)	MSNF (lb)	Sugar (lb)	Stabilizer (lb)	TS (lb)	Cost ($)
Stabilizer	4.00				3.60	3.60	
Corn syrup	67.02			31.50		64.68	
Sweetened condensed whole milk	185.60	14.85	42.69	77.95		135.49	
Liquid sugar, 67%	24.70			16.55		16.55	
Cream, 40%	190.01	76.00	10.17			86.17	
Milk, 4%	428.67	17.15	37.68			54.83	
Total	900.00	108.00	90.54	126.00	3.60	361.32	—
Calculated %		12.00	10.06	14.00	0.40	40.15	
Check with desired wt.	900.00	108.00	90.00	126.00	3.60	327.60	
desired %		12.00	10.00	14.00	0.40	36.40	

Fig. 9.3. Completed proof sheet for Problem 8.

Ingredients	Ingredient weight (lb)	Calculated constituents					
		Fat (lb)	MSNF (lb)	Sugar (lb)	Stabilizer (lb)	TS (lb)	Cost ($)
Cream, 30%	50.00	15.00	3.12			18.12	
Milk, 3%	100.00	3.00	8.33			11.33	
Gelatin	2.33				2.10	2.10	
Cane sugar							
Sweetened condensed whole milk							
Cream, 40%							
Water							
Total	—	—	—	—	—	—	—
Calculated %							
Check with desired wt.	700.00	98.00	63.00	105.00	2.10	268.10	
desired %		14.00	9.00	15.00	0.30	38.30	

Fig. 9.4. Partially completed proof sheet for Problem 9.

MSNF, and 105 lb sugar remains to be prepared by mixing cream, sugar, sweetened condensed whole milk, and water.

Step 4. The amount of milk and cream needed can be calculated in two ways, both of which depend on the following two formulas. The amount of condensed milk is given by

$$\frac{F_{cr} \times MSNF_{tot} - MSNF_{cr} \times F_{tot}}{F_{cr} \times MSNF_{mi} - F_{mi} \times MSNF_{cr}} \times 100 \tag{IV}$$

and the amount of cream is given by

$$\frac{MSNF_{mi} \times F_{tot} - F_{mi} \times MSNF_{tot}}{MSNF_{mi} \times F_{cr} - F_{mi} \times MSNF_{cr}} \times 100 \tag{V}$$

where the following abbreviations have been used:

F_{cr} percentage of fat in cream
F_{mi} percentage of fat in the condensed product
F_{tot} amount of fat required
$MSNF_{cr}$ percentage of MSNF in cream
$MSNF_{mi}$ percentage of MSNF in condensed product
$MSNF_{tot}$ amount of MSNF required

If we combine the two formulas, then for the total amount of cream and condensed product, we obtain

$$\frac{MSNF_{tot} \times (F_{cr} - F_{mi})}{F_{cr} \times MSNF_{mi} - F_{mi} \times MSNF_{cr}} \times 100$$

Using the latter formula,

$$\frac{51.55 \times (40 - 8 \times 100}{40 \times 23 - 8 \times 5.35} = \frac{3061.60}{877.20} \times 100 = 349.02 \quad lb$$

of cream and sweetened condensed whole milk.

Step 5. To find the amount of cream needed, we substitute the appropriate figures into formula (III):

$$\frac{80 - (349.02 \times 0.08)}{0.40 - 0.08} = \frac{52.08}{0.32} = 162.75 \quad lb$$

We then enter in their respective columns the weight, fat, MSNF, and TS supplied by the cream.

Step 6. The amount of sweetened condensed whole milk needed is calculated by subtracting the amount of cream from the total amount of cream and milk: $349.02 - 162.75 = 186.27$ lb of sweetened condensed whole milk needed.

We enter in their respective columns the weight, fat, MSNF, sugar, and TS supplied by the sweetened condensed whole milk.

Step 7. The amount of sugar needed is calculated by subtracting the amount of sugar supplied by the sweet condensed whole milk from the total sugar desired: $105 - 78.23 = 26.77$ lb of sugar to be supplied by the cane sugar. We enter this on the proof sheet.

Step 8. To find the amount of water needed, we subtract the total weight of all ingredients from the total weight of the mix: $700 - 528.12 = 171.88$ lb.

Returning to step 4, we can also determine the amounts of cream and milk directly by substituting into formulas (IV) and (V). The amount of cream needed is given by

$$\frac{40 \times 51.55 - 5.35 \times 80}{40 \times 23 - 8 \times 5.35} \times 100$$

$$= \frac{2062 - 428}{920 - 42.80} \times 100 = \frac{1634}{877.20} \times 100 = 186.27 \quad \text{lb}$$

Similarly, the amount of sweetened condensed whole milk needed is given by

$$\frac{23 \times 80 - 8 \times 51.55}{23 \times 40 - 8 \times 5.35} \times 100$$

$$= \frac{1840 - 412.40}{920 - 42.80} \times 100 = \frac{1427.60}{877.20} \times 100 = 162.75 \quad \text{lb}$$

The rest of the calculations remain the same. The completed proof sheet is shown in Fig. 9.5.

CALCULATING A MIX TO BE MADE IN THE VACUUM PAN

Some dairy plants manufacture condensed whole milk, which they later use in making ice cream mix. Nearly half the time and labor required for these two operations can be eliminated by mixing the ingredients before condensing in the vacuum pan. This process of making the mix in a vacuum pan may be desirable whenever the necessary equipment, a sufficient supply of milk, and a large outlet for the mix are available.

These vacuum pan mixes are readily calculated as follows:

1. List the available ingredients and the number of pounds of each constituent of the desired mix.

Ingredients	Ingredient weight (lb)	Calculated constituents					
		Fat (lb)	MSNF (lb)	Sugar (lb)	Stabilizer (lb)	TS (lb)	Cost ($)
Cream, 30%	50.00	15.00	3.12			18.12	
Milk, 3%	100.00	3.00	8.33			11.33	
Gelatin	2.33				2.10	2.10	
Cane sugar	26.77			26.77		26.77	
Sweetened condensed whole milk	186.27	14.90	42.84	78.23		135.97	
Cream, 40%	162.75	65.10	8.71			73.81	
Water	171.88						
Total	700.00	98.00	63.00	105.00	2.10	268.10	—
Calculated %		14.00	9.00	15.00	0.30	38.30	
Check with desired wt.	700.00	98.00	63.00	105.00	2.10	268.10	
desired %		14.00	9.00	15.00	0.30	38.30	

Fig. 9.5. Completed proof sheet for Problem 9.

2. Make a proof sheet as described earlier and enter the information obtained in step 1.

3. Compute the needed amount of each nonmilk product (egg, stabilizer, etc.) and enter it in the proof sheet.

4. Calculate the needed total pounds of milk and cream by using the following formula:

$$\frac{(\text{total mix}) \times [(\text{MSNF test of mix}) + (\text{fat test of mix} \times 0.09)]}{9.0} \quad (\text{VI})^2$$

5. Calculate the amount of cream needed by using the following formula:

$$\frac{(\text{fat needed}) - [(\text{milk and cream needed}) \times (\text{fat per pound of milk})]}{(\text{fat per pound of cream}) - (\text{fat per pound of milk})} \quad (\text{VII})^3$$

and enter it in the proof sheet.

6. Subtract the amount of cream needed from the total amount of milk and cream to obtain the amount of milk needed. Enter this in the proof sheet.

7. Total each column in the proof sheet and check for accuracy. The total weight of all ingredients will be greater than the desired weight of the mix, and this excess is the amount of water to remove in the condensing process. The total of each of the other columns in the proof sheet should agree with the corresponding figure of the desired mix.

Problem 10.   A vacuum pan will be used in making a 5400 lb mix testing 12% fat, 11% MSNF, 14% sugar, 0.5% egg solids, and 0.3% stabilizer. The available ingredients are stabilizer, fresh eggs, Sweetose (43° Baumé) to furnish 25% of the total sugar, liquid sugar (67° Brix), cream (35% fat), and milk (3% fat). How much of each ingredient is needed?

Solution.   This mix is smaller and contains a larger variety of ingredients than most mixes made in a vacuum pan. Therefore, it will not only illustrate the procedure of calculating simple vacuum pan mixes, but will also serve as a guide in calculating the most complex ones.

Step 1.   Make a list of available ingredients and the constituents desired (Table 9.2).

Step 2.   Make a proof sheet and enter the information from step 1.

Step 3.   Compute the amount of nonmilk products. There is only one source of stabilizer, and it contains 90% TS. Therefore, the 16.2 lb of needed stabilizer will require 16.2/0.90 = 18.00 lb of stabilizer product. Enter this figure in the weight column of the proof sheet; also enter 16.2 lb in the stabilizer and TS columns.

---

[2]This formula assumes that skim milk tests 9% MSNF. However, skim milk obtained from 3% (fat) milk contains only 8.6% MSNF. Therefore, in the next problem, substitute 0.086 and 8.6, respectively, for 0.09 and 9.0.

[3]Amount of milk and cream is obtained from formula (VI).

Table 9.2. Available Ingredients/Desired Composition Table for Problem 10

Available ingredients		Desired mix composition		
Ingredient	Constituent (%)	Constituent	Proportion (%)	Weight (lb)
Stabilizer	TS (90%)	Fat	12	648
Fresh eggs	Fat (10.5%)	MSNF	11	594
	Egg solids (21.6%)	Sugar	14	756
	TS (26.3%)	Egg solids	0.5	27
Corn syrup	Sugar (67%)	Stabilizer	0.3	16.20
	TS (83%)			
Liquid sugar	Sugar (67%)			
	TS (67%)			
Cream	Fat (35%)			
	MSNF (5.69%)			
Milk	Fat (3%)			
	MSNF (8.33%)			

The fresh eggs are the only source of egg solids, and they contain 21.6% egg solids. Therefore, 21.6% of the eggs must equal 27 lb, the desired amount of egg solids. Thus 27/0.216 = 125 lb. Since the edible portion of a dozen eggs weighs 1.17 lb (see Table 5.16) it follows that the number of eggs needed is 125 lb/1.17 lb = approximately 107 dozen eggs. Since 107 dozen eggs weigh $107 \times 1.17 = 125.19$ lb, we enter this figure in the weight column of the proof sheet.

We also enter in their respective columns the fat, egg solids, and TS contained in the eggs. These figures are obtained by multiplying the weight of the eggs by the respective percentages:

$$125.19 \times 0.105 = 13.14 \quad \text{lb fat}$$
$$125.19 \times 0.216 = 27.04 \quad \text{lb egg solids}$$
$$125.19 \times 0.236 = 32.92 \quad \text{lb TS}$$

The amount of corn syrup needed can now be calculated. Since 25% of the total desired sugar equals 756/4 or 189 lb and since the corn syrup has 67% sugar equivalent, it follows that 189/0.67 = 282.09 lb of corn syrup needed. This number is put in the weight column of the proof sheet. We also enter in their respective columns the sugar and the TS contained in corn syrup, which are obtained by multiplying the weight of corn syrup by the respective percentages:

$$282.09 \times 0.67 = 189.00 \quad \text{lb sugar}$$
$$282.09 \text{ lb} \times 0.83 = 234.13 \quad \text{lb TS}$$

To find the remaining amount of sugar needed, we subtract the 189 lb of sugar supplied by corn syrup from the 756 lb of total sugar desired in the mix, which leaves 567 lb of sugar to be obtained from liquid sugar. The liquid sugar contains 67% sugar and therefore 567/0.67 = 846.27 lb of liquid sugar is needed. This number is entered in the weight column of the proof sheet. We also enter 567 lb in the sugar and TS columns.

Step 4.   To calculate the amount of milk and cream needed, we use formula (VI) substituting the figures obtained as follows:

From step 1, the amount of mix is 5400 lb, the MSNF test of mix is 11 (note that the decimal point is *not* moved to the left), and the fat test of mix is 12 (note that the decimal point is *not* moved to the left). In this problem, the milk tests 3.0% fat, and skim milk obtained from it will contain 8.6% MSNF. Therefore, we use 0.086 and 8.6 in place of 0.09 and 9.0, respectively. Substituting these figures in the formula gives

$$\frac{5400 \times (11 + 0.086 \times 12}{8.6}$$

$$= \frac{5400 \times (11 + 1.03)}{8.6} = \frac{5400 \times 12.03}{8.6} = 7553.72 \quad \text{lb}$$

the amount of milk and cream needed.

Step 5.   To find the amount of cream needed, we use formula (VII), substituting the figures obtained as follows:

The amount of fat needed from the milk and cream is obtained by subtracting the amount of fat in the fresh eggs (13.14 lb, step 3) from the amount of fat in the mix (648 lb, step 1), which gives 634.86 lb. The amount of milk and cream is 7553.72 (step 4), the amount of fat in 1 lb of 35% cream is 0.35 lb and the amount of fat in 1 lb of 3% milk is 0.03 lb. Substituting these figures in the formula gives

$$\frac{634.86 - (7553.72 \times 0.03)}{0.35 - 0.03}$$

$$= \frac{634.86 - 226.61}{0.35 - 0.03} = \frac{408.25}{0.32} = 1275.75 \quad \text{lb}$$

the amount of 35% cream needed. We enter this in the weight column of the proof sheet.

We also enter in their respective columns the fat, MSNF, and TS contained in the cream. These figures are obtained by multiplying the 1275.75 lb by the respective percentages:

$$1275.75 \times 0.35 = 446.51 \quad \text{lb fat}$$
$$1275.75 \times 0.0569 = 72.59 \quad \text{lb MSNF}$$
$$1275.75 \times 0.4069 = 519.10 \quad \text{lb TS}$$

Step 6.   To find the lb of 3% milk needed: Since in step 4 it was found that 7553.72 lb of milk and cream are needed, and in step 5 that 1275.75 lb of cream are needed, then subtracting the 1275.75 lb from the 7553.72 lb leaves 6277.97

| Ingredients | Ingredient weight (lb) | Calculated constituents | | | | | | |
		Fat (lb)	MSNF (lb)	Sugar (lb)	Egg Solids (lb)	Stabilizer (lb)	TS (lb)	Cost ($)
Stabilizer	18.00					16.20	16.20	
Fresh eggs	125.19	13.14			27.04		32.92	
Corn syrup	282.09			189.00			234.13	
Liquid sugar	846.27			567.00			567.00	
Cream, 35%	1275.75	446.51	72.59				519.06	
Milk, 3%	6277.97	188.34	522.95				711.29	
Total	8825.27	648.00	595.54	756.00	27.04	16.20	2080.66	
Calculated %		12.00	11.00	14.00	0.50	0.30	38.53	
Check with desired wt.	5400.00[a]	648.00	594.00	756.00	27.00	16.20	2041.20	
desired %		12.00	11.00	14.00	0.50	0.30	37.80	

[a]This figure does not include the water removed in the vacuum pan, 3425.27 lb.

Fig. 9.6. Completed proof sheet for Problem 10.

lb, the amount of 3% milk needed. This figure is entered in the weight column of the proof sheet.

We also enter in their respective columns the fat, MSNF, and TS contained in the milk. These figures are obtained by multiplying the 6277.97 by the respective percentages:

$$6277.97 \times 0.03 = 188.34 \quad \text{lb fat}$$
$$6277.97 \times 0.0833 = 522.95 \quad \text{lb MSNF}$$
$$6277.97 \times 0.1133 = 711.29 \quad \text{lb TS}$$

Step 7. Each column of the proof sheet is totaled and checked for correctness (see Fig. 9.6). It is apparent that the amount of fat contained in all of the ingredients is equal to the amount of fat desired in the mix. The same is true for the sugar, egg solids, and stabilizer. The total MSNF (595.54 lb) is larger than the desired 594 lb of MSNF. Therefore, we compute the MSNF test of the calculated mix:

$$\frac{595.54 \text{ lb total MSNF}}{5400 \text{ wt of desired mix}} = 11.03\%$$

This is slightly higher than the desired 11.00%, but the difference is less than 0.1. It follows that the error is not significant and that the mix is accurately calculated.

The TS test of the mix is computed by dividing 2080.66 lb total solids by 5400 lb, the weight of the finished mix: 2080.66/5400 = 38.53% TS.

The amount of water to be removed in the vacuum pan is obtained by subtracting the weight of the finished mix (5400.00 lb) from the total weight of all ingredients (8825.27 lb), which leaves 3425.27 lb, the weight of water to remove.

Turnbow *et al.* (1946) and Sommer (1951) showed that restandardization generally involved supplying additional fat, additional MSNF, or both. Although the restandardization of mixes may be easily calculated, the mechanics of testing for mix composition and the introduction of additional ingredients into the mix when the continuous automated system is utilized poses difficult time and processing problems for the production supervisor. Aspects of these problems are dealt with in Chapters 11 and 20.

10

Calculating Cost and Percentage of Overrun

CALCULATING COST OF THE MIX

The cost of ingredients in a mix is determined after the mix has been calculated. The simplest procedure is to multiply the price per pound by the amount, for each ingredient, and enter the result in the cost column of the proof sheet. When the cost of each ingredient has been entered in the proof sheet, the column is added to obtain the total cost of all ingredients in the entire batch of mix. When comparing costs one should, of course, be careful to compare the costs of equal amounts of mix.

The cost per pound of mix is a good basis for comparing costs of different mixes and is obtained by dividing total cost by total weight of mix.

Problem 11 demonstrates how to calculate the cost of ingredients used in Problems 3 and 4 (Chapter 8). The cost for Problems 5, 6 (Chapter 8), and 9 (Chapter 9) can be calculated in the same manner. The prices of the ingredients are based on July 1983 figures.

Problem 11. Calculate and compare the costs of the mixes in Problems 3 and 4 (Chapter 8).

Solution. The purchase price of the ingredients used in both problems is assumed to be as shown in Table 10.1. By using these figures, the total cost of the ingredients used in Problem 3 (see proof sheet) can be calculated. Table 10.2 shows that the cost per pound of mix in Problem 3 is $159.24/450 = $0.3538. At this point, we enter the cost of each ingredient in the cost column of the proof sheet for Problem 3.

We then repeat the procedure, using the ingredients in Problem 4. Table 10.3 gives the cost per pound of mix in Problem 4 as $77.68/200 = $0.3884. Again, we enter the cost of each ingredient in the cost column of the proof sheet for Problem 4.

A comparison shows that the mix in Problem 4 costs $0.0345/lb more than the mix in Problem 3.

Table 10.1. Cost of Ingredients Used in Problems 3 and 4

Ingredient	Purchase price ($)[a]	Cost/lb ($)
Stabilizer	—	1.70
Dried egg yolk	—	2.00
Cane sugar	—	0.31
MSNF	—	0.92
Cream, 30%	52.93 for 40-qt can, weighing 83.5 lb	0.6339
Cream, 40%	68.08 for 40-qt can, weighing 83.28 lb	0.8175
Condensed skim milk, 27% TS	22.98 for 40-qt can, weighing 92.5 lb	0.2484
Milk, 4%	12.56 for 100-lb can	0.1256
Water		0.002

[a] The purchase price is given for ingredients that are not priced by the pound.

Table 10.2. Total Cost of Ingredients in Problem 3

Ingredient	Quantity (lb)	Cost/lb ($)	Total cost ($)
Stabilizer	2.50	1.70	4.25
Dried egg yolk	2.39	2.00	4.78
Cane sugar	63.00	0.31	19.53
Cream, 30%	145.02	0.6339	91.93
MSNF	41.70	0.92	38.36
Water	95.38	0.002	0.39
Total	450.00		159.24

Table 10.3. Total Cost of Ingredients in Problem 4

Ingredient	Quantity (lb)	Cost/lb ($)	Total cost ($)
Stabilizer	1.11	1.70	1.88
Cane sugar	26.00	0.31	8.06
Condensed skim milk, 27% TS	27.56	0.2484	6.84
Cream, 40%	61.63	0.8175	50.39
Milk, 4%	83.70	0.1256	10.51
Total	200.00		77.68

COMPARE FOR COSTS AND QUALITY

A comparison of the cost of either ingredients or mixes should receive careful consideration because many factors are closely related to cost. The use of less expensive ingredients is often good business because it lowers the cost of the mix. However, substitutions must be made wisely or they may result in the appearance of defects and a low-quality product. For example, the mix in

Problem 3 is less expensive than the mix in Problem 4, but it would probably have a more pronounced "condensed" or "serum solids" flavor. Sometimes these defects can be avoided by properly balancing the mix. However, care must be taken not to throw the mix out of balance when the ingredients are changed. For example, in the more expensive mix of Problem 4 the condensed skim milk and whole milk cannot be replaced by nonfat dry milk solids and water unless egg yolk solids are added, as in Problem 3.

Since any change of ingredients will frequently throw a mix out of balance, it seems better to balance a mix properly for each group of ingredients before it is calculated and costs are considered. However, once the standard mixes are decided on, it is a good policy to purchase the ingredients from the most economical source, provided that this will not lower the quality, palatability, or other desired characteristics of the finished ice cream.

From a practical point of view, since butterfat is nearly always one of the principal items as well as the most expensive one that enter into the ice cream, the cheapest source of good quality butterfat should be selected.

CALCULATING PERCENTAGE OVERRUN

England (1968) defined overrun in the ice cream plant as the increase in volume of the ice cream over the volume of the mix due to the incorporation of air. When expressed as a percentage of the volume of the mix, this is known as percentage overrun. There are two basic ways to calculate percentage overrun: by volume and by weight. Each way has three variations.

Calculation by Volume

1. Simple formulation. When calculating the percentage overrun for plain ice cream or when an approximation is all that is required for a flavored ice cream, this simple formulation can be used:

$$\text{overrun \%} = \frac{\text{volume of ice cream} - \text{volume of mix}}{\text{volume of mix}} \times 100$$

Here the overrun is expressed as a percentage of the unflavored mix. This method is perhaps the most widely used. For example, if 5 gal of mix is frozen to make 9.5 gal of ice cream,

$$\frac{9.5 \times 5.0}{5.0} \times 100 = 90\% \quad \text{overrun}$$

2. Plant overrun formulation. This variation, which expresses the overrun as a percentage of the flavored mix, is more accurate and thus more useful in cost studies:

$$\text{overrun \%} = \frac{\text{volume of ice cream} - (\text{volume of mix} + \text{volume of flavor})}{\text{volume of mix} + \text{volume of flavor}}$$

For example, when 40 gal of unflavored mix is colored and flavored with 1 gal of coffee extract and frozen to 77.9 gal of ice cream,

$$\frac{77.9 - (40 + 1)}{40 + 1} \times 100 = 90\% \quad \text{overrun}$$

3. Overrun on plain mix. This variation is used for determining the overrun as a percentage of the plain mix. It recognizes the fact that flavorings and colorings add little overrun:

$$\text{overrun } \% = \frac{\text{volume of ice cream } - \text{ (volume of mix + volume of flavor)}}{\text{volume of plain mix}}$$

For example, when 17 gal of plain mix is colored and flavored with 3 gal of maple nut and frozen to 40 gal of ice cream,

$$\frac{40 - (17 + 3)}{17} \times 100 = 117.6\% \quad \text{overrun}$$

Calculation by Weight[1]

The three variations of calculating percentage overrun by weight are similar to those by volume.

1. Simple formulation. When calculating the percentage overrun for plain ice cream or when an approximation is required:

$$\text{overrun } \% = \frac{\text{weight of 1 gal mix } - \text{ weight of 1 gal ice cream}}{\text{weight of 1 gal ice cream}} \times 100$$

2. Plant overrun formulation. This variation expresses the overrun as a percentage of the flavored mix:

$$\text{overrun } \% = \frac{\text{weight of 1 gal flavored mix } - \text{ weight of 1 gal ice cream}}{\text{weight of 1 gal ice cream}} \times 100$$

For example, when the flavored and colored mix weighing 8.85 lb/gal is frozen into ice cream that weighs 5.06 lb/gal,

$$\frac{8.85 - 5.06}{5.06} \times 100 = 74.9\% \quad \text{overrun}$$

---

[1]These examples use weight per gallon, but it is equally correct to use the weight of any other volume, so long as the same measure is used throughout the calculations. The important quantity in these calculations is the density.

3. *Overrun on plain mix.* This variation is useful in determining the overrun as a percentage of the plain mix:

$$\text{overrun \%} = \frac{\text{weight of 1 gal flavored mix} - \text{weight of 1 gal ice cream}}{\text{weight of 1 gal ice cream}}$$

$$\times \frac{\text{volume of plain mix} + \text{volume of flavor}}{\text{volume of plain mix}} \times 100$$

For example, 17 gal of plain mix is flavored and colored with 3 gal of maple nut to give a flavored mix weighing 8.85 lb/gal. When this is frozen into ice cream weighing 5.06 lb/gal,

$$\frac{8.85 - 5.06}{5.06} \times \frac{17 + 3}{72} \times 100 = 0.749 \times 1.176 \times 100 = 88.1\% \quad \text{overrun}$$

Filled-Package Weight

Practical control of overrun demands frequent weighing of filled packages. For example, assume ice cream, at 80% overrun, weighs 5.08 lb per gal and pint packages weighing 0.84 oz each are being filled with a desired overrun of 80%. To find the weight of each pint package,

$$\frac{5.08 \text{ lb/gal}}{8 \text{ pt/gal}} = 0.635 \text{ lb/pt} \times 16 \text{ oz/lb} = 10.16 \text{ oz/pt}$$

net weight (i.e., weight of the contents of the package). The gross weight (contents plus container) is

$$10.16 \text{ oz} + 0.84 \text{ oz} = 11 \text{ oz}$$

Overrun Chart

An overrun chart is useful for establishing the weight of a cup of ice cream at various overrun percentages. First, assemble all of the tools necessary for overrun testing (weights, scales, cups, and striker). The size of the cup should be between 1/4 and 1 pint. To calculate the gross weight of a cup of ice cream, use the formula

$$\frac{\text{gross weight at}}{\text{desired overrun}} = \frac{\text{net weight of cup of mix}}{100 + \text{desired overrun}} \times 100 + \text{weight of cup}$$

For example, for a desired overrun of 80%, a net weight of one cup of mix 12 oz, and the weight of the empty cup at 1.3 oz,

$$\frac{12}{100 + 80} \times 100 + 1.3 = 7.96 \text{ oz}$$

By making the same calculation at each 5% overrun from 60 to 100%, we can prepare the overrun chart shown in Table 10.4.

Calculation of Overrun on Fruit Ice Cream

Problem 12.   Fruit added to ice cream mix.   If 20 gal of fruit weighing 10 lb/gal is added to 100 gal of mix weighing 9.15 lb/gal, and 200 lb of ice cream is produced, what is the overrun in the ice cream?

Solution

Variation 1.   Ignoring the fruit in the mix,

$$\frac{200 - 100}{100} \times 100 = 100\%$$

Variation 2.   Considering the fruit as part of the mix, there are 120 gal of mix:

$$\frac{200 - 120}{120} \times 100 = 66.6\% \text{ apparent overrun}$$

Variation 3.   Actual overrun on the mix is given by

$$\frac{200 - (100 \times 20)}{100} \times 100 = 80\% \text{ actual overrun}$$

considering no overrun on the fruit.

Table 10.4.   Overrun Chart for Plain Ice Cream

Overrun (%)	Weight of cup and ice cream (oz)
60	8.80
65	8.57
70	8.36
75	8.16
80	7.96
85	7.79
90	7.62
95	7.45
100	7.30

Problem 13.   Weight of the ice cream per gallon.   What should the ice cream in Problem 12 weigh per gallon?

Solution.   At 9.15 lb/gal, the mix will wiegh $100 \times 9.15 = 915$ lb. At 10 lb/gal, the fruit will weigh $20 \times 10 = 200$ lb. The total weight will then be $915 + 200 = 1115$ lb. The weight of the ice cream (200 gal) per gallon will then be

$$\frac{1115 \text{ lb}}{200 \text{ gal}} = 5.577 \text{ lb/gal}$$

Problem 14.   Overrun of fruit ice cream based on mix overrun.   It is desired to add 18 gal of strawberries to each 100 gal of mix. To what overrun should the ice cream be frozen so that 85% overrun on the mix is obtained?

Solution.   The formula for the apparent overrun is

$$\frac{\text{volume of mix}}{\text{volume of mix} + \text{volume of fruit}} \times \text{actual mix overrun desired}$$

In this example,

$$\frac{100}{100 + 18} \times 85 = 72\%$$

At 72% apparent overrun, each gallon of flavored mix yields 1.72 gal of fruit ice cream, and so 118 gal of mix yields 203 gal of fruit ice cream. To calculate the weight per gallon, we assume the weight of the mix is 9.15 lb/gal and that of the fruit is 10 lb/gal. Then

$$\frac{915 + 180}{203} = 5.39 \text{ lb/gal}$$

To check the accuracy of our overrun calculations, 100 gal of mix at 85% overrun gives 185 gal of ice cream. This 185 gal plus 18 gal of fruit gives 203 gal of fruit ice cream, which agrees with our calculation.

Overrun Chart for Fruit Ice Cream

To prepare an overrun chart for fruit ice cream, for each overrun figure on the chart (as before, every 5% from 60 to 100%), we use the following formula:

$$\frac{\text{net weight of cup of mix}}{100 + \text{apparent overrun desired}} \times 100 + \text{weight of empty cup} \qquad \text{(IX)}$$

which gives the weight of the fruit ice cream and its container (gross weight).

We find the apparent overrun for 100 gal of mix and 25 gal of fruit for a 75% overrun by using formula (VIII):

$$\frac{100}{100 + 25} \times 75 = 60\% \quad \text{apparent overrun}$$

We use the 60% figure in formula (IX) to calculate the weight of the ice cream and cup for the chart (with the weights of mix and cup the same as before):

$$\frac{12}{100 + 60} \times 100 + 1.3 = 8.8 \quad \text{oz}$$

This figure is entered into the chart on the line with 60% overrun and 75% apparent overrun. The completed chart is given in Table 10.5.

Special Overrun Problems

(A) If the law requires that ice cream contain 1.6 lb of food solids per gallon and that it shall weigh at least 4.5 lb/gal, what is the minimum percentage of TS of the mix that can be made and the maximum overrun that can be taken on the ice cream? Mix weight is 9 lb/gal.

The TS percentage is given by

$$\frac{1.6}{4.5} \times 100 = 35.56\%$$

and the maximum overrun is

$$\frac{9.0 - 4.5}{4.5} \times 100 = 100\%$$

At 38% TS, what is the maximum overrun that could be taken, and what is food solids content per gallon? Mix weight is 9.1 lb/gal.

Table 10.5. Overrun Chart for Fruit Ice Cream

Actual mix overrun(%)	Apparent overrun(%)	Weight of cup and ice cream(oz)
6	48	9.41
65	52	9.19
70	56	8.93
75	60	8.80
80	64	8.62
85	68	8.44
90	72	8.28
95	76	8.12
100	80	7.96

The maximum overrun is calculated as above,

$$\frac{9.1 - 4.5}{4.5} \times 100 = 102\%$$

and the food solids per gallon is

$$38\% \times 4.5 = 1.71 \quad \text{lb}$$

(B)   An ice cream manufacturer wishes to know the maximum legal over-run that can be taken on the ice cream. Specifications call for a minimum of 1.8 lb of food solids per gallon. The mix contains 37% TS and weighs 9.1 lb/gal. The weight of the ice cream per gallon is

$$\frac{1.8}{37} \times 100 = 4.85 \text{ lb}$$

and substituting this into the overrun formula, the maximum overrun that can be taken is

$$\frac{9.1 - 4.85}{4.85} \times 100 = 87.6\%$$

(C)   What is the weight of food solids per gallon in ice cream containing 40% total solids? The overrun is 90% and the mix weight 9.15 lb/gal.

First we find the weight of 1 gal of ice cream: 9.15/1.9 = 4.81 lb. Then the weight of the TS per gallon is given by 40% × 4.81 = 1.92 lb.

CALCULATING THE DESIRED OVERRUN FOR BULKY-FLAVOR ICE CREAM

The overrun at which to draw ice cream is discussed in Chapter 12. That discussion aids in establishing the correct overrun at which to draw plain ice cream and emphasizes the importance of the right amount of incorporated air in proportion to the amount of plain mix and the solids in the mix. When the most desirable overrun, or ratio of incorporated air to plain mix, has been established for plain ice cream, then the correct or corresponding overrun for composite ice cream can be calculated.

Bulky-flavor ice cream drawn with too much overrun generally has body and texture defects described as "weak" and "fluffy," a common criticism of fruit and nut ice cream. This can be corrected by drawing a sufficiently lower overrun to obtain the same ratio of incorporated air to plain mix as is obtained in plain ice cream. This desired overrun for bulky-flavor ice cream is calculated as follows:

$$\% \text{ overrun for plain ice cream} \times \frac{\text{gallons of plain mix}}{\text{gallons of flavored mix}} \times 100$$

Problem 15.   What is the correct overrun at which to draw a bulky-flavor ice cream containing 3.0 gal of coloring and flavoring material added to 17 gal of plain mix, if 90% is the desired overrun for plain vanilla ice cream?

Solution.   The total amount of mix is 17 + 3 = 20 gal of flavored mix. We substitute into the above formula:

$$(0.90) \times \frac{17}{20} \times 100 = 76.5\%$$

which is the overrun at which to draw the ice cream.

CALCULATING THE WEIGHT PER GALLON OF A MIX

When 10 or more cans are carefully filled with mix and weighed, the approximate weight per gallon can be obtained. However, a more accurate value can be calculated from the composition of the mix as illustrated by Problem 15.

Table 10.6.   Weight per Gallon of Mixes of Varying
Composition at 60°F

Fat (%)	MSNF (%)	Sugar (%)	Weight per gallon (lb)
8	10	14	9.14
8	11	14	9.17
8	12	14	9.21
8	13	14	9.25
8	14	14	9.29
9	10	14	9.132
10	10	14	9.124
11	10	14	9.116
12	10	14	9.109
13	10	14	9.102
14	10	14	9.095
8	10	15	9.18
8	10	16	9.22
12	10	15	9.15
12	11	15	9.19
14	10	15	9.14
15	9.5	15	9.11
16	9.0	15	9.08
18	8.5	15	9.05

Although temperature greatly influences the accuracy of this calculation, the following formula for weight per pound of mix based on composition is considered sufficiently accurate at ordinary mix storage temperatures:

$$\frac{8.33585}{\text{fat \%} \times (1.07527) + (\text{TS \%} - \text{fat \%}) \times (0.6329) + \text{water \%}} \quad \text{(X)}$$

Problem 16. Calculate the weight per gallon of a mix containing 12.0% fat, 11.0% MSNF, 15.0% sugar, 0.30% stabilizer, and 38.3% TS.

Solution. Using formula (X), substitute the following:

$$\frac{8.33585}{0.12 \times 1.07527 + (0.383 - 0.12) \times (0.6329) + 0.617}$$

$$= \frac{8.33585}{0.12903 + 0.263 \times 0.6329 + 0.617} = \frac{8.33585}{0.12903 + 0.16645 + 0.617}$$

$$= \frac{8.33585}{0.91248} \times 9.135 \quad \text{lb}$$

Turnbow *et al.* (1946) stated that the weight per gallon of mixes in the temperature range 5–15.6°C could be obtained by first calculating the specific gravity by the formula

$$1 + [(4.87 \times \text{sucrose \%}) + (4.41 \times \text{MSNF\%})$$

$$- (0.88 \times \text{fat\%} - 6.26) - T\ (°C) - 5) \times (0.0003)]/1000$$

Then the weight per gallon can be calculated by the relationship (see Table 10.6) weight/gal = specific gravity × 8.34

Hilker and Caldwell (1961) gave a formula and example for calculating weight per gallon of fluid dairy products using specific gravity tables for density of fat at various temperatures and factors for solids not fat as follows:

$$W = \frac{A + B + C}{100} \times D$$

where W is the weight in pounds per gallon, A the percentage of fat × specific gravity of fat at a given temperature (value from a specific gravity table), B the percentage of total solids-not-fat (TSNF) × factor for solids corresponding to (TSNF % × 100)/(TSNF % + water %), C the percentage of water × the density of water at given temperature (value from a specific gravity table), and D the weight of 1 gal of water at 40°F, or 8.345 lb.

Problem 17. Calculate the weight per gallon of ice cream mix held 4 hr or longer at 40°F, and of composition (%) as follows:

Fat	11.2	
MSNF	11.0	
Sugar	12.0	TSNF 27.3%
Corn syrup		
solids	4.1	
Stabilizer	0.2	
TS	38.5	

Solution. The calculation uses the formula of Hilker and Caldwell (1961) and the composition of the mix given above.

For fat (A in the formula) the weight per gallon is given[2] by $11.2 \times 0.958 = 10.7296$. For TSNF, we first find the factor for solids corresponding to

$$\frac{27.3 \times 100}{27.3 + 61.5} = 30.74\%$$

The factor for 30.74% is[3] 1.4246. The weight per gallon of TSNF (B in the formula) is then given by $27.3 \times 1.4246 = 38.8916$. For water[3] ($C$ in the formula), we have $61.5 \times 1 = 61.5$.

Substituting these values into the formula, we have

$$W = \frac{10.7296 + 38.8916 + 61.5}{100} \times 8.345 = 9.273 \quad \text{lb/gal}$$

CALCULATING WEIGHT PER PACKAGE

Frequently it is important to know the correct weight of a package of ice cream when the ice cream contains the desired amount of overrun. This is readily obtained by adding the weight of the empty package to the calculated weight of the ice cream per package. The formula assumes a 1-gal package, but any other size may be substituted. The weight of ice cream per gallon is given by

$$\frac{\text{weight of 1 gal of mix}}{1 + \text{desired overrun \%}} \tag{XI}$$

Problem 18. For a mix that weighs 9.135 lb/gal with a desired overrun of 90%, calculate the weight of a 1-gal package that weights 0.5 lb when empty.

---

[2]From Table 1 of Hilker and Caldwell (1961).
[3]From Table 3 of Hilker and Caldwell (1961).

Solution. Use formula (XI) and substitute:

$$\frac{9.135}{1 + 0.90} = \frac{9.135}{1.90} = 4.808 \quad \text{lb}$$

If we add to this the weight of the package, we have 4.808 + 0.50 = 5.308 lb, the gross weight of the full package.

Weight per Package of Bulky-Flavor Ice Cream

When making bulky-flavor ice cream, it is desirable to take a lower overrun, which will ensure the same proportion of air to plain mix as is used in plain ice creams. The desired weight per gallon of bulky-flavor ice cream necessary to maintain this same proportion of air to plain mix can be calculated as follows:

$$\frac{\text{weight of 1 gal of flavored mix}}{1 + (\text{desired overrun } \%) \times \dfrac{\text{volume of plain mix}}{\text{volume of flavored mix}}} \qquad \text{(XII)}$$

Problem 19. The overrun used on plain ice cream is 90%. Maple nut ice cream is to be made using 3 gal (24 lb) of coloring and flavoring material to every 17 gal of plain mix (9 lb/gal). What should be the weight of a 1-gal package of the finished maple nut ice cream if the empty package weighs 0.526 lb?

Solution

Step 1. Find the weight of 1 gal of flavored mix as follows: Since 3 gal of flavor is 24 lb, and 17 gal of plain mix is 17 × 9 = 153 lb, then adding gives 20 gal of flavored mix, which is 24.0 + 153.0 = 177 lb. The weight of 1 gal of flavored mix is then 177/20 = 8.85 lb.

Step 2. Substitute into formula (XII):

$$\frac{8.85}{1 + 0.90 \times 17/20} = \frac{8.85}{1.765} = 5.014 \quad \text{lb}$$

the net weight per package. The total or gross weight is then obtained by adding: 0.526 + 5.014 = 5.54 lb.

CALCULATION OF MILKFAT AND TOTAL MILK SOLIDS REDUCTION IN FRUIT, NUT, AND CHOCOLATE ICE CREAMS

The USDA requires that ice cream contain not less than 10% milkfat and 20% total milk solids. However, in bulky-flavored ice creams, the weights of milkfat and total milk solids are allowed to be 10% and 20%, respectively, of the mix after subtracting the weight of the bulky flavorings. In calculating this reduction, in order to allow for the additional sweetening ingredients needed when these bulky flavorings are used, the weight of the chocolate or cocoa solids is multiplied by 2.5, the weight of fruit or nuts is multiplied by 1.4, and the weight of dried fruits of fruit juices is multiplied first by a factor to obtain the original weight before drying and then multiplied by 1.4. In any case, the content of the finished product by weight must not be less than 8% milkfat and 16% total milk solids.

IAICM (1961a) gave a detailed procedure of how to calculate the reduction of milkfat and total milk solids in bulky-flavored ice creams. It is necessary to know the percentage of fruit, nuts, or chocolate in the syrup or the fruit pack level in the final product; the fat level in the unflavored mix; and the weight per gallon of the bulky ingredient. The following problem demonstrates the method for determination of milkfat level.

Problem 20.   Milkfat in strawberry ice cream.   Given 100 lb of strawberry mix, containing 15 lb of strawberry syrup weighing 10 lb/gal and testing 33% fruit, determine the allowable test of the plain mix, to conform with USDA standards.

Solution.   The 15 lb of syrup contains 5 lb of strawberries, and the factor for fruits is 1.4. Therefore, the amount by which the total mix may be reduced is 5 × 1.4 = 7 lb. According to USDA standards, the remaining 93 lb of mix must test no lower than 10% milkfat, which yields 9.3 lb of milkfat. However, since 15 lb of syrup was used, the original mix weighed only 85 lb. Therefore, the original 85-lb mix must test

$$\frac{9.3}{85} \times 100 = 10.9\%$$

milkfat in order to be a legal ice cream for interstate shipment.

METHODS FOR CALCULATION OF
THE FREEZING POINT

In the manufacture of ice cream, it is necessary to know at what point a mix will freeze and how the freezing point of the mix is lowered from that of water by sucrose and by milk salts. Leighton (1927) developed a relatively accurate method for calculation of the freezing point of ice cream. It is based on the percentage of lactose in MSNF, the freezing point curve of the sucrose–lactose mixture, and the amount the freezing point is lowered by the milk salts.

Doan and Kenney's (1965) method of calculating the freezing point of an ice cream mix makes use of the sum of the freezing point depression value for the sugars and for the salts. For the sugars (lactose and sucrose), the following formula is utilized to determine the parts of disaccharide sugar (expressed as sucrose equivalent) to 100 parts of water in the mix:

$$\frac{[(\text{MSNF} \times 0.545) + S]100}{W} \tag{XIII}$$

where MSNF is expressed as a percentage, 0.545 is the amount of lactose in the MSNF, S is the percentage of sucrose in the mix, and W is the percentage of water in the mix. The freezing point lowering due to the sugars (sucrose equivalent) is then obtained by interpolation from the data in Table 10.7.

The freezing point depression due to the milk salts is calculated from the formula

$$\frac{\text{MSNF} \times 2.37}{W} \tag{XIV}$$

where 2.37 is a constant based on the apparent molecular weight of the salts (78.6)

Table 10.7. Freezing Point Lowering of Sucrose Solution

Parts sucrose per 100 parts of water	Sucrose (%)	Lowering	
		(°C)	(°F)
3.59	3.47	0.21	0.37
6.85	6.41	0.40	0.71
10.84	9.78	0.65	1.16
15.83	13.67	0.95	1.69
19.80	16.53	1.23	2.20
22.58	18.42	1.37	2.45
25.64	20.41	1.58	2.52
28.51	22.19	1.77	3.16
32.22	24.37	1.99	3.55
35.14	26.00	2.15	3.84
37.86	27.46	2.33	4.16
43.72	30.42	2.71	4.82
45.62	31.33	2.82	5.03
50.02	33.35	3.13	5.89
54.74	35.37	3.47	6.19
59.46	37.29	3.81	6.80
64.55	39.23	4.22	7.54
69.74	41.09	4.60	8.21
75.91	43.15	5.07	9.05
82.35	45.16	5.65	0.08
88.67	47.00	6.11	10.91
95.94	48.97	6.76	12.07
102.70	50.65	7.38	13.18
111.30	52.67	8.06	14.39
121.00	54.75	9.02	16.10
131.60	56.82	9.93	17.73
143.10	58.86	10.90	19.46
153.80	60.60	11.69	20.87
165.60	62.35	12.72	22.71
181.70	64.49	13.80	24.64

The freezing point lowering due to the sucrose equivalent plus the lowering caused by the milk salts gives the freezing point of the mix.

Problem 21.   Find the freezing point of a mix with 12% fat, 10% MSNF, 15% sugar, and 0.5% stabilizer.

Solution
Step 1.   The parts of sucrose per 100 parts of water is calculated from formula (XIII):

$$\frac{[(10 \times 0.545) + 15]100}{62.5} = 32.88$$

The value of 62.5% for the water is obtained by subtracting from 100% the combined percentages of the other ingredients:

$$100 - (12 + 10 + 15 + 0.5) = 62.5$$

Step 2.   This 32.88 parts sucrose per 100 parts water, by interpolation from Table 10.7, lowers the freezing point by 2.03°C.
Step 3.   To calculate the lowering of the freezing point caused by the salts, we use formula (XIV):

$$\frac{10 \times 2.37}{62.5} = 0.38°C$$

Step 4.   The total lowering of the freezing point is then 2.03 + 0.38 = 2.41°C (4.34°F).
Step 5.   The freezing point of the mix is then obtained by subtracting this value from the freezing point of water:

$$0° - 2.41° = -2.41°C \text{ (or } 32° - 4.34° = 27.66°F)$$

Wolff (1982) and Bradley (1984) gave calculations pertaining to frozen products and plotting freezing curves for frozen desserts. These calculations involve several assumptions and do not yield exact freezing points.

CALCULATION OF SUCROSE EQUIVALENT FOR FREEZING POINT DEPRESSION OF SWEETENERS (BASED ON MOLECULAR WEIGHT)

1.   Calculate the lactose content of mix: Assume MSNF is 54.5% lactose and whey solids 76.5% lactose. Establish percentage of total lactose hydrolyzed.
2.   Calculate sucrose equivalent for freezing point depression by multiplying the percentage of sweetener times the freezing point equivalence factor. Assume disaccharides (sucrose) as 1.0, monosaccharides as 1.9. Refer to Table 5.12 for appropriate factors for other sweeteners.

3.   Calculate total sucrose equivalent by multiplying the percentage of each sweetener by the appropriate factor and then totaling.

4.   Calculate the percentage sucrose equivalent (SE) in the H_2O portion of mix using the formula

$$SE = \frac{\text{total SE (\%)}}{H_2O \text{ in mix (\%)} + \text{total SE (\%)}} \times 100$$

where

$$H_2O \text{ (\%)} = 100\% - TS \text{ of mix}$$

and

$$\frac{\text{parts SE}}{100 \text{ parts } H_2O} = \frac{\text{total SE \%}}{\text{water in mix \%}} \times 100$$

5.   Determine the freezing point depression by reference to Table 10.7.

6.   Determine the freezing point depression (of) due to milk salts by the formula

$$\frac{MSNF \% \times 4.26}{H_2O \text{ (\%)}}$$

7.   Calculate the freezing point of mix by subtracting the results of step 5 and 6 from 32°F.

11
Mix Processing

In order to make good ice cream, the milk products and other ingredients must first be selected and combined so as to produce the desired body and a delicately blended flavor. Then they must be skillfully processed. Obviously, the selection of good wholesome ingredients and calculation of a satisfactory composition, as discussed in previous chapters, precede the mixing of the ingredients in a vat where they can be heated to facilitate dissolving, blending, and pasteurizing.

The basic steps of production in the manufacturing of ice cream are composing the mix, pasteurization, homogenization, cooling, aging, flavoring, freezing, packaging, hardening storage, loading-out products, and cleaning equipment. The flow diagram given by Arbuckle (1968) remains typical of the processes used in the manufacture of different frozen dairy foods (Fig. 11.1).

The first step of processing is composing the mix. This procedure may range in scope from the small batch operation, where each ingredient is weighed or measured into a pasteurizing vat, to the large, automatic, continuous operation where many of the ingredients are metered into the batch. Continuous mix-making procedures may be quite variable and some such operations may actually be modifications of the batch operation. Liquid stabilizers and product-blending equipment have been developed to facilitate the continuous operation. (The sequence in which the products are blended into the mix is the same for both types of operation.)

Automated and highly mechanized operating methods and plant layouts are being utilized as a means of reducing costs for ice cream plants. One study grouped the size of dairy plants manufacturing ice cream and ice cream novelties as those annually manufacturing 200,000 gal of ice cream and those manufacturing 1,000,000 gal of ice cream and 250,000 gal of novelties. Illustrations and details of how an automated plant operates are provided later in this chapter.

PREPARATION OF THE MIX[1]

Preparing the mix involves moving the ingredients from the storage area to the mix preparation area, weighing or metering and mixing them, and pasteurizing, homogenizing, cooling, and storing of the mix.

---

[1]Readers interested in early techniques of preparing ice cream mixes should refer to the work of Sherfey and Smallwood (1928), who give a good account of methods reported in the early literature.

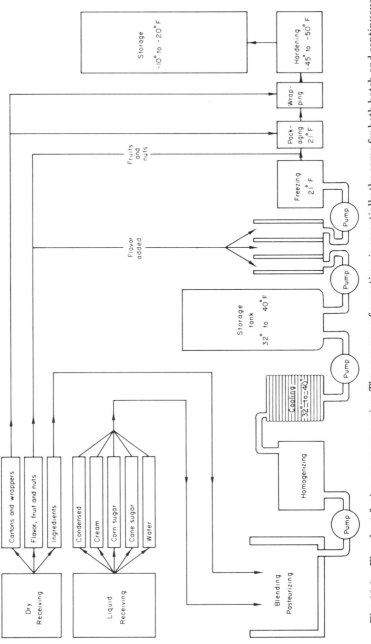

Fig. 11.1. Flowchart for ice cream processing. The sequence of operations is essentially the same for both batch and continuous processing. For batch, pasteurizing takes place for 30 min at 155°F. For continuous HTST, pasteurizing is done at 175°F for 25 sec.

Taylor (1961) studied ice cream manufacturing plant methods, equipment, and layout and found that four methods are used for processing mix: (1) bulk ingredients and continuous high-temperature-short time (HTST) pasteurization; (2) ingredients in cans and HTST pasteurization; (3) bulk ingredients and batch pasteurization; and (4) ingredients in cans and batch pasteurization. All four methods are commonly used, depending upon the size of the plant. The smaller operations (<250,000 gal/year) tend to use method (4). Medium-sized plants (250,000–1,000,000 gal/year) tend to use method (2) or (3). Larger plants (>1,000,000 gal/year) tend to use method (1). The lowest-cost method for preparing mix is method (4), due to the low cost of equipment involved.

Computers can be used to control the cost and quality of ice cream mixes by the mathematical technique known as linear programming. Kreider and Snyder (1964) showed that linear programming can be effective even for small plants:

- to determine the sensitivity of least-cost formulas to changes in ingredient costs
- to determine the sensitivity of formula cost to quality specifications
- to determine the cost of individual quality specifications
- to obtain computer-generated reports of least-cost information

Order of Adding Ingredients

All liquid ingredients (cream, milk, condensed milk, syrup, etc.) are placed in the vat, and the agitation and heating started at once. The dry ingredients, including MSNF, dried eggs, cocoa, sugar, and stabilizer (with a few exceptions), are added while the liquid material is agitated and before the temperature reaches 120°F (see Fig. 11.1). Proper suspension to avoid lumpiness of the dry ingredients may be obtained by (1) mixing the dry material thoroughly with part of the sugar before slowly adding it to the liquid, or (2) sifting or otherwise slowly adding these substances to the liquid. MSNF, cocoa, and similar products should be sifted on top of the liquid and always while the agitated liquid is still cool (under 80°F). If gelatin is the stabilizer used, it is best to add it after it is thoroughly mixed with an equal volume of sugar and before the liquid reaches 120°F. It can also be sprinkled on the surface of the cold liquid and allowed to soak before the mixture is heated. Another method is to soak the gelatin in water and then heat the mixture to dissolve the gelatin completely. This gelatin suspension is usually added to warm (100–120°F) mix. Many other stabilizers such as Krageleen and CMC (sodium carboxymethylcellulose) can be added in a similar manner. However, sodium alginate should not be added until the temperature of the liquid material has reached at least 150°F; it is not allowed to soak but is stirred up with cold water and immediately dumped into the hot mix. When butter, plastic cream, frozen cream, or other frozen products are used, they should be cut into fairly small pieces and added in time to allow complete melting before the pasteurizing temperature is reached. With a few exceptions, coloring and flavoring materials are added at the time the mix is frozen.

PASTEURIZATION OF THE MIX

Pasteurization of all mixes is compulsory because this process destroys all pathogenic or disease-producing bacteria, thereby safeguarding the health of the consumer. Pasteurization requires only slight additional expense, since the mix is usually heated to facilitate solution, and since the homogenization process can be accomplished best at the pasteurization temperature level.

Most states and many cities specify certain definite temperature regulations when pasteurization is required, but these generally apply only to the dairy products used. Usually it is permissible to use higher temperatures for pasteurization than are required for market milk, and in many instances it is legal to repasteurize products that have already been pasteurized once. Every manufacturer should be acquainted with the legal regulations that apply in the market area and make special note of the following:

1. What dairy products, if any, may be used without being pasteurized.
2. The maximum bacterial count of ingredients used even when followed by pasteurization.
3. The pasteurization time and temperature requirements.
4. The maximum permitted bacterial count of the finished product. (Usually it is different for ices, ice cream, etc. It also differs for products that are not pasteurized, as opposed to those which are pasteurized.)
5. Whether the product must be frozen on the premises where it is pasteurized.

Proper pasteurization consists in rapidly heating to a definite temperature, holding at that temperature for a definite minimum of time, and then rapidly cooling to below 40°F. Mix pasteurization is required by law in most states and cities. The recommendations of the U.S. Public Health Service for the batch method, HTST, or other approved procedures are shown in Table 11.1.

Pasteurization (1) renders the mix substantially free of pathogenic bacteria, (2) brings into solution and aids in blending the ingredients of the mix, (3) improves the flavor, (4) improves keeping quality, and (5) produces a more uniform product. There is a trend toward the higher temperature processes: The introduction of high-temperature pasteurization equipment suitable for processing ice cream mix and the establishment of the additional pasteurization standards of 175°F for 25 sec for ice cream mix has created considerable

Table 11.1. Public Health Service Recommended Times and Temperatures for Pasteurization of Ice Cream Mixes

Method	Time	Temperature (°F)
Batch	30 min	155
HTST	25 sec	175
Vacreation	1–3 sec	194
Ultrahigh temperature	0–40 sec	210–263

Source: U.S. Public Health Services (1965).

interest in the potentials of this method of pasteurization in the ice cream industry during recent years.

Pasteurization equipment is available and is being used which is capable of heating the mix to a temperature much higher than is required for pasteurization standards.

Reasons for high-temperature pasteurization of ice cream mix include (1) greater bacterial kill resulting in lower bacterial count in ice cream, (2) better body and texture, (3) better flavor, (4) protection against oxidation, (5) saving of stabilizer, (6) saving of time, labor, and space, (7) increased capacity.

Some studies indicate that cooked flavors result above 250°F. This naturally will depend on the type of equipment, but for maximum benefits the mix probably should be processed at 210–220°F.

The reduction in stabilizer needed may be 25–35%, as compared with that used in batch pasteurization. Stabilizers suitable for high-temperature processing usually contain CMC and carrageenan, or algins with additional materials.

Continuous and automatically controlled high-temperature units are almost always more economical than batch methods. The differences between various high-temperature pasteurizing systems depend on (1) incorporation of regenerative heating and cooling, (2) amount of regeneration utilized, (3) ability to maintain long continuous operation without loss in efficiency, (4) adaptability to circulation cleaning, (5) pressures maintained in equipment, which affect pumping efficiencies, (6) effectiveness of control, which affects properties of finished products, (7) adaptability to small batches.

The continuous-mix process can still vary widely. When it was first initiated there were almost as many different arrangements of equipment as there were plants using the process. This is not so much the case at present but there is still no standard arrangement of equipment for the continuous operation. The process is generally considered continuous if the blended raw mix is available during the entire run. Blending should be at a temperature of 50°F or below.

High-temperature mix pasteurization systems also vary considerably. Some so-called continuous operations may actually be modified batch operations. Liquid stabilizers or product-blending equipment have been promoted to facilitate the continuous operation. Pressure or vacuum control valves, metering pumps, and vacuum vaporizing cylinders may occur in the system. Heat regeneration may approach 85%. Greater standardization of the typical system featuring more accurate controls may be expected in the continuous high-temperature pasteurization installation of the future. (Currently, the circular-recording graph controller is still widely in use; see Fig. 11.2.)

In the batch system, the mix is usually heated and held before going to the homogenizer and from there passes over a cooler. The heating and holding may be accomplished in the vat used for mixing the ingredients. Many large factories make use of continuous pasteurizers and profitably incorporate the regeneration principle. This principle employs the use of the cool mix, which is being heated, as a cooling medium for the hot mix coming from the homogenizer.

Speck *et al.* (1954) studied HTST pasteurization of ice cream mix and found that the standard of 175°F for 25 sec appeared to be more stringent than that of

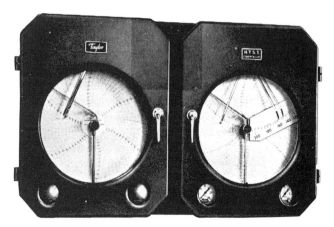

Fig. 11.2. Taylor HTST controller for pasteurization. This instrument controls continuous pasteurization and diverts milk or mix flow within 2 sec if temperature falls below the legal limit. (Courtesy of Taylor Instrument Co.)

batch processing, 155°F for 30 min. They made preliminary studies using *Micrococcus* sp. (MS 102) with the vacreator, which showed adequate pasteurization to occur at a first-chamber temperature of 191.5°F. Similar studies with tubular equipment gave proper pasteurization when set at 172.2°F.

Tobias *et al.* (1955) also used *Micrococcus* sp. (MS 102) and studied HTST pasteurizing equipment with no intended holding time. They found a holding time derived from the lethal effect of the heat-up, discharge, and cooling times. The destruction of *Micrococcus* equivalent to that resulting from laboratory pasteurization at 155°F for 30 min was obtained at 187.2 or 181.3°F with effective holding times of 0.8 and 3.8 sec, respectively.

Mitten (1958) stated that ultrahigh-temperature (UHT) pasteurization of ice cream mix assured greater bacterial kill and produced desirable physical and chemical changes in the mix. Mixes so processed generally had greater water-binding characteristics, required less stabilizer, and had slightly more dryness when frozen, greater stability against oxidization, and excellent flavor. He stated that stabilizers for continuously made mixes should give the desired stabilizing effect, disperse readily, and be soluble in the cold mix.

Arbuckle and Nisonger (1951) conducted early studies on the effect of high-temperature pasteurization of ice cream mix using temperatures of 170, 180, 190, and 200°F. They reported that the temperature of pasteurization had no effect on acidity or pH and little effect on surface tension.

As pasteurization temperature increased in this range, there was a tendency for mix viscosity to decrease; and mixes pasteurized at 170 and 180°F for 15 sec developed off-flavors during the storage period. The melting rate was greatest at the lowest pasteurization temperature. Pasteurization temperature had little effect on the body and texture characteristics.

Later studies showed improvement in body and texture at 215–220°F and again near 260°F.

England (1953) reported favorable results in the use of the vacreator equipment for pasteurization of ice cream mix. The vacreator is a recognized pasteurization method that provides heat treatment under reduced pressure. The treatment is helpful in removing volatile flavors. The equipment was developed in New Zealand and Australia, where it is extensively used to pasteurize cream. It is used only to a limited extent in pasteurizing ice cream mixes, but it is a legally recognized method in the United States.

HOMOGENIZING THE MIX

The main purpose of homogenization is to make a permanent and uniform suspension of the fat by reducing the size of the fat droplets to a very small diameter, preferably not more than 2 μm. This means that when a mix is properly homogenized, the fat will not rise and form a cream layer. Other advantages are also obtained, such as a more uniform ice cream with a smoother texture and improved whipping ability, a shorter aging period, less opportunity for churning to occur in the freezer, and the use of slightly less stabilizer. Butter, butter oil, plastic cream, and frozen cream can be used in the mix only when the mix is homogenized.

Homogenization is usually accomplished by forcing the mix through a small orifice under suitable conditions of temperature and pressure, using a positive-displacement plunger pump to furnish the pressure. The orifice consists of a valve and seat in which the two adjacent surfaces are parallel and lapped smooth and is surrounded by an impact ring against which the mix impinges as it leaves the valve. The breakup of fat particles is caused by the shear forces set up in a thin stream of mix traveling at high velocity (approximately 30,000 fpm) between the closely adjacent surfaces of the valve and seat and then by a shattering effect as it impinges on the impact ring upon leaving the valve.

There is also a third factor in the breakup of the fat globules, which is called cavitation. This is caused by the sudden release of pressure, which momentarily lowers the vapor pressure of the milk to a point where vapor pockets are formed. The fat globules bounce back and forth inside these vapor bubbles and are shattered by the impacts against the bubble walls. Two typical homogenizers and close-ups of their internal parts are shown in Figs. 11.3–11.6.

Jenness and Patton (1959) stated that there appears to be adequate evidence that the valve assembly during homogenization is completely filled with liquid. It seems quite possible that the flow of liquid leaving the valve under high pressure may act like a water aspirator, where residual bubbles of air cause the formation of vacuoles, which would be filled almost instantaneously with water vapor. If these subsequently collapse, some shattering might be expected. In any event it would appear worthwhile to attempt securing some evidence on whether a gaseous phase of any sort exists beyond the homogenization valve, since three of the four proposed theories predict such a state (see, for example, Sommer, 1951).

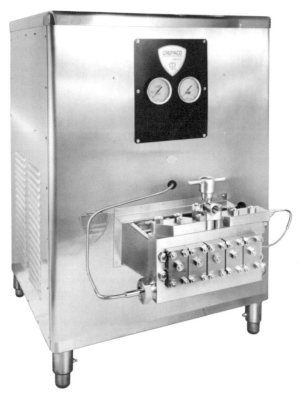

Fig. 11.3. Stainless steel Multi-Flo Homogenizer. Single-stage homogenizing valve is shown, but two-stage valves are available. (Courtesy of Crepaco, Inc.)

The effects of homogenization on mix properties have been recorded by Sommer (1951), Reid and Garrison (1929), Reid and Russell (1930), and Turnbow *et al.* (1946).

Physical Effects of Homogenization

The process of homogenization is assumed to affect the mix only physically. The fat globules are reduced to about 10% of the normal size, which increases the total surface of the globules about 100 times. Therefore, it is easy to see why homogenization produces effects that differ considerably with varying composition, acidity, temperature, pressure, etc. The substances in colloidal suspension and true solution tend to be concentrated on the fat globule surfaces. Varying conditions will have different effects on the films forming at these surfaces. There is a tendency for fat globules to form in groups as the mix passes away from the homogenizing valve. This is particularly true of the butter and frozen cream types of mixes, of cold mixes, or of acid mixes. This clumping of the fat globules, if marked, causes excessive viscosity and slow

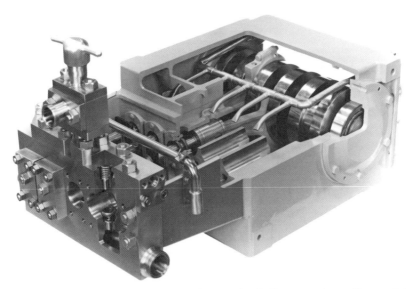

Fig. 11.4. Homogenizer crankcase and pump head. Cutaway view of heavy-duty gearless model with five cylinders. (Courtesy of Crepaco, Inc.)

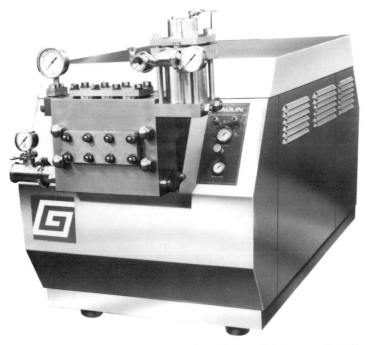

Fig. 11.5. Gaulin low-pressure homogenizer. This model features the Micro-Gap homogenizing valve and low-pressure cylinder for increased homogenizing efficiency. (Courtesy of APV Gaulin Inc., Everett MA.)

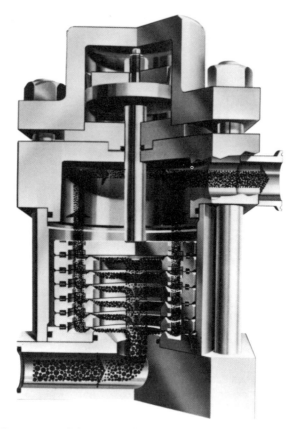

Fig. 11.6. Cross-sectional diagram of the Micro-Gap homogenizing valve. The product enters at the bottom of the valve assembly, is homogenized as it passes through the microgaps between the circular valve and seats, and then exits at the top of the valve body. (Courtesy of APV Gaulin Inc., Everett MA.)

shipping. For this reason some homogenizers are equipped with a second valve to break up the clumps; in other words, the mix passes through one valve (called the first stage) under a high pressure (above 1000 lb) where clumping may occur and then through another valve (called the second stage) under a low pressure (500–1000 lb is sufficient) where the clumps are broken up. Then the mix passes out of the homogenizer toward the cooler (see Fig. 11.7).

Homogenizing Temperatures

The mix is usually homogenized at 145–170°F because at low temperatures (120–130°F) homogenization increases the formation of clumps of fat globules, increases the viscosity, and increases the freezing time in batch freezers. When using a high pasteurizing temperature (170°F) with the batch system, the mix may be cooled to 150°F for homogenization, a desirable practice to reduce the

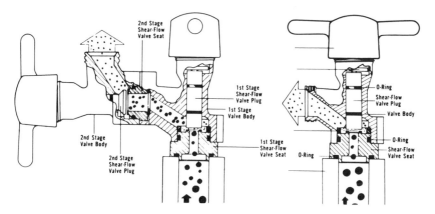

Fig. 11.7. Diagram of single- and two-stage homogenizer valve assemblies. (Courtesy of Crepaco, Inc.)

intensity of the cooked flavor and the length of time the mix has to be held at the high temperature, especially when homogenization is not completed in 30 min. However, within certain limits, better homogenization is obtained with each increase in the temperature used, and sometimes the mix is pasteurized at 145°F and then heated to 160–170°F for homogenization. The use of these high temperatures results in less clumping of the fat globules, a lower viscosity, and a shorter freezing time in batch freezers.

Pressures for Homogenization

The pressure to use for homogenization depends upon several factors: desired viscosity, composition of the mix, stability of the mix, temperature used, and construction of the homogenizing machine. Because of the influence of each of these factors, one can recommend only a range of pressures, realizing that a specific case may require pressure above or below the range. A pressure of 2000–2500 lb with one valve or 2500–3000 lb on the first stage and 500 lb on the second stage will usually give good results for an average mix.

Chocolate mixes and other high-solids mixes usually have sufficient viscosity if the pressure is reduced about 500 lb (i.e., 1500–2000 lb for single stage and 1500–2000 lb on the first valve with 500 lb on the second valve for two-stage homogenization). The same is true for mixes using butter, plastic cream, etc., as the only source of fat; or concentrated products as the only source of MSNF. The pressures in Table 11.2 are suggested only as an approximation for mixes containing different percentages of fat.

Causes of Fluctuating Pressures

When operating a homogenizer, the needle of the pressure gauge should be steady and should not oscillate, should not change markedly unless the valve

Table 11.2. Approximate Homogenization Pressures for Mixes of Different Fat Contents

Fat (%)	Single stage (lb)	Two stage	
		First valve (lb)	Second valve (lb)
8–12	2500–3000	2500–3000	500
12–14	2000–2500	2000–2500	500
15–17	1500–2000	1500–2000	500
18	1200–1800	1200–1800	500
>18	800–1200	800–1200	500

is opened or closed, and should change whenever the valve is adjusted. Failure of the pressure gauge to respond to the adjustment of the wheel on the homogenizer valve may be caused by a plugged line to the gauge, by slipping of the belt, by packing or similar material being caught under the homogenizing valve, or by a worn valve. When the gauge pressure changes without the valve turning, one should look for a slipping belt, material such as packing under the homogenizer valve, or a loose spring under the valve. Sometimes the change in gauge pressure may be caused by heat expanding the metal and producing a change in the space between the valve and valve seat. Oscillation of the gauge pressure may be due (1) to an uneven amount being pumped by each valve because of the strainer being clogged or air leaks in the suction line, or (2) to anything that allows mix to pass back by the valves into the machine head (such as slipping belt, pumping valves opening too wide and not closing promptly, or valve surfaces damaged by wear or scores). Air leaks in the suction line may be caused by scratches on the surface of the joints in the pipe lines, and therefore the pipes should be carefully handled. Moving parts such as pump pistons passing through packing may be slightly grooved or the packing may become old and bits of it breaking off into the mix and eventually sticking in the small valve openings. Thus extreme care is needed in handling equipment.

Factors that lead to high viscosity and the clumping of the fat globules are (1) high pressures with a single valve, (2) low temperature of mix when homogenized, (3) low stability of the mix due to high acidity or improper salt balance, and (4) a high ratio of fat content to MSNF content. The easiest and most convenient way to reduce the viscosity produced by homogenization is to use lower pressures, especially when homogenizing mixes of low stability. The use of higher temperature during homogenization will also reduce the viscosity and fat clumping. Standardizing the acidity will help when the viscosity is due to high acidity in the mix. The use of a second valve is especially effective in reducing the clumping of the fat globules and reducing the excessive viscosity produced by this phenomenon.

Defective or improper homogenization can be detected by examining a sample of the mix with a microscope. This enables an experienced technician to measure the size of the fat globules and detect clumping. Another method such as that used for homogenized milk is simpler but less accurate, and requires less experience on the part of the operator. In this method, a quart milk bottle is filled with mix and stored at 40°F for 48 hr. Then without agitation the top 80–100 ml are quickly poured off into a graduated cylinder. Each portion (the portion poured off and the portion remaining in the milk bottle) is separately mixed and tested for fat content. The difference between the tests of the two portions should be less than 0.7% if the mix has been properly homogenized.

Care of Working Parts of the Machine

Since the working parts of the homogenizer are enclosed, special care of the machine is necessary to prevent bacterial contamination by the homogenizer. It should be taken apart frequently, preferably after each use, and left apart until reassembled for immediate use. In this way the parts remain dry. The machine should be flushed out thoroughly with hot water before it is used. The valves should be ground occasionally and kept free from scores.

MAKING THE MIX IN A VACUUM PAN

A vacuum pan is sometimes used in making extremely large quantities of ice cream mixes and also in making condensed and powdered ice cream mix. These procedures require large investments and present a few special problems. Discussion of these problems is omitted here because of the relatively small amount of product handled in this manner.

COOLING THE MIX

Many studies show that slow cooling of the mix from 80–100°F down to 40°F imparts increased viscosity to the mix.

Cooling the mix immediately after homogenization to 32–40°F is essential, after which it should be held in aging tanks until used. Unless the mix is cooled to a temperature of 40°F or lower, it will become very viscous and the ice cream will not melt down smoothly. Also, temperatures below 40°F retard the growth of bacteria (see Fig. 11.8).

Coolers of the surface or cabinet types are generally used for ice cream mix, as the product is too viscous to be cooled effectively in the internal tubular cooler. The surface cooler should be so constructed that moisture condensation forming on the ends of the tubes cannot flow into the mix or drop into the lower trough. The cabinet cooler, which is essentially a battery of small surface coolers, works very satisfactorily with ice cream mix. In some factories that handle mixes of lower viscosity, modern plate coolers are being used successfully.

AGING THE MIX

Experimental work shows that appreciable benefits result from an aging period, although little is gained by aging longer than 4 hr.

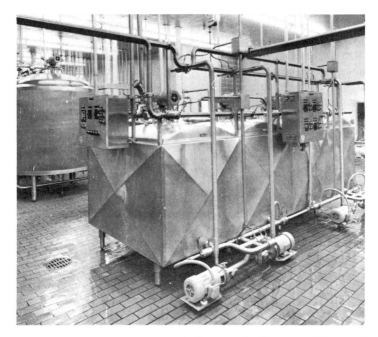

Fig. 11.8. A multicompartment mix flavor tank. (Courtesy of Crepaco, Inc.)

Aging the mix before freezing has been practiced since the inception of the ice cream industry. The following changes undoubtedly occur during aging:

1. The fat is solidified.
2. If gelatin has been used as a stabilizer it swells and combines with water.
3. The proteins of the mix may change slightly.
4. The viscosity is increased, largely due to the previously mentioned changes.

There is no question but that smoothness of body and texture, resistance to melting, and ease of whipping are improved by aging. How much time is necessary for the realization of these advantages is the question. Until recently, the generally accepted time for aging the mix was about 24 hr. Recent experimental work seems to prove that under the average commercial conditions 3–4 hr of aging is all that is essential unless batch-type freezers with limited whipping mechanisms are used. Then a longer aging period seems to give better results. With high-fat mixes that have been homogenized at very low pressures, 24 hr of aging produce good results.

The aging temperature should not exceed 40°F. Many plants age the mix around 36°F or a little lower. At these temperatures, the bacteria count will not increase during aging. Aging temperatures as low as 28–30°F are some-

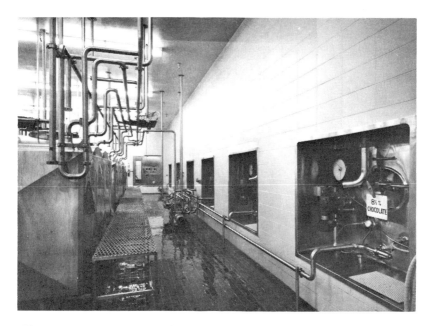

Fig. 11.9. Processing room showing alcoves (right) leading to storage tanks foi pasteurized mixes. These tanks have refrigerated surfaces to hold the mix temperature at the temperature of entry for extended periods, if desired. Air-operated valves, valve clusters, and pumping stations permit freezing room personnel to move mix from storage to the flavor tanks (left) and to the ice cream freezers from a control panel. (Courtesy of Crepaco, Inc.)

times used. There seems to be no advantage in this; in fact, there is the danger that the first of the mix to enter the freezer might freeze fast to the cold walls of the freezer and tend to damage the dasher.

When the mix has been properly aged it is ready for the freezing process, which generally follows immediately. Holding the mix for more than about five days is likely to cause at least some deterioration in both flavor and quality (see Fig. 11.9).

AUTOMATION IN ICE CREAM PROCESSING

The processing procedures in the manufacture of ice cream have become fully mechanized, and various degrees of automation which is the bringing of mechanized systems under automatic control, is now widely taking place. This means several pieces of equipment are unified and work together. Some applications may include any one or more of the automatically controlled procedures: batch operations, mix processing, packaging, equipment cleaning, inventory, and mix computing. The goal of automation is increased labor productivity. The potentials for adaptation of automation are great but careful planning is always important and the extent of efficient adaptation may vary considerably among different operations.

The following description of an automated plant installed in Boston is adapted from information provided to the author by H. P. Hood & Sons, Boston.

Example of a Large Automated Plant

H. P. Hood & Sons initiated its automated system at its Boston ice cream plant in 1960. The system, described by the company as "the world's first fully automatic batching process for ice cream mix," was conceived by the dairy company and application-engineered by Brown Instruments Division of Minneapolis-Honeywell Regulator Company.

Recipes for bulk production of America's favorite dessert are calculated by a computer far more quickly and accurately than possible by any human.

Electronic equipment "masterminded" by coded punch cards opens valves sending basic ice cream ingredients from storage to blending tanks, measures their flow with electrical impulses from metering devices, and then closes the valves when the predetermined amount is reached.

Instruments watch over the pasteurization, homogenization, and cooling processes to see that nothing goes wrong. Even the cleaning of lines, valves, and tanks, once a time-consuming chore, is pushbutton programmed from a master control panel that portrays the entire ice cream making process (see Fig. 11.10).

Advanced Control Concepts

"To the best of our knowledge, this system incorporates automatic control concepts believed to be the most advanced in the ice cream industry, and the improvement in mix batching over conventional methods borders on the miraculous. It takes the guesswork out of making ice cream and assures a product of uniformly high quality."

Hood credits the automatic equipment with eliminating much of the heavy manual labor normally involved in batching—the combining of dairy and other products to make fluid ice cream mix.

In addition, integration of the automatic system with new equipment has enabled the company to increase production capacity at this plant approximately 70%.

"In an industry noted for low profit margins, and in which there is a continuing trend toward a larger number and variety of items to meet consumer demands, it is essential to attain maximum productivity of labor and facilities."

It should be pointed out that the installation of the automatic equipment was accomplished without any decrease in the work force, which was in line with company policy.

Mix—A Complex Problem

Mix proportioning of the dairy ingredients is highly complex. Butterfat and nonfat content, called serum solids, fluctuate daily, requiring changes in basic recipes. Seasonal availability and raw materials costs, as well as maintenance

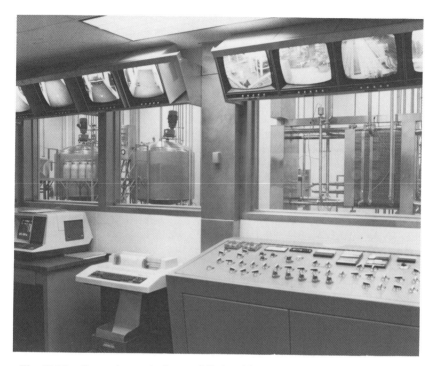

Fig. 11.10.   Processing control room. Mix batching, pasteurizing, product flow routing, and cleaning in place of storage tanks, processing equipment, and pipe lines are
controlled from this room. All operations are computer controlled with manual back-up
capability. The printer provides a complete record of each step, including time of event,
the number of the equipment piece operated, and routing and processing data such as
amount, temperature, and type of products. There is also video observation of various
areas of the plant. (Courtesy of Crepaco, Inc.)

of quality of the finished ice cream, also are important considerations. Furthermore, different types of mix vary widely in combinations and proportions of
dairy ingredients.

The computer, separate from the control system, selects the two or three
dairy ingredients required for a mix from among a number available and
decides how much of each is needed for a specific mix. In a fraction of a second
the analog-type computer has the answer. If it is impractical, it says so.

Recipe Coded on Punch Card

The recipe is digitally coded on a punch card that also may be used for
production control and accounting purposes. It is "read" by instrumentation
that opens and shuts valves and measures and controls the simultaneous flow
of all liquid ingredients from storage to blending tanks. All the operator need
do is to set switches that will determine the flow sequence of ingredients for
batching called for by the punch card.

Key to the measuring process is a flow-sensing device known as a Potter-meter, which records the flow rate of ingredients with a turbine-type rotor imbedded with a powerful magnet. As liquids pass through the meters, the rotor generates a pulse train proportional to the rate of flow. These automatically drive totalizers, recorders, and other controls in the control room.

The overall system includes a graphic programming console from which the entire mix operation, including automatic cleaning of batching equipment, can be controlled by a single person. The console, with more than three miles of hidden wiring, includes pushbuttons for starting and stopping pumps, indicators showing tank liquid levels, and integrators that total the amount of ingredients used in batching operations.

A pushbutton programmed clean-in-place (CIP) system with built-in cost savings refinements is an integral part of the automated mix operation at the Boston plant.

The automatic CIP system—actually five systems in one, each operating independently—is incorporated in a console, which graphically represents the entire mix process, including tank levels, flow totals of ingredients, valve positions, and pump operations.

A unique feature of the system is the recycling, in sequential cleaning of tanks, of the final rinse for uses as the prerinse for the next tank to be cleaned.

Sequential Cleaning

All individual CIP circuits have high- and low-level tank probes, temperature controllers, adjustable cam timers for governing sequence and length of cleaning operations, and cycle circuit steppers. The cam timer is equipped with a microswitch whose on–off action causes valves to pulsate. This agitation dislodges hard-to-remove solids from the valves.

Another system feature is a series of interlocks that prevent start-up if improper manual field connections are made.

All mix process equipment at the ice cream plant is cleaned in place in five steps: (1) raw product pipelines, (2) HTST, (3) pasteurization lines, (4) raw product tanks, and (5) mix storage tanks. Two solution tanks permit simultaneous cleaning of any two steps.

Normally, pipelines and HTST CIP is performed at the end of each day's batching operations while tank cleaning may be done during batching.

Six basic three-way valves—three for each solution tank—control cleaning cycles. Automatic regulation of the valves permits these functions to be performed:

(1) Filling of solution tanks with water.
(2) Prerinse.
(3) Wash and final rinse. These follow the necessary pattern until all lines are cleaned. Timing is preset to adequately clean the system.
(4) Control of process valves from graphic console.

The Hood CIP system is also equipped with a selector switch for periodic cleaning of tank with an acid wash instead of a detergent wash.

Automated and highly mechanized operating methods and an improved layout can reduce costs for ice cream plants. The principles of plant layout and methods of operation for an automated ice cream plant handling 200,000 gal of ice cream annually are illustrated next by assuming that 90% of the production is ice cream and 10% ices and sherbets and that the plant handles 30,000 gal of novelties purchased from outside sources. The following is based on Tracy (1966) and covers operating schedule, ingredients, freezing rates, plan of operation, receipt of products, mix assembly, control panel, mix assembly, product flow, processing methods, load out, and cleaning procedures for such a plant.

Example of a 200,000 gal Annual Production Plant

The volume of ice cream manufactured varies by seasons of the year and from month to month. Based on national averages, production is smallest during November, December, January, and February and largest during June, July, and August. The peak production month is July. During this month 11% of the annual production is manufactured. Thus, a plant producing 200,000 gal annually would manufacture about 22,000 gal of ice cream during July.

The equipment and the layout of a plant should be adequate to meet the peak operating requirements. Assuming that the July production is evenly divided into weeks, the peak weekly production would be 5500 gal. It is assumed that the plant would prepare mix ingredients on Monday and Thursday and manufacture ice cream on Tuesday and Friday. Thus, ice cream for the week's needs is produced in two days—2750 gal each day, of which 2475 gal is ice cream and 275 gal sherbets and ices.

To manufacture this volume efficiently, a weekly operating schedule is necessary. Table 11.3 shows the assumed operating schedule for the plant. The plant would operate five days a week—Monday, Tuesday, Thursday, Friday, and Saturday. On Monday and Thursday the mix-making, loading-out, cleaning, and maintenance operations would be performed. The receiving of mix ingredients, freezing, packaging, storing, loading-out, cleaning, and maintenance operations would be performed on Tuesday. All these operations, with the exception of receiving mix ingredients, would be repeated on Friday. On

Table 11.3. Operating Schedule by Day of Week for Performing Major Operations in an Ice Cream Plant Manufacturing 5500 gal of Ice Cream a Week

Operation	Mon.	Tues.	Wed.	Thurs.	Fri.	Sat.	Sun.
Receiving mix ingredients		×				×	
Mix-making	×			×			
Freezing		×			×		
Packaging		×			×		
Storing		×			×		
Loading-out	×	×			×	×	
Cleaning	×	×		×	×	×	
Maintenance	×	×		×	×	×	

Saturday, such operations as loading-out, cleaning, maintenance, and receiving mix ingredients would be performed.

The ice cream will have an average overrun of 85% and sherbets and ices 50%. The ingredients used in preparing 1000 gal of ice cream mix, sherbet mix, and water ice mix, for the purpose of this study, are shown in Table 11.4. The amount of ice cream mix required on a day when 2475 gal of ice cream are manufactured is 1337 gal; for 275 gal of ices and sherbets, 183 gal of mix are required.

It is also assumed that the plant would manufacture 12 different flavors of ice cream, sherbets, and ices: vanilla, chocolate, chocolate ripple, strawberry, butter pecan, coffee, pineapple, peach, and banana ice cream, and orange, raspberry, and pineapple ice and sherbet. However, not all flavors would be produced each manufacturing day.

Twenty-four percent of the ice cream, sherbets, and ices would be packaged in 2-1/2 gal cans, 62% in 1/2-gal cartons, and 14% in pint cartons.

Novelties purchased from other manufacturers would consist of stick items, such as water ice and chocolate-coated bars, chocolate-coated ice cream bars, and 4-oz cups of ice cream. All novelties would be received in the plant in bags—12 items to each bag.

The rate for freezing ice cream, sherbets, and ices and filling containers would average about 372 gal/hr, but would vary by container sizes. The total time required for freezing 2750 gal of ice cream, sherbets, and ices, and for filling containers the sizes of those assumed herein is 7 hr and 24 min (Table 11.5).

How the Plant Operates

The major operations involved in manufacturing ice cream are (1) receiving raw products; (2) assembling mix; (3) pasteurizing, homogenizing, and cooling; (4) freezing, packaging, and storing; (5) loading-out products; and (6) cleaning the equipment. Assembling and processing mix and cleaning and sanitizing certain items of equipment are automated operations handled from the control panel (Fig. 11.11). Other operations are mechanized or manually controlled.

Table 11.4.   Ingredients for 1000 gal of Ice Cream, Sherbet, and Water Ice Milk

Ingredient	Ice cream mix (lb)	Sherbet mix (lb)	Water ice milk (lb)
Cream, 40%	2288		
Concentrated skim milk, 30%	3096		
Corn syrup (40% solids)	384	1000	1000
Liquid sugar (67% solids)	1748		
Stabilizer	27.5	22	22
Emulsifier	5		
Sugar syrup (67% solids)		3000	3000
Ice cream mix (10%)		915	
Citric acid		43	43
Water	1601.5	4520	5350
Total	9150	9500	9415

Table 11.5.   Freezing and Filling Rate by Type of Product and Container for a Peak
Day of 2750 gal of Ice Cream, Sherbets, and Ices

Product and container size	Freezing and filling rate (gal/hr)	Containers filled (no.)	Total production (gal)	Filling time required (hr)
Ice cream				
2-½ gal containers	460	238	595	1.29
½-gal cartons	350	3068	1534	4.38
Pint cartons	350	2776	346	0.99
Subtotal		6082	2475	6.66
Sherbet and ices				
2½-gal containers	460	26	65	0.14
½-gal cartons	350	340	170	0.49
Pint cartons	350	320	40	0.11
Subtotal		686	275	0.74
Total		6768	2750	7.40

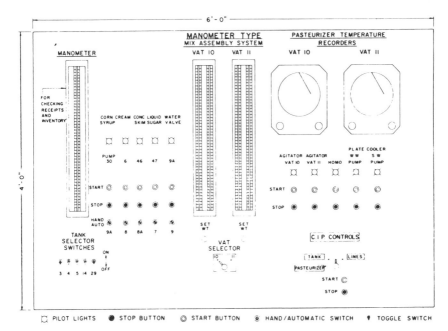

Fig. 11.11.   A suggested control panel for an automated ice cream plant manufacturing 200,000 gal of ice cream annually. (From USDA 1966.)

The flow of mix ingredients and ice cream from receiving through filling is shown in Fig 11.12.

Receiving Raw Products. To save labor, the receiving of raw products follows a definite schedule. The cream and condensed skim milk are received in a two-compartment tank truck on Tuesday and Saturday. The maximum amount of cream received in 1 day is about 420 gal during July, the peak production month; the maximum amount of concentrated skim milk is 570 gal. In the periods of low production, such as January, approximately 2/3 as much milk products will be received.

The two-compartment tank truck containing the milk products backs into the unloading area under the projecting roof. One of the plant workers takes samples of the cream and concentrated skim milk for testing. A sanitary pipeline that extends through the wall connects the tank truck with receiving pump (no. 2 in Fig. 11.12) located adjacent to the milk products storage tanks (nos. 4 and 5). Since the capacity of the unloading pump is 100 gal/min, a 1200-gal delivery of products can be unloaded in about 12 min. About 5 min are required to collect the sample, connect the pipeline, and start the pump.

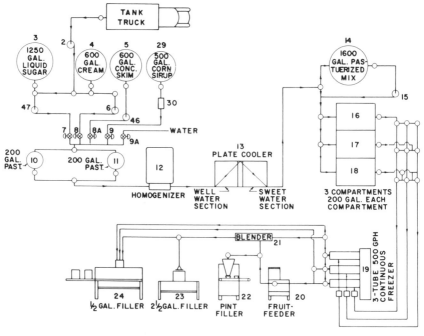

Fig. 11.12. Flow of mix ingredients and ice cream from receiving through filling. (From USDA 1966.)

Cream and concentrated skim milk are tested in the laboratory to determine whether the milk solids are in the proper ratio and concentration. If variation from the standard is significant, a change in the formula will be necessary when the mix is made.

The sweetening agents—liquid sugar and corn syrup—are received in separate tank trucks on Saturday. The amount ordered is determined by reference to the production schedule and mix formulation chart. The trucks unload in the same way as the milk products trucks. The corn syrup truck has its own pump for unloading. Corn syrup is pumped into a 500-gal tank (no. 29) and the liquid sugar is pumped into a 1250-gal tank (no. 3).

At the control panel, the amount of product received or the amount remaining in the tank can be determined by pressing the tank selector switch for the desired storage tank. The manometer, mounted on the left of the control panel, is connected to level transducers located in the bottom of the tanks. A calibration chart serves as a ready reference in converting the manometer reading from inches to pounds or gallons.

Novelties are received every Saturday during the peak summer season and about once each three to four weeks in the winter.

Mix Assembly. The maximum amount of ice cream mix and sherbet and ice mix to be prepared in one month (July) is 12,160 gal. Assuming that this load is distributed evenly over the eight mix-making days (Monday and Thursday of each week) in the month, the average amount to be made in one day is 1520 gal (1337 gal of ice cream mix and 183 gal of sherbet and ice mix). The ingredients are mixed in the two pasteurizing vats (nos. 10 and 11), each of which holds 200 gal.

The mix assembly system on the control panel (Fig. 11.11) consists of two manometers, labeled VAT 10 and VAT 11, two set weight knobs mounted directly below the manometers, a vat selector switch, and to the left of the manometers, pushbuttons (start and stop) and pilot lights for the pumps (nos. 30, 6, 46, 47, and 9a) and automatic valves (nos. 9a, 8, 8a, 7, and 9).

Before mix assembly, the lines are flushed with a sanitizing solution. (See description of CIP system in the section on Cleaning Equipment.)

In assembling a batch of ice cream mix in pasteurizing vat 10, the operator throws the vat selector switch to vat 10 (Fig. 11.11), sets the weight of the cream (first ingredient) on the right-hand scale of the manometer, and pushes the start buttons for the cream pump (no. 6) and cream tank valve (no. 8). The pilot light comes on; cream is pumped into the vat until the manometer trips the switch, indicating that the desired weight has been reached; this deactivates the cream pump and shuts off the tank valve automatically. Then the operator sets the weight of the next ingredient (concentrated skim milk) plus the weight of the cream on the manometer and pushes the start buttons for the concentrated skim milk pump (no. 46) and valve (no. 8a). Again, the manometer indicates when the desired weight has been reached, deactivates the skim milk pump, and shuts off the tank valve automatically. The same procedure is followed to add liquid sugar, corn syrup, and water to the mix. The stabilizer and emulsifier (preweighed and bagged) are added manually to the vat. The total weight of the mix can be read on the right-hand scale of the manometer as a check on the formulation of the batch.

Water ice, which is made from a mixture of sugar syrup, corn syrup, stabilizer, and water, is assembled in vat 10 or 11 in the same manner as ice cream mix. Sherbet, which is made of the same ingredients as water ice, except that about 10% ice cream mix is added, is also assembled in the same manner. The desired amount of ice cream mix is pumped from the mix storage vat (no. 14). Citric acid is added just before freezing.

Pasteurizing, Homogenizing, and Cooling. The mix is now ready to be pasteurized. Immediately below the recording thermometers, which are in the upper right-hand corner of the panel board are pushbuttons for controlling the agitators on the pasteurizing vats (nos. 10 and 11). Pushbuttons for starting and stopping the homogenizer (no. 12) and the well water and sweet water pumps for the plate cooler (no. 13) are also in this section. The operator pushes the button for starting the agitator in either vat 10 or 11; the steam valve is then manually opened to heat the mix to 160°F. The steam is automatically controlled by a self-acting regulator. When the predetermined temperature (160°F) is reached in the mix, the steam valve closes. The desired temperature is then automatically maintained during the 30-min holding period. The bulb of the recorder, located in the jacket of the vat, indicates on the recorder the temperature of the mix and the time it has been held. After the 30-min holding period, the operator opens the pasteurizer valve, pushes the homogenizer start button, and regulates the homogenizer valves to the desired pressure— ordinarily 2000 lb on the first valve and 500 lb on the second, when a two-stage homogenizer is used. The purpose of the second stage valve is to break up the clumps of fat produced in the mix by the first stage and thereby prevent excessive mix viscosity.

At the same time the homogenizer is being started, the operator pushes the buttons to start the well water and refrigerated sweet water circulating through the plate cooler (no. 13). Homogenization adds about 5° of frictional heat to the mix. If the mix has been pasteurized at 160°F, it then enters the well water section of the plate cooler at 165°F. The mix is cooled in this section to approximately 70°F, assuming the well water is 65°F. The mix then passes through the second section of the plate cooler, where the temperature is reduced to 40°F by the 34°F sweet water.

After the mix pasteurizing vat (no. 10) has been emptied and the discharge valve closed, the operator pushes the stop buttons on the homogenizer, vat agitator, well water pump, and sweet water pump. The pasteurized mix is now homogenized and ready for storage in the pasteurized mix tank (no. 14), where it is maintained at 40°F.

Mix must be flavored before it enters the freezer. It is first pumped from the pasteurized mix storage vat (no. 14) by the mix pump (no. 15) into one of the three compartments of the flavoring vat (nos. 16, 17, 18), and the flavor is added manually. The valves at the three-compartment flavoring vat are so arranged that the mix from any compartment can be fed to any one of the three positive mix pumps on the freezer (no. 19). A second pump, revolving faster than the mix pump (no. 15), not only handles mix from the first pump but sucks air into the system.

The freezer lowers the mix temperature from about 40° to about 21°F; at the same time, air is pumped into the freezing chamber to obtain the desired overrun. The speed of the air pump determines the amount of air incorporated into the mix in the freezer.

The piping and valves beyond the freezer are so arranged that the output of any freezing tube can be sent to any one of the three filling devices either through or around the first feeder (no. 20) or blender (no. 21).

Freezing, Packaging, and Storing. As indicated in Table 11.3, freezing days are Tuesday and Friday. The amount of ice cream, sherbet, and ices frozen each of the eight freezing days in the peak month (July) is approximately 2750 gal. The three-cylinder freezer (no. 19) has a rated capacity of 500 gal/hr at 100% overrun. With lower overrun the capacity is less. Bulk ice cream is usually drawn at 90–100% overrun and package ice cream at 80–85% overrun. In this report, 85% overrun is assumed for all ice cream. Sherbets and ices are normally drawn at about 50% overrun.

Processing the amounts of ice cream, sherbets, and ices needed on a peak day requires approximately 7.5 hr operating time. It is therefore advisable that some duties preparatory to processing be performed on the mix-making days: withdrawal of empty containers from storage, makeup of bulk containers, and preparation of fruits, nuts, and flavorings. In this way only the operation of the freezer, the handling of the filled packages at the filling machines, and the transfer of packages into the hardening room need be attended to on freezing days.

The fruit feeder is provided with a 12:1 variation in capacity by a combination of a two-speed motor and a 3:1 variable drive, and by halving the piston displacement. The liquid capacity of the fruit feeder varies from 12 to 140 gal/hr. Large pieces of fruit or whole cherries reduce the top capacity to 90 gal/hr. For fruit ice cream, the amount of fruit added is 10–15% of the weight of the mix. When the same fruit ice cream is made in all three cylinders of the freezer at one time, the ice cream from one cylinder is passed through the fruit feeder, where sufficient fruit is added for the total capacity of the freezer. The discharges from the other cylinders and the fruit feeder are then uniformly mixed in the blender (no. 21).

Valves in the discharge line from the freezer, fruit feeder, or blender regulate the flow of ice cream into the filling machines. There are two package fillers, one for pints (no. 22) and one for 1/2-gal (no. 24), and one filler for bulk ice cream in 2-1/2 gal cans (no. 23). The pint filler is completely automatic; it forms, fills, and closes about 2800 pt packages per hour (350 gal/hr). One operator is needed to keep the carton hopper supplied with folded cartons. The 1/2-gal filler also has a capacity of 350 gal/hr. It requires one person to set up cartons and one to close the cartons after they have been filled. Both filler speeds are automatically synchronized to the speed at which the ice cream is discharged from the freezer, fruit feeder, or blender.

The operator of the 2-1/2 gal can filler (no. 23) must set up the paper cans and also place the lids on the filled cans. This filling operation proceeds at about 500 gal/hr.

The 1/2-gal and pint packages are placed in paper sacks, making 1-gal bundles labeled with flavor and size of package. Bagging and labeling aid in storing the ice cream in the hardening room, in taking inventory, and in making delivery. About half of one worker's time is required to place the packages in gallon bags and place the bags in wire cases. Both 1/2-gal and pint containers leave the package fillers on a chute, on which several gallons can accumulate. The 1-gal bags are placed over the end of the chute, and the worker pushes 2-1/2 gal or 8-pt packages into a bag, tapes it shut, and places it in the wire case. While a few gallons are accumulating, there is time to attend to other phases of the operation.

The wire cases hold six 1-gal packages; they are of lightweight construction and can be stacked 10 high in the hardening room. The open construction of the cases permits free air circulation around the ice cream and produces faster hardening.

After being placed in the wire cases, the bundles of ice cream are moved by belt conveyor into the hardening room where a worker stacks them on the floor, keeping different flavors and sizes separate.

Loading-Out. Since ice cream deliveries are usually made in the morning, the trucks are loaded the previous afternoon. Loading can be done by one plant worker and the truck driver. Using the driver's load sheet, the plant worker in the hardening room places the items called for onto the loading cart and pushes it out to the loading dock. The truck driver checks the items against his copy of the load sheet and places them in the truck.

Two wholesale delivery trucks are suggested for this plant. Each has the capacity of about 1200 gal. Daily deliveries vary with the season, averaging about 800 gal.

On returning to the plant, the driver checks in at the office, accounts for the day's sales, and prepares a load sheet for the next day. After reloading, the driver parks the truck in the enclosed truck parking area and plugs in the truck compressor at the electrical connection.

Cleaning the Equipment. All plant equipment that comes in contact with ice cream or ice cream ingredients must be cleaned immediately after use. A sanitizing solution is run through the system before startup. The pasteurizing vats (nos. 10 and 11), cream and concentrated skim milk storage tanks (nos. 4 and 5), pasteurizing mix storage vat (no. 14), and connecting pipelines and automatic valves are cleaned by the CIP system immediately after use. All other equipment is cleaned manually.

There are three essential parts to the CIP system: the solution tanks and circulating pump, located in the dry storage room where chemicals are kept; the connecting station located in the processing room on the other side of the wall from the solution tanks; and the controls on the control panel in the processing area for operating the system. One of the tanks is used for acid solution, one for alkaline solution, and one for the sanitizing solution (chlorine). Chemicals should be changed each operating day. The connecting station directs the cleaning, rinsing, and sanitizing solutions into the circuits desired.

The indicator knob for CIP controls is set for the desired equipment and the automatic control is provided for the various steps in cleaning, rinsing, and sanitizing, which include the following: (1) A complete wash, which consists of an acid and an alkali wash and three rinses, (2) an alkali or acid wash, which consists of a prerinse, the wash, and final rinse, (3) the sanitizing cycle, which is only a water rinse to which a sanitizer such as chlorine is added.

A predetermined time cycle for each cleaning operation is selected at the controls on the solution tanks. Once set, the time period will be selected each time the master switch is turned to the desired operation. The time setting, however, can be varied by a simple adjustment of the controls.

A horn sounds when a cleaning cycle has been completed.

The following is an example of the CIP system showing the various steps in cleaning and sanitizing a pasteurizing vat:

(1) prerinse, 75 sec
(2) drain vat
(3) delay, 30 sec
(4) wash (acid) at 145°F, 20 min
(5) drain vat
(6) delay, 30 sec
(7) rinse, 75 sec
(8) drain vat
(9) delay, 30 sec
(10) wash (alkaline) at 145°F, 20 min
(11) drain vat
(12) delay, 30 sec
(13) rinse, 75 sec
(14) drain vat
(15) sanitize with chemical sterilizer (200 ppm), 10 min
(16) drain vat, leaving lines open
(17) stop cycle.

Since acid cleaning is needed only on heated surfaces, such as pasteurizers, the controller omits this cycle on such equipment as raw milk storage vats and the pasteurized mix storage tank.

Both the temperature and the time of circulation of any solution can be changed quickly by adjusting the rheostat controlling these operations. This is located on the back of the panel board.

During the circulation of each solution, a pulsator wired into the CIP circuit closes the automatic outlet valve on the tank every 45 sec and holds it closed for 15 sec. This cleans the seals and stems of the valve. In pipeline cleaning, the circuits are arranged in such a way that the solution path is alternated through all parts of a three-way valve to provide stem cleaning and sanitizing. If a second circuit cannot be used with an automatic valve, a pulsator opens and closes the valve a sufficient number of times to clean the stem and seals.

All vats and tanks are provided with spray balls or devices to distribute the cleaning, rinsing, and sanitizing solutions under pressure to all surfaces to be treated.

The homogenizer, fruit feeder, freezer, fillers, pumps, and packaging machines are washed manually. Warm (120°F) water containing 4 oz of washing powder per 10 gal of water is first pumped through the equipment for rinsing. The machines are then disassembled and washed and rinsed in wash sinks.

It is also customary to wash the milk products truck tanks. Since there will be only two of these truck tanks to be cleaned each week during the peak season, CIP cleaning is not economical. Washing, therefore, is done by hand. Hot and cold water facilities and hose connections are provided in the unloading area for this purpose.

Labor Requirements

In this plant during the peak month two full-time plant workers plus the foreperson and one half-time worker can handle all operations. Running this plant without automation would require three full-time workers four days a week. The extra labor (equivalent to 1.1 full-time workers) for operating the nonautomated plant would be required for hand washing the raw cream, concentrated milk, and mix storage tanks, the connecting pipelines and valves, and the flavoring tanks. Extra labor also would be needed for the manual assembling and processing of the mix ingredients and for hand packaging. Two workers would be needed four days a week to perform these operations. They would not work on Saturday.

Assuming that during July, three workers in the automated plant worked 20 days of 8 hr each and the fourth worked half-time, they would work 560 hr (3.5 × 8 × 20) to produce 22,000 gal of ice cream.[2] Productivity per man-hour would then equal 39.3 gal. However, on a yearly basis the figure would be much less, since efficiency decreases during low production months.

Yearly productivity for the three full-time workers and one half-time worker is calculated as follows:

$$\text{total hours worked} = 52 \text{ weeks} \times 5 \text{ days/week}$$
$$\times 8 \text{ hr/day} \times 3.5 \text{ workers}$$
$$= 7280$$

$$\text{gallons per hour} = 200,000 \text{ gal}/7280 \text{ hr}$$
$$= 27.5$$

For the nonautomated plant, using three full-time workers plus two additional workers four days a week (the equivalent of 1.6 full-time workers) the productivity during July would be 30 gal/hr, and for the year it would be 21 gal/hr. These figures show the importance of sustaining production at a high level throughout the year to maintain productivity of labor.

The operating schedule shows on what day the various plant operations are performed. For example, on Monday mix is made, requiring approximately 6.5 hr; the rest of the time is spent in maintenance, receiving materials for dry storage, preparing packages for the next day's freezing, loading-out, plant

---

[2]These calculations disregard the time necessary to receive and store novelties.

cleaning, and laboratory work. On Tuesday all operations except mix-making are performed. Wednesday the plant is closed. Thursday is a repeat of Monday. Friday is a repeat of Tuesday except that no milk products are received. Saturday is spent in cleaning and maintenance work, laboratory testing, receiving mix ingredients, and loading-out. Sunday, the plant is closed. Records are kept by the foreperson throughout the week.

The work schedule on mix-making days (Monday and Thursday) is as follows:

Worker no. 1
8:00–12:00	Sanitizing equipment and mix-making
12:00–12:30	Break for lunch
12:30–1:00	Mix-making
1:00–4:30	Plant cleanup, maintenance

Worker no. 2 (foreperson)
8:00–12:30	Sanitizing equipment and mixmaking
12:30–1:00	Break for lunch
1:00–4:30	Laboratory, plant records, checking-in and loading-out trucks

Worker no. 3
8:00–11:30	Receiving items for dry storage; preparing fruits and flavors for ice cream; preparing packages
11:30–12:00	Break for lunch
12:00–1:00	Mix-making
1:00–4:30	Plant cleanup, maintenance

The work schedule on freezing days (Tuesday and Friday) is as follows:

A fourth worker (assumed to be half-time) will be added on these two days. Worker no. 1 reports for duty at 7:15 A.M. and works until 3:15 P.M., assembling and sanitizing the freezing and packaging equipment. This requires about 0.75 hr. Workers no. 2, 3, and 4 check in at 8 A.M. and proceed without stopping until about 3:30 P.M. Breaks for lunch (30 min) are allowed the four workers between 11:30 A.M. and 1 P.M.

From 3:15 to 4:15 P.M. worker no. 4 checks in and loads out the delivery trucks. A half-time worker, this worker generally works more than 8 hr per day on these two days.

At the completion of freezing, workers no. 1 and 3 clean the freezers and packaging equipment. Worker no. 2 receives the milk products on Tuesday and works on plant records on Friday. Worker no. 4 cleans the bulk tank trucks that deliver the cream and condensed milk.

It requires about 5 min to start and adjust an ice cream freezer; after the freezer is operating, it requires very little attention. A total of about 5 min/hr is enough for making minor adjustments necessary to control the weight of the ice cream and the degree it is frozen, and to add flavor to tanks of mix and change tanks feeding the freezer. Each of the three compartments of the mix tank supplies the freezer for nearly 1 hr if a full tank of flavor is required. The foreperson handles the freezers.

The remaining 55 min of the foreperson's time is used in filling packages, and with two assistants, performing the freezing, packaging, and bagging. A fourth worker brings packaging material to the filler, places the bags in wire cases, and stacks the cases in the hardening room. The four-worker team is flexible, and each can, for a short time, do any job or substitute for any other during breaks.

The work schedule on Saturday involves receiving milk products, liquid sugar and corn syrup, novelties, fruits, and flavors; cleaning milk products trucks; checking-in and loading-out delivery trucks; and maintenance. One worker checks in at 7 A.M. and two workers at 8 A.M. Their schedule is as follows:

Worker no. 1
    7:00–9:30   Receiving, weighing, and sampling cream and condensed milk; washing and sanitizing tank trucks
    9:30–10:30   Weighing and receiving liquid sugar and corn syrup
    10:30–11:45   Receiving, recording, and storing novelties
    11:45–12:15   Break for lunch
    12:15–3:30   Cleaning windows and walls in plant

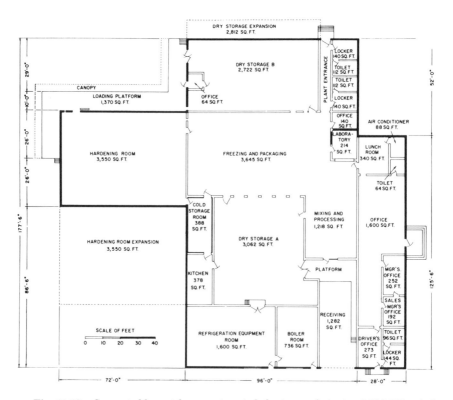

Fig. 11.13. Suggested layout for an automated plant manufacturing 1,000,000 gal of ice cream and 250,000 gal of novelties annually. (From USDA 1966.)

Worker no. 2 (foreperson)
   8:00–12:00   Laboratory tests, hardening room and dry storage
                         inventory, plant records
12:00–12:30   Break for lunch
12:30–4:30   Maintenance
Worker no. 3
   8:00–10:30   Assisting no. 1 in washing and sanitizing tank trucks, and
                         weighing and receiving liquid sugar and corn syrup
10:30–11:45   Receiving, recording, and storing novelties
11:45–12:15   Break for lunch
12:15–3:00   Cleaning platform and premises outside of building
   3:00–4:30   Checking in and loading out trucks

Similar operating criteria for automation of dairy plants manufacturing 1,000,000 gal of ice cream and 250,000 gal of novelties yearly are available from equipment manufactures. A suggested layout for this size of plant is shown in Fig. 11.13.

12
The Freezing Process

Freezing the mix is one of the most important operations in making ice cream, for upon it depend the quality, palatability, and yield of the finished product. The freezing process may, for convenience, be divided into two parts: (1) The mix, with the proper amount of color and flavoring materials generally added at the freezer, is quickly frozen while being agitated to incorporate air in such a way as to produce and control formation of the small ice crystals that are necessary to give smoothness in body and texture, palability, and satisfactory overrun in the finished ice cream. (2) When ice cream is partially frozen to the proper consistency, it is drawn from the freezer into packages and quickly transferred to cold storage rooms, where the freezing and hardening process is completed without agitation. Changes that take place in the hardening room are discussed in Chapter 13.

The general procedure of the freezing process is easily learned since it only involves accurate measurement of the ingredients, which are placed in the freezer and then removed. However, the correct handling of the details to produce a uniform product requires expert judgment and almost split-second timing—a technique acquired only through experience guided by continual, careful study. In fact, it is very seldom that any two people execute the details in exactly the same manner. Therefore, they obtain different ice creams even when using the same ingredients, formulas, and equipment. The effect of slight variations in the amount of coloring and flavoring materials, which are usually added at the freezer, readily is observed, but equally important are the variations in details of operation.

CHANGES THAT TAKE PLACE DURING
THE FREEZING PROCESS

The function of the freezing process is to freeze a portion of the water of the mix. This involves lowering the temperature of the mix from aging temperature to the freezing point, freezing a portion of the water of the mix, incorporating air into the mix, and cooling the ice cream from the temperature at which it is drawn from the freezer to hardening room temperature. The temperature of the mix that is put into the freezer drops very rapidly while the sensible heat (which thermometers measure) is being removed and before any ice crystals are formed. This process should take less than 1–2 min. Meanwhile, the rapid agitation reduces the viscosity by partly destroying the gel structure and by breaking up the fat globule clusters. The gel structure may partially reform during the hardening process in the hardening room. Also, the rapid agitation hastens incorporation of air into the mix.

When the freezing point is reached, the liquid water changes to ice crystals, which appear in the mix. The ice crystals are practically pure water in a solid form, and thus the sugar, as well as other solutes, become more concentrated in the remaining liquid water. Increasing the concentration of these solutes causes the freezing point of the liquid portion to be slightly lower so that the temperature (or sensible heat, as it is called) must be lowered before more ice crystals will form. However, the heat called latent heat of fusion that must be removed to change liquid water into solid ice crystals is not measured by the thermometer, so that the temperature of the mix would not change noticeably while ice crystals are forming. This actually happens when pure water is frozen, but in freezing ice cream the freezing point is continually being lowered by the formation of the ice crystals, so that the temperature continues to drop but at a slower rate than during the first minute or two while approaching the initial freezing point. As the temperature drops, more ice crystals are formed, increasing the concentration of sugar and other solutes in the remaining liquid water until the concentration is so great that freezing will not occur. Thus all of the water is not frozen even after long periods in the hardening room (see Table 12.1).

As Table 12.1 shows, the first phase of the freezing process accounts for freezing 33–67% of the water depending on the drawing temperature. The hardening process then may account for an additional 23–57%, depending on the drawing temperature.

During the period in the freezer while ice crystals are forming, more air is incorporated into the mix, and such ingredients as acid fruit juices, fruits, or nuts may be added without any danger of coagulating the mix. Also, at this time the refrigerant may be shut off from the batch freezers. In hand or home freezers, agitation is usually stopped when the product has reached a certain consistency or stiffness, which depends upon the amount of water already changed into ice crystals and the amount of air incorporated into the mix. In commercial freezers, when this point is reached the ice cream is drawn out of the freezers into packages to be placed in the hardening room. At this time, the

Table 12.1. Approximate Percentage of Water Frozen in Ice Cream Mix at Various Drawing Temperatures

Temp. (°F)	Water frozen (%)	Temp. (°F)	Water frozen (%)
25	33	20	59
24	41	19	62
23	47	18	64
22	52	17	67
21	56	−15	90

ice cream contains the desired amount of air, but not all of the desired amount of ice crystals.

The results of the freezing process can best be explained by examining the internal structure of the frozen product. The texture of ice cream is known to be affected by many factors but depends principally upon the presence of ice crystals, air cells, and unfrozen material.

The physical structure of ice cream represents a complicated physicochemical system. Air cells are dispersed in a continuous liquid phase with embedded ice crystals. The liquid phase also contains solidified fat particles, milk proteins, insoluble salts, lactose crystals in some cases, stabilizers of colloidal dimension, and sucrose, lactose, other sugars, and soluble salts in true solution. Such a material consisting of liquid, air, and solid is called a three-phase system (see Fig. 12.1).

The general description of ice cream structure and the way in which the components are built up was clearly displayed by Berger et al. (1972), in a series of electron micrographs obtained by the freeze-etching technique (Figs. 12.1–12.4). Figure 12.2 shows two structural elements of ice cream in relation to each other: the small air cell is coated by fat globules, which constitute most of the continuous phase. Figure 12.3 shows crystallized fat and casein micelle agglomerates. The cell mix interface is a continuous layer of unstructured material, coated by a layer of discrete fat globules, which go through to the inside of the air cell, indicating that the interfacial layer is relatively thin and easily distorted.

The form of the ice mix interface (Fig. 12.4) shows a lamella of continuous phase between ice crystals and air cells. The continuous phase contains some

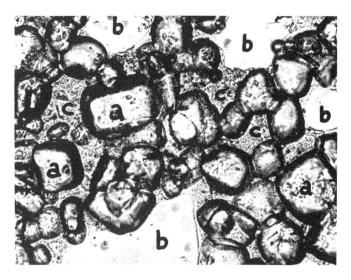

Fig. 12.1. The internal structure of ice cream. (a) Ice crystals, average size 45–55 μm. (b) Air cells, average size 110–185 μm. (c) Unfrozen material. Average distance between ice crystals or between ice crystals and air cells, 6–8 μm. Average distance between air cells, 100–150 μm.

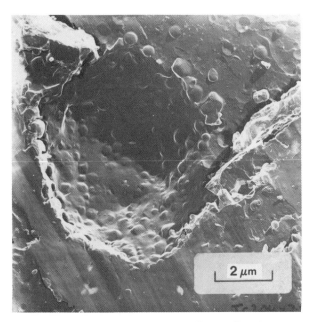

Fig. 12.2. Electron micrograph of interior of small air cell in frozen ice cream. The small projections are fat globules. [Reproduced from Berger *et al.* (1972), by permission.]

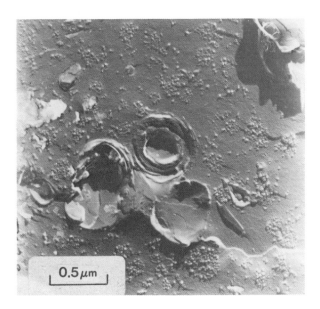

Fig. 12.3. Electron micrograph of fat globules fractured in the freezing process and cemented together by liquid fat. Note the shell of high-melting triglycerides. [Reproduced from Berger *et al.* (1972) by permission.]

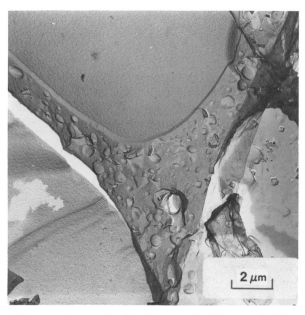

12.4.   Electron micrograph of wall separating ice crystals. [Reproduced from
et al. (1972) by permission.]

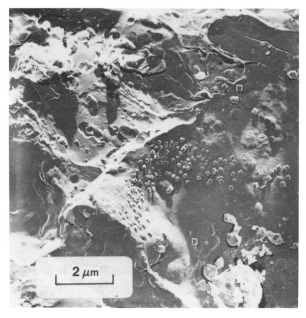

Fig. 12.5.   Electron micrograph of sucrose microcrystals in ice cream. [Reproduced
from Berger *et al.* (1972) by permission.]

clumps of fat and some individual fat globules and, in addition, the characteristic structured appearance of casein micells.

The disposition of sucrose microcrystals in ice cream is shown in Fig. 12.5.

REFRIGERATION REQUIREMENTS FOR
ICE CREAM FREEZING

Heldman and Hedrick (1968) state that the heat to be removed from an ice cream mix during freezing is a function of several variables with composition the predominant factor. They obtained experimental results with mix composition in which the sugar content was varied from 100% sucrose, to 79% sucrose and 21% corn syrup solids, to 50% sucrose and 50% corn syrup solids. The findings showed that refrigeration requirements for freezing to 15°F increased from 71 BTU/lb for the 100% sucrose mix to 87 BTU/lb for the mix with 50% sucrose mix.

Tracy (1966) calculated the heat removal necessary in freezing novelties, using the quantities products sensible heat and products latent heat, with the sum of the two equaling the total refrigeration load. He used the following formulas:

(a) Products sensible heat (BTU/hr)
   weight of product (lb/hr) × temperature range × specific heat (0.90)
(b) Products latent heat (BTU/hr)
   weight of product (lb/hr) × water frozen (%) × water in product (%) × latent heat of fusion of water (144 BTU)

The specific heat of water is 1 by definition; the specific heat of ice is 0.492; the latent heat of fusion of ice is 144 BTU/lb (or 80 cal/g in the metric system). Sommer (1951) cited references giving the specific heat as 0.30 for carbohydrates, 0.34 for proteins, and 0.40 for fats at 32°F. Specific heat can be calculated by the formula

$$\text{specific heat} = a + (1 - a)W$$

where a is the specific heat of the dry matter and W the percentage of water divided by 100.

A mix containing 12.5% fat, 10% MSNF, 16% sugar, 0.3% stabilizer, and 61.2% water has a specific heat of 0.8176 and requires 4905.84 cal/100 g to heat or cool at 0–60°C.

FREEZING TIME AND THE IMPORTANCE
OF THE FREEZER

Fast freezing is essential for a smooth product, because ice crystals that are formed quickly are smaller than those formed slowly. Therefore, it is desirable to freeze and draw from the freezer in as short a time as possible. The freezing time and temperature are affected by the type of freezer used (see Table 12.2). Freezers fall into three main groupings:

Table 12.2. Freezing Times and Drawing Temperatures

Kind of freezer	Freezing time to 90% overrun	Drawing temperature (°F)
Batch freezer	7 min	24–26
Continuous freezer	24 sec	21–22
Low-temperature continuous freezer	26–36 sec	16–18
Soft-serve freezer	3 min	18–20
Counter freezer	10 min	26

1. Batch freezers, in which each batch must be measured, colored, and flavored separately. They consist of the brine type (now obsolete); the salt and ice type (obsolete except in some small home freezers); direct-expansion type (using ammonia or Freon as refrigerant), including vertical (for some counter freezers), horizontal (now mostly replaced by continuous freezers), and single-, triple-, and quadruple-tube freezers).

2. Continuous freezers, in which the ingredients are fed continually into the freezer and ice cream is continually produced. They consist of horizontal and direct-expansion types, and are widely used in commercial production.

3. Soft-serve freezers, which are direct-expansion type batch or continuous freezers.

The freezing time is affected by both mechanical factors and the properties of the mix. The mechanical factors are

1. Type and make of freezer
2. Condition of freezer walls and blades
3. Speed of dasher (consisting of blades and beater—this scrapes the walls free of ice crystals, beats in air, keeps mix in contact with freezer wall, and moves the mix forward for unloading
4. Temperature of refrigerant
5. Velocity of refrigerant as it passes around the freezing chamber
6. Overrun desired
7. Temperature at which the ice cream is drawn
8. Rate of unloading freezer

The mix characteristics that affect the freezing time are

1. Composition
2. Freezing point
3. Acidity content of ingredients
4. Kind of ingredients, especially those carrying fat)
5. Methods of processing
6. Kind and amount of flavoring materials

Taylor (1961) noted that freezing is characterized by short production runs, necessitated by frequent changes in flavors and container sizes. The two most common types of freezers found in ice cream plants are the single-tube freezer and the triple-tube freezer. Plants with an annual volume of 150,000 gal would require and justify either two single-tube freezers or one triple-tube freezer. The three-tube freezer consists of three separate tubes, fed by a three-compartment flavor tank. Three flavors may be frozen at the same time. In the single-tube method, two single-tube freezers are usually used to give operational flexibility when producing two or more flavors. Taylor found that the freezing rate of both types of freezers varies widely and that plants often operate the freezers at less than full capacity. In the freezing of ice cream, he found the method employed for freezing by the triple-tube method was essentially the same as that for the single-tube; namely, mixes were pumped from the storage tank to the flavor tank, flavored and colored, then pumped through the freezer, and fruit added as the ice cream left the freezer. Equipment costs were approximately the same for the two methods.

THE CONTINUOUS FREEZER

The continuous freezer process was first patented in 1913 but did not become widely used until the early 1930s. Briefly described, the process consists of continually feeding a metered amount of ice cream mix and air into one end of the freezing chamber. As the mixture passes through the freezing chamber it is agitated and partially frozen and then discharged in a continuous stream of about the same consistency usually obtained from a batch freezer. This partially frozen stream is delivered into packages, which are then placed in the hardening room to complete the freezing process. The modern machines for this purpose are known as "continuous" or "instant" freezers.

Figure 12.6 shows a plant that uses continuous-freezer operation. A diagram of the continuous freezing process is shown in Fig. 12.7, and two examples of currently used continuous freezers are shown in Figs. 12.8 and 12.9. (The dashers for the freezer in Fig. 12.8 are shown in Fig. 12.10.)

Some important advantages of the continuous method are

1. Less stabilizer is needed, because a larger amount of the ice crystals can be formed in the freezer instead of in the hardening room where slow freezing gives larger crystals, and because less viscosity is needed in the mix.

2. A shorter aging time is possible because less viscosity is needed and the incorporation of air is less dependent upon the character of the mixture.

3. Less flavoring material is needed because the smaller ice crystals melt more rapidly in the mouth and make the flavor slightly more pronounced.

4. Smoother ice cream is obtained because the ice crystals are much smaller and more uniformly small, and fewer larger crystals are formed in the hardening room.

5. There is less tendency toward sandiness because rapid freezing favors small lactose crystals.

6. A more uniform yield is obtained with less variation between packages, especially when small packages are filled.

7. Continuous freezing facilitates the making of specialties such as center

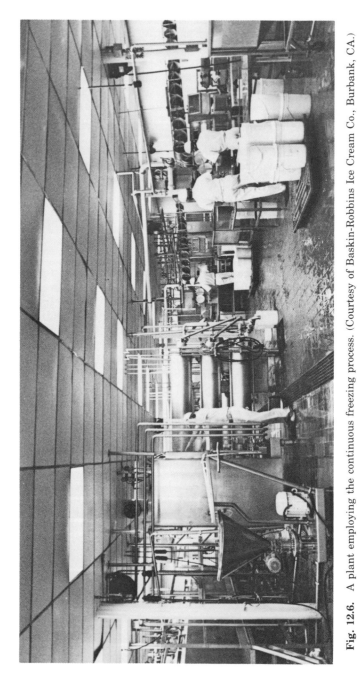

Fig. 12.6. A plant employing the continuous freezing process. (Courtesy of Baskin-Robbins Ice Cream Co., Burbank, CA.)

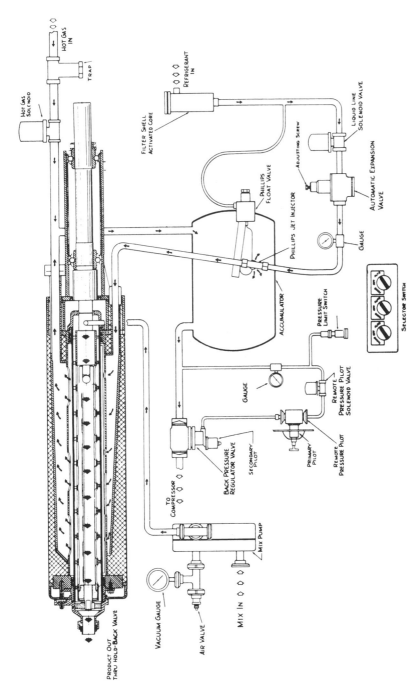

Fig. 12.7. Diagram of a continuous freezer operation.

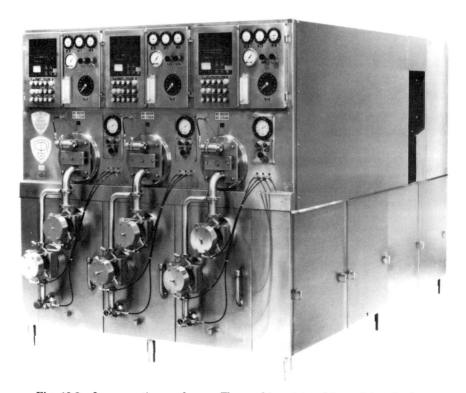

Fig. 12.8. Large continuous freezer. The machine pictured is a triple-tube, large-capacity model with microprocessor control of start-up and shut-down procedures (both routine and emergency), overrun, product-drawing stiffness, cylinder pressure, and CIP sequencing. Three different types of dasher are available for soft products for filling molds, standard products, and low-temperature extrusions. This model has an 800 gal/hr capacity for 100% overrun ice cream, drawn at $-22°F$. (Courtesy of Crepaco, Inc.)

molds, special shapes, combinations of different flavors or colors in one package, variegated ice creams, or individual serving-sized package.

8. The volume of ice cream frozen per worker-hour of labor is increased. This is most pronounced in packages of the 1-pt or 1-qt size.

9. There is less opportunity for contamination when filling packages and specialties.

Some disadvantages of the continuous method are inherent in the process while others may eventually be eliminated by better engineering:

1. Great care must be taken in handling the parts of the machine that fit with very small clearances.

2. Operators and mechanics must have special experience and training in order to avoid operational difficulties and damage to equipment.

3. It is easy to obtain excessive overrun.

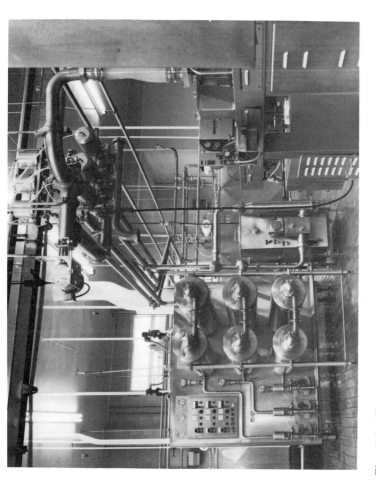

Fig. 12.9. Vogt instant freezer operation. (Courtesy of Cherry Burrell, Cedar Rapids, IA.)

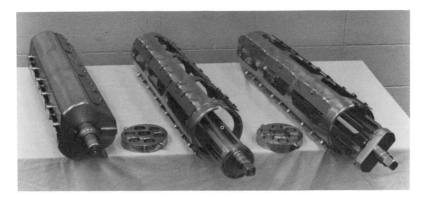

Fig. 12.10. Dashers for the Crepaco continuous freezer of Fig. 12.7. These dashers give the freezer considerable flexibility, each giving optimum results for a specific range of products. The open-frame dashers are partially disassembled to show construction of the beater assemblies.

4. There is a greater tendency for ice cream to shrink in volume after hardening. However, research on this problem may indicate that changing the composition of the mix will correct this difficulty.

5. More help is needed to supply containers and carry packages.

6. Initial cost of the more elaborate equipment is high.

Addition of Bulk-Flavoring Ingredients

Fruit and nut flavors can be frozen in the continuous freezers by finely grinding or chopping the fruit or nuts and adding to and mixing thoroughly in the ice cream mix before freezing. The mix with fruit and nuts added may be thoroughly mixed in the flavor tank of the freezer. This procedure is convenient for small batches of 5 or 10 gal. If larger batches are to be made, the most convenient method is to mix and prepare the fruit or nut mixes in a 50- or 100-gal flavor vat, with the outlet connection piped to the pump inlet at the freezer.

When fruit or nut ice cream is desired with large particles of fruit showing, the fruit juice flavoring and color are added to the mix prior to freezing, and a fruit feeder for the large particles must be used connected to the outlet of the freezer (see Fig. 12.11).

Low-Temperature Continuous Freezers

Low-temperature freezing of ice cream and related products was introduced to the ice cream industry some time ago. This process delivers the semifrozen product from the freezer at approximately 16–17°F. This delivery temperature is 5–6° lower than the 21–23°F usually possible in the continuous freezers that were widely in use. Smith (1963) stated that the low-temperature freezer requires a higher pressure, 200–300 lb/in.^{2}, as compared to about 50 lb/in.^{2} It

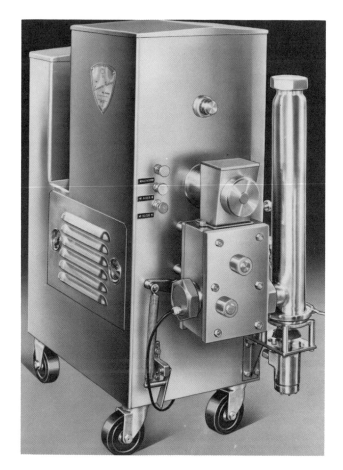

Fig. 12.11. A continuous ingredient feeder. (Courtesy of Crepaco, Inc.)

consists of a freezing barrel similar to a conventional continuous freezer (see Fig. 12.12) from which the partly frozen mix is conducted into a second freezing barrel that uses a dasher consisting of a rotating eccentrically mounted mutator shaft containing a series of short blades. It is different in design from the freezers that it replaced. The mix is subjected to more rigorous treatment in the freezing chamber than in other freezers.

In low-temperature freezing the ice crystal size may be reduced as much as 40%, e.g., from 45–55 μm to 18–22 μm. The air cell size seems to remain about the same or become a little larger, but the number of air cells increases slightly in number. The air cell wall thickness is reduced considerably, such as from 100–150 μm to 50–100 μm. The nature of the cell wall is also different as the unfrozen material becomes more dominant since the ice crystals are very small. Arbuckle (1964) stated that low-temperature frozen ice cream is more resistant to adverse handling conditions than regular frozen ice cream.

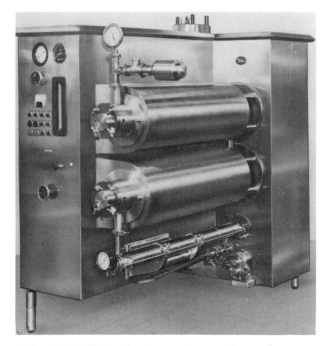

Fig. 12.12.   Votator low-temperature continuous freezer.

Operating the Continuous Freezer

The operator's principal work is (1) to regulate the amount of air being introduced into the mix to give the desired overrun, and (2) to regulate the temperature of the refrigerant on the freezing chamber. Once the machine is started, the refrigerant is shut off from the freezing chamber only when the machine is to be stopped. Usually the refrigerant is shut off a few minutes before the last mix enters the machine, so that the rinse water (100°F), which follows the mix, will pass through the freezing chamber without being frozen. The temperature of the refrigerant on the freezing chamber is adjusted to give the desired consistency when the product leaves the machine. While these two variables require frequent checks, changes in adjustments are not frequent and thus a large quantity of ice cream can be made with comparatively slight variations in quality.

The operation of the continuous freezer demands care and management on the part of the operator. The following are the chief requisites for keeping the freezer operating properly:

1. Keep the ammonia jacket clean and free from oil, water, and nonvolatile ammonia fractions. (Check oil trap for oil, water, etc.) Drain as needed.

2. Keep the scraper blades sharp and straight. (Be careful in handling and

cleaning. Do not drop this piece of equipment and never bend any parts to clean it better.)

3. Keep the mix pumps in proper working condition. (Check pump motor for proper lubrication and tightness of pulley belts.)

4. Make certain that there is always a plentiful supply of ammonia at the freezer. (Proper ammonia supply ensures proper freezing.)

5. Provide a steady suction pressure at all times, 1 lb or so lower than that at which the freezer must operate to give ice cream of the proper temperature. (The continuous freezer makes a continual drain on the liquid ammonia line and refrigeration system. Any lack of liquid or great rise in the suction pressure will soon make itself evident by softness of the ice cream on being discharged.)

The proper method for cleaning the continuous freezer is the same as for most equipment:

1. Remove all conveyor pipes that carry ice cream mix to the freezer.

2. Remove the front of the freezer unit, and pull out the freezer dasher. Rinse all parts of machine that come in contact with ice cream mix, with a warm wash water about 90–110°F. Flush the freezing tube with cold water, followed with warm and then hot. Thoroughly wash and clean all parts of the freezer and sanitary piping.

3. Rinse parts with warm water and check for cleanliness.

4. Rinse with scalding hot water and allow to dry. Wipe outside surfaces of freezer with chamois cloth.

5. Do not assemble unless directed to do so.

Precautions to Be Remembered

1. Have all mix line connections tight to prevent mix leaking out and air leaking in.

2. Check controls frequently to ensure proper operation.

3. Drain oil trap frequently to ensure that all oil, water, etc., has been removed from the system.

4. Never bend scraper blades. Never drop the freezer dasher. Be careful when removing it from the freezing cylinder.

5. Allow freezing chamber to warm up prior to rinsing with hot or warm water.

6. Check the pump motor to ensure proper lubrication and proper tightness of pulley belts.

7. Use extreme care in handling dasher in assembling or in dismantling the freezer in order to prevent personal injury.

Cleaning the Continuous Freezer

When the freezer is not going to be used for 2 hr or more, it should be taken ·apart, cleaned, and sanitized. This is most easily and efficiently done immediately after the last ice cream is drawn. The rinse water should not be over 100°F to rinse out the ice cream, and the dasher during this process should be turned only a few revolutions. The dasher and other removable parts should be removed to a sink and thoroughly scrubbed with a hot (120°F) washing solution, rinsed, sanitized, and stored where they may dry. The freezing chamber and other parts that cannot be placed in a sink must be scrubbed with a hotter (130°F) washing solution using special care to remove the greasy film left on the surface and in the corners (all places difficult to reach) especially at the rear of the chamber. These parts should also be thoroughly rinsed and left open to dry. The freezer should not be assembled until it is to be used.

Freezers are cleaned by the same CIP procedures used for pasteurizing equipment, except milk stone remover needs to be used only twice per month if the equipment is cleaned properly each day. The steps that should be taken in the CIP cleaning of freezers are (1) rinse with water (100°F or less) until rinse water runs clear, (2) flush for 20–30 min with 150–160°F water containing 1–1.5 lb of alkali detergent for each 10 gal of water, (3) rinse until equipment is cooled. When acid cleaner is used, circulate cleaning solution containing sufficient acid (phosphoric and hydroxy-acetic) to give 0.15–0.6% acidity, at 150–160°F and 5–7.5 ft/sec velocity for 20–30 min. Drain and rinse with water at 145°F for 5–7 min.

During the cleaning cycle all dead ends, air valve connections, and the like should be bled and the freezer run 10 sec each 10 min.

While the circuits are assembled the sanitation crews can run 180–200°F water through the entire system each time after cleaning, and then, before starting the operation again, 100–200 ppm chlorine solution can be run through the entire system.

PROGRAMMED ICE CREAM FREEZER OPERATION

A programmed ice cream freezer operation is designed for economy through the elimination of many costly manual operations and through the improvement of production efficiency. Basic functions can be performed in the simplest way by the use of a manual selector switch and air-operated valves as illustrated in Fig. 12.13. Greater degrees of automated operation than are shown in Fig. 12.13, with more sophisticated controls, can be built into each system at the option of the ice cream manufacturer. Such a system is shown in Fig. 12.14.

Advantages of Such a System

1. Quality control
   (a) All conditions for operation will be met before actual ice cream production can begin.
   (b) There will be proper sanitizing of equipment before production.
   (c) There will be no intermixing of flavors.
2. Quick changeover
   (a) A flavor change can be made in minutes.
   (b) There are product savings with air blow to rerun.
   (c) Quality control is maintained through proper rinsing and sanitizing with no flavor intermixing.

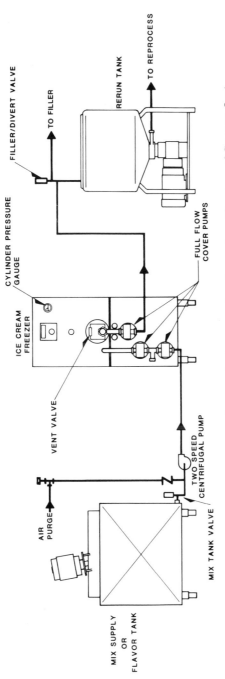

Fig. 12.13. Basic programming elements for ice cream freezing system. (Courtesy of Crepaco, Inc.)

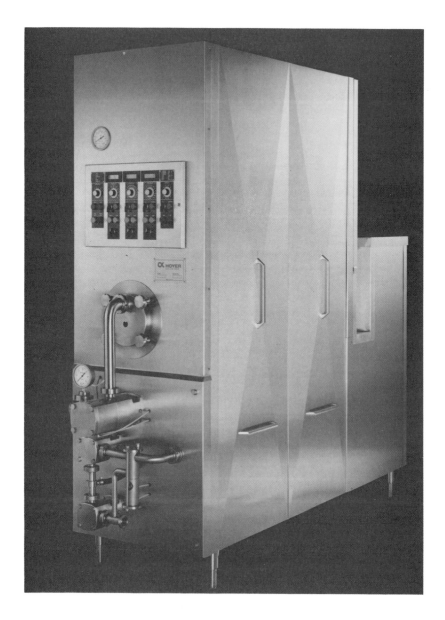

Fig. 12.14. A Hoyer microprocessor controlled freezer. These units are fully equipped with automatic controls for stop/start, viscosity, and overrun. (Courtesy of Hoyer—Alfa Laval Group.)

3. Product and labor savings
   (a) There is a minimum loss of mix with the bypass to rerun system.
   (b) The rerun system handles rerun as it is produced so that it can be added to the mix vat without disrupting the operation of the freezer with no carryover or reprocessing cost.
   (c) There are further savings and improved performance with CIP washing, rinsing, and sanitizing.

Sequence of Operation

1. Sanitizing
   (a) Sanitizing solution is in the mix tank and operator turns the program selector switch to the sanitize position and actuates the start switch: (1) mix tank valve opens; (2) two-speed pump runs at fast speed; (3) mix and mix-air pump bypasses open; and (4) ice cream pump bypass opens.
   (b) Automatic divert valve is switched from the filler position to the rerun position so that both lines are sanitized.
   (c) When the solution has run for a predetermined time, the operator actuates the stop switch: (1) mix tank valve closes; (2) two-speed pump stops; (3) mix and mix-air pump bypasses close; (4) ice cream pump bypass closes. The sanitize cycle must be followed by the air purge cycle to force the sanitizing solution out of the lines and the freezer.
2. Air purging
   (a) The operator turns the program selector to the air purge position and actuates the start switch: (1) mix tank valve closes; (2) air purge valve opens; (3) bypasses on pumps are open.
   (b) When product is clear of lines, operator presses stop button.
3. Filling
   (a) The operator turns the program selector to fill and actuates the start switch: (1) mix tank valve opens; (2) two-speed pump runs at fast speed; (3) mix and mix-air pump bypasses open; (4) ice cream pump bypass closes; and (5) the vent valve remains open for predetermined time, then closes and the freezer cylinder pressurizes. When the operator observes the correct pressure on the sanitary gauge, the operator actuates the stop switch.
4. Freezing:
   The operator turns the program selector to freeze and acuates the start switch
   (a) Mix tank valve opens.
   (b) Two-speed pump starts at low speed.
   (c) The pump bypasses are closed and the freezer is ready to be operated in its normal manner for both freezing and shutdown. The air purge cycle is now available for evacuation of the freezer after shutdown.
5. Rinsing:
   The rinse cycle is a repetition of the sanitizing cycle except that rinse water is used instead of sanitizing solution.

6. CIP:
    This system is so designed that the application of cleaning solutions can be integrated with the rinsing and sanitizing functions.

Changing Flavors

Darker flavors should follow lighter ones without shutting down. In case strawberry or any other flavor containing seeds or particles of fruit or nuts has been frozen, it is necessary to stop the freezer, open the pumps, and wash pumps, lines, freezing tube and tank in order for fruits and seeds to be removed before freezing the next flavor. Practically all the mix, of which there will be only a small quantity, can be saved by draining before washing out the equipment.

Preparing Fruits and Nuts

The juice should be drained from fruit and the fruit placed into the hopper as dry as possible. This prevents undesirable ice formation in the ice cream from the introduction of unfrozen fruit juice. The fruit juices and flavoring materials must be added to the mix before the mix is frozen.

The nuts are usually dry and can be put into the hopper without further preparation.

Specially prepared fruits and nuts should be drained if they come packed in syrup or juice and the syrup or juice added to the mix. It may be found desirable with canned nuts packed in heavy syrup to dissolve the syrup with a small amount of mix before draining the nuts.

Mixtures of fruit and nuts should be mixed together in the fruit hopper and not before. Do not fill the hopper full of a mixture because the fruits and nuts will then mix slowly and may not mix as completely as desired. It is better to fill the hopper about half full and add the fruit and nuts to the hopper a little more frequently.

Candy must be well broken up into pieces that are to show in the ice cream and should not be larger than 3/8 in. square. Large pieces of candy are likely to cause jamming in the equipment, and so the candy should be screened to take out large pieces. The hopper should not be filled, but small portions should be added at frequent intervals since, if large amounts are put in, the candy is likely to stick together and form balls. It is very desirable, where possible, to put any nuts together with candy as would be the case with walnut and pecan crunch. The higher the percentage of nuts in the mixture, the better the operation, since some of the moisture in the candy is absorbed by the nuts and the tendency of the candy to stick together is minimized. An alternative method of using candy, which gives good results, is to add just enough mix to it to give it a slight flow. This helps prevent the candy from sticking and aids materially in feeding it into the ice cream.

Any product to be fed into the ice cream, particularly nuts and firm-bodied fruits in large pieces should not be fed into the freezer or fruit feeder. Break or cut the pieces to some extent, but they should remain large enough to show well in the finished ice cream.

THE BATCH FREEZER

The batch freezer, in which each batch must be measured, flavored, and colored separately, is the one most used in small plants, and in large plants for special sherbets and ices (see Fig. 12.15).

The dasher, which fits into the freezing chamber and can be easily removed for cleaning, is an important part of every batch freezer. In the batch freezer it consists of two parts, the scraper blades and the beater. It is, of course, important to have the dasher in proper alignment and the blades sharp.

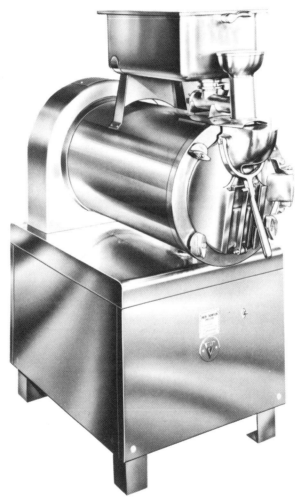

Fig. 12.15. A batch ice cream freezer that makes 40 qt at a time, and has the capacity to produce more than 70 gal/hr.

The temperature of the refrigerant is very important and should be from -10 to $-20°F$ in order to get a rapid formation of ice crystals. This rapid formation favors the development of small crystals and results in a smoother ice cream. However, the freezing should be slow enough to permit incorporating the desired amount of air, since this also affects the body and texture of the ice cream. The most desirable refrigerant temperature to use depends on (1) the efficiency of the freezer, i.e., the heat transfer rate of the walls, (2) the freezing point of the mix (based on the amount of MSNF, sugar, and flavoring material present), (3) the sharpness of the scraper blades, and (4) the amount of refrigerant available.

In the direct-expansion freezers, the freezing chamber is surrounded by liquid ammonia or other refrigerant. Ammonia is the most common refrigerant and has now nearly replaced other types for both the batch and continuous freezers in ice cream factories because it is cheaper due to saving in power and equipment, and it increases refrigeration capacity.

Freezing Procedure for Batch Freezers

The first step in the freezing procedure is to prepare the freezer. Its parts should be inspected to be sure they are clean and dry, and then assembled in accordance with instructions from the manufacturer. The operator's hands should be clean to avoid contamination of the product, which later contacts these parts. When the freezer is assembled, some operators sanitize the machine by running hot water or a cold solution of a chemical sanitizing agent through the machine. In addition to sanitizing, this may also serve to test for leaks and faulty operating condition. While sanitizing, the dasher should not be turned more than a few revolutions, to avoid excessive wear. If hot water is used, it must be at least 180°F to obtain any sanitizing effect, and must be followed by a cold water rinse to cool the freezer. When a chemical sanitizing agent is used, complete draining is essential.

The second step in the freezing procedure is adding the mix. When the freezer has been properly prepared, it is ready for the measured amount of mix, flavoring, and coloring. It is always desirable to have the temperature of the mix below 40°F when it goes into the freezer. Color and flavorings should be accurately measured and poured into the mix rather than carelessly poured on the sides of the vat or freezer. Uniform drainage of the measuring cups is essential for accurate measurement. The total volume of the mix, flavor, and color should be about half the total capacity of the freezing chamber. Thus, in vanilla and similar ice creams flavored with 1 pt or less of extract and color, it is customary to use 20 qt of mix in a 40-qt freezer; while in fruit or nut ice creams 18 qt of mix with about 2 qt of fruit or nuts make up the 20 qt of mixture for a batch.

The flavoring and coloring materials must be added so as to become uniformly distributed, but the actual moment or order of adding them may be varied. Special precautions apply when adding acid fruits, nuts, etc.; these should be added only after some ice crystals have formed. Acid fruits will coagulate the milk in the mix if they are added before the ice crystals start to form. Nuts, candy, and cookies will be less likely to dissolve if added late, and fruits will remain in larger pieces. Therefore, such materials should be added as late as possible and still give time enough to have them uniformly distributed; it is best to determine the exact time for each machine, since some machines are more efficient in carrying the nuts back into the freezer; but generally it is safe to accept the manufacturer's directions as a basis. When using a continuous freezer, the solid materials (nuts, fruit, etc.) must be added as the ice cream is being discharged from the freezing chamber and all liquid material including fruit juices must be added to the mix before it passes into the freezing chamber.

Finally, the freezer should be operated uniformly as to speed, refrigerant, temperature, etc. The refrigerant temperature should be well below 0°F.

The mix is run into the freezer, the dasher started, and then the refrigerant is turned onto the freezing chamber. This sequence must be preserved to avoid damage to the machine. To avoid rapid dulling and wearing of the scraper blades, the dasher must never be operated when there is no mix in the freezer. The refrigerant must never be turned on unless the dasher is in motion because even a drop of water may freeze the dasher to the wall of the freezer and cause the dasher to be bent or twisted when attempting to start the machine. This order of operation and these precautions apply to all freezers regardless of size, type, or installation.

Operating the Batch Freezer

The use of batch freezers makes it difficult to prevent undesirable variations and burdens the operator with many more details to get uniform quality. Each batch of mix must be measured, colored, and flavored separately, requiring the measurement of smaller quantities which presents many more chances for errors with resulting lack of uniform quality of finished ice cream. A carefully prepared work plan will avoid many errors (such as forgetting to add color).

Using the sequence previously described, the machine is started, and then the operator must determine largely by observation, through the peephole, the correct time to shut off the refrigerant. At this correct time, only a small part of the water in the mix is frozen, giving it a certain luster and consistency that must be recognized.

Shutting off the refrigerant too soon results in (1) longer time to obtain overrun, (2) possible failure to obtain the desired overrun as the softer condition will repel overrun, (3) too high a temperature when drawn from the freezer, (4) soft ice cream, and (5) a tendency toward coarse ice cream since the ice crystals formed slowly in the hardening room will be larger. When the refrigerant is not shut off soon enough, the mixture is too hard and results in (1) difficulty in obtaining overrun, (2) longer time in the freezer, as stiff ice cream repels whipping (even if it is allowed to soften in an effort to incorporate air), (3) usually a lower temperature when drawn from the freezer, and (4) a smoother ice cream provided it does not become soft in obtaining overrun.

After the refrigerant is shut off, the machine within certain limits continues to operate, incorporating air and freezing more of the mixture until the product attains both the desired overrun and the desired consistency. Then the operator allows the product to be drawn from the freezer. Since the air is incorporated during the freezing process and by the whipping action of the dasher, the operator must adjust the refrigerant to allow the right amount of time for whipping. This time will vary with the composition of the mix, the construction of the freezer, the rate of cooling or freezing, and the consistency, temperature, etc., in the freezer. These latter conditions change so rapidly in the freezer that they can only be estimated by the operator's observation and this requires study as well as considerable experience. While there is some loss of air, in general it can be said that up to a certain point air is being continually whipped into the ice cream mix. However, after that point is reached it loses air faster than it gains it, if the whipping is carried on too long. Therefore the operator must adjust the refrigerant so that the ice cream can be drawn at the moment the desired overrun and consistency of the ice cream are obtained. When the ice cream is drawn from the freezer it should be stiff enough to "ribbon" or almost hold its shape, and yet soft enough to "settle" or lose its shape within a minute or two.

Filling the Containers

The container or package into which the ice cream is drawn should be cooled sufficiently to prevent melting the ice cream. When such melting around the edges does occur, it will be frozen again later in the hardening room and the ice crystals formed will be large, giving a coarse and icy condition at the edge of the package. Furthermore, this melting will cause a loss of overrun. Another precaution to take is against the formation of air-pockets, which leave the container partly filled. This can be avoided easily if the ice cream is not too stiff when drawn. Precaution should also be taken to see that chocolate ice cream, acid fruit-flavored ice cream, sherbets, and ices are placed either in well-tinned containers or more safely in paper or paper-lined containers, since the acid in these products will react with the iron to cause undesirable defects.

The freezer should be emptied as rapidly as possible to prevent wide fluctuations in overrun in the packages. Therefore, avoid filling small packages directly from the batch freezer. When a 40-qt freezer is emptied into 2-1/2 gal containers, the first one may have 90% overrun, the second 100%, the third 80%, and the fourth 70% overrun. The variation will follow this general up and down trend, the extent of variation depending on the length of time required for filling each container.

If metal containers are filled it is usually desirable to put a parchment paper over the top under the cover. This paper protects the metal cover and may also be used to designate the flavor of the ice cream, date made, and possibly a key number to identify the operator, the batch of mix, and freezer batch— information that aids in handling inventories, records, and tracing the cause of defects.

While the ice cream is being drawn from the freezer it gradually becomes softer and should not be "drained" out when it gets too soft. A possible exception to this rule is to drain the freezer completely when it is to be taken apart and cleaned. At other times the small amount left in the freezer goes into the next batch, which can follow immediately without stopping the dasher. However, if the next batch is of a different flavor or color, i.e., one that will not cover up or blend with the previous batch, it is necessary to take out the dasher and clean the freezer. This is especially true of nut and fruit ice creams, since pieces of nuts and fruit cannot be removed from the dasher without taking the freezer apart, but if left in the freezer they will appear in the next batch of ice cream.

HOW TO OBTAIN AND CONTROL OVERRUN

Overrun is usually defined as the volume of ice cream obtained in excess of the volume of the mix. It is usually expressed as percentage of overrun. This increased volume is composed mainly of air incorporated during the freezing process. The amount of air that should be incorporated depends upon the composition of the mix and the way it is processed, and is regulated so as to give the percentage of overrun or yield that will give the proper body, texture, and palatability necessary to good-quality ice cream. Too much air will produce a snowy, fluffy, unpalatable ice cream; too little air, a soggy, heavy product. Generally, mixes with a high TS content justify the incorporation of a higher percentage of air—a higher overrun—than mixes lower in TS. Although no definite percentage can be stated, some authorities indicate as most desirable an overrun between two and three times the percentage of TS content of the mix. For example, a mix with a TS content of 40% might justify an overrun of as high as 100%. Formulas for determining the overrun and solving problems in overrun are discussed in Chapter 10.

Five factors that are usually considered when determining the amount of overrun are

1. Legal regulations enforced in the market area.
2. TS content of the ice cream. Higher TS may permit use of a higher overrun.
3. Bulky-flavor ice creams (such as fruit and nut) require a lower overrun than plain ice cream in order to obtain an equally desirable body and texture. The correct overrun to take may be estimated as described in Chapter 10.
4. Selling price of ice cream.
5. Type of package. So-called "bulk" packages, which are sold for "dipping," usually contain 90–100% overrun, while packages of the carry-home type (not dipped before reaching the consumer) usually are most satisfactory if they contain 70–80% overrun.

The ability to obtain overrun at the freezer depends partly on the concentration and type of ingredients in the mix (see discussion in Chapter 11 on influence of sugars, TS, etc.) and on the freezing process itself. Sharpness of scraper blades, speed of dasher, volume of refrigerant passing over freezing chamber and temperature of refrigerant are important, as described previously, to produce rapid freezing and favor overrun. The stiffness of the product at the time refrigerant is shut off and the fullness of the freezer are two of the most important factors and perhaps the two most likely to fluctuate under careless operation.

England (1968) outlined the factors of overrun control as factors that depress overrun and factors that enhance overrun with factors specific for continuous freezers. The factors that depress overrun included

- fat content
- MSNF content
- corn syrup solids content
- increased amount of stabilizer
- fruits, cocoa, and chocolate
- excessive calcium salts
- poor homogenization
- amount of mix in batch freezer
- insufficient refrigeration
- mix too warm
- dull freezer blades
- freezing the mix too stiff

Factors specific for continuous freezers included

- slow freezer speed
- slow pump speed
- pumps worn or need adjusting
- pump spring bent
- fruit feeder operation

The factors listed as enhancing overrun included

- sodium caseinate
- whey solids
- egg yolks
- emulsifiers
- certain stabilizers
- certain salts
- pasteurization of mix at a higher temperature

Those factors specific for continuous freezers included

- air leaks in mix intake line
- erratic springs in air intake valve
- height of flavor tank
- volume of mix in the flavor tank
- distance of flavor tank from freezer
- worn second-stage air pump.

To secure uniform overrun and yield, the following points should receive attention:

1. Uniformity in refrigerant temperature and rate of flow of refrigerant.
2. The use of overrun testers, Draw-Rite or Willman controls.
3. Uniform make, etc., of freezers for the freezer person.
4. Not too many freezers per worker.
5. Hopper systems for filling containers if batch freezers are used. This allows freezers to be emptied rapidly into a hopper where there is less agitation while filling packages. Higher overrun at the freezer is necessary to compensate for some loss in overrun in the hopper.
6. The use of a system of checking the weight of packages or containers as they enter the hardening room.

Table 12.3. Percentage Overrun for Different Products

Product	Overrun (%)
Ice cream, packaged	70–80
Ice cream, bulk	90–100
Sherbet	30–40
Ice	25–30
Soft ice cream	30–50
Ice milk	50–80
Milk shake	10–15
Superpremium ice cream	0–20

The control of overrun is very important and should be maintained as nearly constant as possible from batch to batch and from day to day. A variation of 10% in overrun represents a sizable difference in profit to the manufacturer. Lack of uniformity is also frowned upon by the retailer and the consumer. The experienced, intelligent operator, with the aid of an overrun tester or laboratory checks, should not have much trouble with the control of overrun.

The correct overrun percentage depends upon the kind and composition of product and freezing equipment. The overrun on different products may normally range as shown in Table 12.3.

13
Packaging, Hardening, and Shipping

PACKAGING

When ice cream is drawn from the freezer, it is put into containers that give it the desired form and size for convenient handling during the hardening, shipping, and marketing processes. The packaging of ice cream is of two types: bulk packaging for the sale of dipped ice creams, and packaging for direct retail sale.

Bulk Packaging

Bulk packaging of ice cream was originally done entirely in reusable, or multiservice, containers, which had to be cleaned and sanitized before refilling. These were steel cans that had been tinned with lead solder. Now that throwaway, or single-service, containers have become standard in the industry, the reusable can is not used much any more, but the steel can remains the main type of reusable container.

The vast improvement of the highway system after World War II, the development of reliable refrigerated delivery trucks and mechanically refrigerated cabinets, and the now widespread use of continuous freezers and automatic packaging equipment all hastened the appearance of the single-service container. Consumer tastes and purchasing habits also favored this type of ice cream package. These containers are generally made of fiberboard, either paper or cardboard, which has been treated to make it impervious to moisture.

The developments that led to the single-service package also created the potential for greatly increased production. The many different types of automatic packaging devices allow for handling a wide variety of sizes and shapes, but for the most part, bulk ice cream is packaged in 5-, 3-, and 2-1/2-gal fiberboard containers. The forming and filling of these containers is done in one of two ways: the single-spindle conveyor or the manual single spindle. In the former, using a single-spindle can former, the worker moves the cans on a conveyor for filling, closing, and labeling (see Fig. 13.1). In the latter, all of the operations are done manually. Because the cost of equipment remains high, the manual system is still the less expensive.

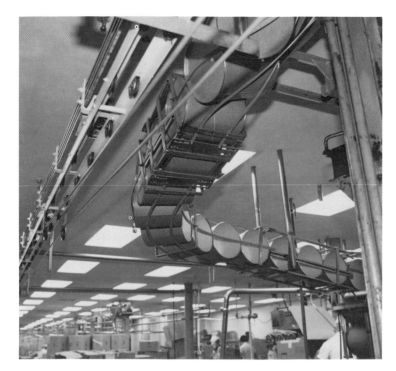

Fig. 13.1. Conveying cartons of ice cream in a processing room. Two types of overhead conveyor are shown: the cable type on the left carries filled cartons at relatively high speed; the gravity-flow type on the right feeds bulk containers to a bulk filler. (Courtesy of Dean Foods Company.)

Packaging for Direct Retail Sale

Ice cream for direct retail sale is packaged in containers of several sizes, depending on the type of market outlet and local consumer preferences. Some plants concentrate their production on one particular size, while others package only novelties. Many plants also handle two sizes of cups: 5 and 3 oz. Although there are a number of methods of doing this—involving combinations ranging from one worker and an automated system to five or more workers and a manual system—the lowest-cost method will depend on individual plant conditions and production capacity.

The percentage of ice cream packaged in the standard containers is as follows:

Carton size	Amount (%)
Less than 1 pt	0.9
Pint	8.2
Quart	2.8
Half-gallon	81.5
Gallon	5.0
Novelties	1.6

Packaging ice cream involves forming, filling, closing, weighing, and bagging the containers. Containers are bagged to reduce the unit number of packages that have to be handled and to keep the individual containers clean.

The ice cream put into the factory-filled carryout container usually has a lower overrun than the same product put into bulk packages. This difference is commonly 15–20% and partially compensates for the greater weight obtained when the dealer dips a similar package from the retail cabinet.

Economy of Packaging Operation

Getting the most out of a filling operation requires the application of statistical quality control. The problem of how best to schedule production is essentially one of inventory and the most economical length of run. An analysis of this problem can be done by using an optimizing lot size formula, where the number of units produced per run, the number of units required per time unit, the cost of holding a unit in inventory (storage) per unit of time, and the cost of setting up and tearing down for production run are factors (see, for example, Kramer and Arbuckle, 1965).

Fill control is also important and may be determined by examining how much of a variation normally occurs from one filler to another, and from one container to another from the same filler. Relatively simple procedures are available for using this information (Kramer and Arbuckle 1965). Variations of a statistically significant magnitude then provide information that can be used as a basis for control adjustments. A control chart with an upper control limit and a lower control limit provides a guide for closer control.

THE HARDENING PROCESS

When ice cream is drawn from the freezer and put into the container to be placed in the hardening room, it has a semifluid consistency and is not stiff enough to hold its shape. Therefore, the freezing process is continued without agitation until the temperature of the ice cream reaches 0°F or lower, preferably −15°F. Here, as in the freezer, quick hardening is desirable, since slow hardening favors the formation of large ice crystals and a corresponding coarseness of texture.

The time required for hardening has been assumed to be the time necessary for the temperature at the center of the package to drop to 0°F. This hardening time for a still-air operation (described below) may be as short as 30 min for 1/4-pt packages or as long as 24 hr for 5-gal packages. The shorter time always gives a smoother ice cream. A hardening time of 6–8 hr for 5-gal packages is usually considered an excellent operation, but most operators allow at least 12 hr. When hardening tunnels are used (see discussion below) the rate of hardening is several times faster (Fig. 13.2).

Factors Affecting the Hardening Time

Some of the more important factors affecting the hardening time are (Tracy and McCown 1934) as follows:

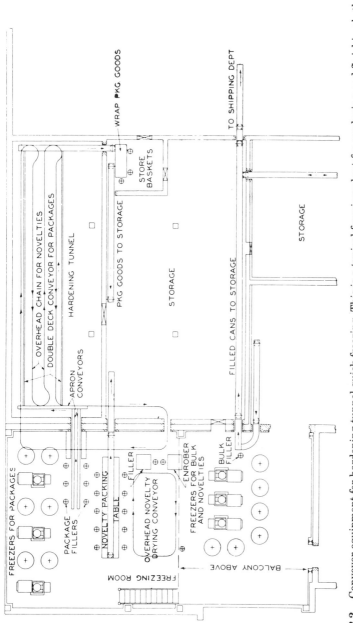

Fig. 13.2. Conveyor equipment for hardening-tunnel quick freezing. This is a typical freezing plant for producing and finishing both bulk and package novelties, either coated or uncoated. A plant of this size can freeze as much as 450 gal in pint cartons and 200 trays of frozen novelties per hour. The mix is prepared elsewhere in the plant and delivered to storage tanks in the freezing room for processing. Conveyors propel the packages of novelties through the hardening tunnels and into the storage room. The conveyors are also arranged to speed delivery to the shipping department. (Courtesy of Alvey Conveyor Manufacturing Co.)

1. *Size and shape of package.*   Doubling the size of the package increases the hardening time by about 50%; when 2-1/2 gal packages require 14 hr, 5-gal packages will require about 22 hr. The shape is important in determining the amount of surface area per gallon of ice cream and also the speed of airflow around the package. Light-colored packages and those having good reflecting surfaces are slower to cool.

2. *Air circulation.*   With forced circulation like an air blast, hardening requires only about 60% of the time required in still air. Of course, the speed of the air blast is also important. Properly stacking the packages facilitates rapid air movement, which also suggests the desirability of hardening each package rather than making bundles of packages.

3. *Temperature of the air.*   Temperatures above $-10°F$ and colder than $-25°F$ are less desirable from the standpoint of quality of product and economical operation.

4. *Section of the room.*   In the still-air type of room, the ice cream hardens about as quickly near the ceiling as on the floor, while directly on the ammonia coils it requires only two-thirds as much time. The center aisle requires twice as long.

5. *Temperature of ice cream drawn from the freezer.*   Each degree higher at which the ice cream is drawn will increase the hardening time by about 10–15%.

6. *Composition of the mix.*   There is a tendency for a shorter hardening time as the fat content decreases and as the freezing point of the mix rises.

7. *Percentage overrun.*   There is a slight tendency for the hardening time to increase as the percentage overrun increases.

When ice cream was frozen in the continuous freezer and was subsequently hardened by contact with $-30°F$ refrigerated plates, by immersion in $-40°F$ brine, or by placing it in a $-20°F$ moving air room, very little difference could be detected in the body and texture scores of the ice cream after storage in a $0°F$ cabinet for 24 or 72 hr. The brine- and plate-hardened samples were both judged to be slightly superior to samples air-hardened at $-20°F$. The results indicated that rapid freezing in both the freezing and hardening phases influenced the texture of ice cream.

The first reported work (Der Hovanesian 1960) on immersion of ice cream packages in liquid nitrogen for hardening indicated that a center temperature of $-30°F$ in pint packages could be reached in less than 5 min with the outer temperature of the product at $-250°F$ or lower. Other studies (Pearson 1963) showed that when individual pint packages of vanilla ice cream were immersed in liquid nitrogen at $-320°F$ for 1 min, bagged together in groups of 8 packages, and placed in a hardening cabinet at $-9°F$, a product possessing good body and texture resulted. The body and texture were comparable to that achieved when individual pint packages were exposed to wind tunnel conditions for approximately 90 min.

The same conditions of body and texture did not result when pint packages were immersed in liquid nitrogen for 1 min and placed separately in the hardening cabinet. The improved body and texture of the overwrapped package of 8 units are probably due to the reserve of refrigeration stored in the hardened shell of each individual unit, which extracts heat from the center of each unit at an ideal rate to produce desirable body and texture characteristics. If the time of exposure to liquid nitrogen of each pint package was extended beyond 1 min, the texture became very smooth to "salvy" and the body became crumbly. Ice cream hardened by liquid-nitrogen immersion was decidedly whiter in appearance than that which was slowly hardened. This phenomenon is probably due to the fact that very rapid hardening, such as occurs by exposure to liquid nitrogen produces many smaller crystals than does the conventional hardening method, resulting in greater light reflection. Although immersion of pint packages in liquid nitrogen for 1 min produced an ice cream with desirable body and texture characteristics immediately after hardening, it also produced pronounced shrinkage in the ice cream after a 2-week storage period. Along with the shrinkage, the surface of the ice cream appeared dry and cracked, became yellow in appearance, and was gummy to the taste. This demonstrated a visible breakdown in the structure of the ice cream at the surface. One-minute immersion per pint was considered the maximum treatment to which ice cream could be subjected without adversely affecting body and texture. It was calculated that 0.56 lb of liquid nitrogen was required per pound of ice cream.

FAST-HARDENING SYSTEMS FOR ICE CREAM

The problems of the fast hardening of ice cream and fast-hardening systems for ice cream have been capably discussed and illustrated by Anderson (1958) and include some of the following suggestions. The ice cream manufacturer may act in three ways to fast-harden ice cream: (1) improve hardening-room design, (2) install fast-hardening system for contact- or blast-hardening, and (3) install fast-hardening systems with controlled handling in a portion of the hardening room.

Hardening Room

In a good hardening room, fast hardening can be accomplished by following these suggested rules: (1) have plenty of refrigeration to maintain temperatures at $-20°F$ or colder, (2) maintain good air turbulence around products, (3) provide sufficient space for a 5- or 6-day inventory based on 14 gal/ft^2 and 8–10 gal/ft^2 for a few large items, (4) recognize the limitations of the hardening room.

Hardening rooms (Fig. 13.3) where the packaged ice cream is placed in dry air maintained at a temperature between 10 and $-50°F$ are used currently by manufacturers. Most factories employ ammonia or Freon as the refrigerant to maintain a temperature of -20 or $-25°F$. For economical operation, the hardening room should be entered through an anteroom, which may be large enough to permit storage of some ingredients at about 30°F.

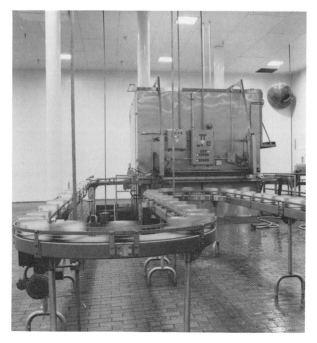

Fig. 13.3. Contact plate hardener. (Courtesy of Crepaco, Inc.)

Precautions to Observe in the Operation of Hardening Rooms

1.   Sometimes the latch on the door fails to operate properly, making it impossible to open the door from the inside and trapping the operator. At such times, a telephone or alarm system for calling for help is necessary and should be installed in such a manner as to attract help from outside when regular workers in the plant are absent.

2.   Keep both an ax and a sledge hammer in a prescribed location just inside the door. These might be needed for breaking through the door as a last resort in case assistance cannot be obtained.

3.   Keep wooden doors, etc., well painted, since moist wood tends to give off odors that are absorbed by unprotected ice cream.

4.   Keep floors, walls, etc., clean. Specialties decorated with whipped cream acquire off-flavors from odors in the air due to dirt.

5.   Do not store nondairy products, wooden boxes, or crates in the hardening room.

6.   Avoid placing ice cream packages close together until hardened.

7.   Avoid placing newly frozen ice cream close to packages that are already hardened.

8.   Have the packages clearly dated and remove the older packages first.

9.   Avoid fluctuations in temperature.

10. Remove frost from the ammonia coils frequently. Frost 1/4 in. thick or more greatly decreases the efficiency of the coils.

11. Whenever feasible avoid keeping the same ice cream in the hardening room for more than 5 days.

12. Take inventory at regular intervals, preferably daily.

Unit Hardening Systems

Numerous types of fast-hardening units are available for pints, half-gallons, single units, or wrapped gallon units. The plate or contact hardeners and blast tunnel hardeners are in general use. Contact hardeners include the plate hardener on the elevating platform and stationary- and rotary-plate types.

Hardening Tunnels

Some manufacturers of larger volumes use hardening tunnels that produce an air blast at -30 to $-50°F$ for fast hardening. These may or may not contain a conveyor belt, and their greatest advantage comes when hardening smaller packages, which can be hardened in 1 hr (Stein *et al.* 1963).

Blast tunnel hardeners have been in use for several years. The conveying systems have been expanded more recently to include the wide flat belt, fixed tray, suspended free tray, and multishelf carrier types of conveyors. The zone hardening tunnel and the ceiling conveyor systems are other types of hardeners. Both of these systems occupy areas within the hardening room. Large volumes of air are discharged in these areas to accomplish fast hardening.

Hardening Cabinet

Hardening cabinets resemble the retail ice cream cabinet and are refrigerated by mechanical refrigeration. The ice cream package is placed in the dry, watertight compartments, each of which will hold one or two 5-gal containers. These are usually operated at a temperature between -10 and $-15°F$, are most economical for a limited volume of business, and avoid exposure of the operator to sudden chilling temperatures.

STORAGE

After the ice cream is hardened it may be immediately marketed, or it may be stored for a week or two at the most. Manufacturers plan on a maximum of 5 days between freezing and marketing, with an average 3-day turnover. At least 12 hr of this time is required for hardening the ice cream which frequently remains in the hardening room until marketed, thus using the same room for both hardening and storage. Since the hardened ice cream can be stored satisfactorily at slightly higher temperatures than are required for hardening, it is sometimes more economical to use special storage rooms. This is particularly true for retailers, who may use one cabinet for storage in addition to the dispensing cabinets.

The operation of storage rooms is the same as for hardening rooms with two exceptions: (1) the temperature should be maintained uniformly at a point between −10 and 0°F, and (2) the packages should be piled very closely to delay changes in the temperature of the ice cream (see Fig. 13.4).

SHIPPING

When the ice cream is marketed, the manufacturer usually ships it to the retailer under refrigeration at the same temperature as is maintained in the retailer's cabinets.

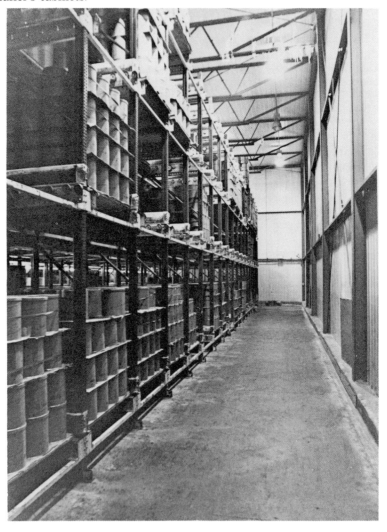

Fig. 13.4. Finished product inventory storage room. After hardening, 3-gal containers are stored on pallets. (Courtesy of Baskin-Robbins Ice Cream Co., Burbank, CA.)

Dry ice (carbon dioxide) is used extensively for package deliveries. This ice is sawed into pieces of appropriate size, which are wrapped in paper to delay rapid evaporation, and then placed around the package of the ice cream inside an insulated packer, or in the single-service type packer. The latter are usually cardboard boxes insulated with corrugated cardboard and are used especially for the carryout packages. This type of refrigeration has several distinct advantages:

1. It is free from moisture and messiness.
2. It requires no salt.
3. Its package is neat in appearance.
4. It does not water-log the insulation.
5. It is very light weight.
6. It is especially good for specialties sold direct to the consumer, where no return trip to pick up packers is required.

The main disadvantages of dry ice are as follows:

1. Present high cost and limited availability.
2. Loss during handling and storage, amounting to 10–15% in many cases, due to the impracticability of providing sufficient insulation in storage boxes.
3. Danger of "burns" to handler: The very low subliming point makes it easy to freeze fingers without the sensation of cold, causing severe damage. Therefore, care must be taken by those who handle it.
4. Necessity for unpacking or removing the ice cream: The ice cream must be unpacked or removed from the dry ice sufficiently long to allow it to soften so as to be easily eaten and so that the delicate flavors may be properly appreciated.
5. The greater opportunity for "heat-shock": When ice cream warms up and then freezes harder again, it receives a heatshock, which may affect the texture. Dry ice freezes the ice cream to lower temperatures than do the usual hardening rooms (the freezing point of dry ice is about $-109°F$).

Mechanical refrigeration, most commonly used for the refrigeration of ice cream during shipping, uses a complete refrigeration system with the expansion coils cooling the packer. These packers are similar to storage rooms, and are mainly truck bodies for trucking large volumes and for long hauls of as much as 48 hr. The subzero temperature is maintained by self-contained diesel temperature control units (usually 41,000 BTU, for control to $-15°F$).

The many problems and the variety of special conditions connected with shipping by truck have made it impossible to standardize the procedure or the truck, and especially difficult to get comparative cost data. For example, costs, efficiency, and depreciation are all influenced by road conditions, the driver, frequency of opening the truck for partial unloading, etc. Therefore, definite limitations and advantages cannot be stated.

Ice cream is loaded directly from the hardening room into refrigerated trucks for shipment to distribution stations near the point of consumption, often many miles from the manufacturing plant. The ice cream is then delivered from the distribution station to the consumer. Manual, conveyor, or pallet handling methods may be used. The temperature of the ice cream during distribution should never rise to a point higher than the temperature of the dealer's cabinet.

14

Soft-Frozen Dairy Products and Special Formulas

SOFT-SERVE PRODUCTS

There is a marked demand for the form of ice cream that has generally come to be known as soft or soft-serve ice cream.[1] This term has been applied largely because these products are marketed in a soft form and are ready for consumption shortly after they are drawn from the freezer.

Stores selling soft-serve products sometimes combine these products with other food items or sell both hard products and handle soft serve products only. Figure 14.1 gives an illustration of a floor plan for a store selling soft-serve products.

Several functional types of soft-serve freezers are available, including floor models, counter-top models, two- or three-flavor models, models combining milk shake and soft serve , low-overrun machines, milk shake machines, and batch or continuous equipment. Some of these are shown in Figs. 14.2–14.5.

Figure 14.6 shows a complete soft-serve system. The machine on the left is a multiflavor shake maker. This machine automatically dispenses flavor and product into the cup when the front gate pedal is raised. At the same time, the mixer motor starts blending the flavor with the product. The operator has the choice of three flavors plus "neutral," and can produce a flavored shake in less than 10 sec. The manufacturer rates the capacity of the machine at 35 gal of finished product per hour, which is the equivalent of approximately six 12-oz (by volume) milk shakes per minute.

The soft-serve fountain in the center incorporates a storage compartment for either 5- or 10-gal mix cans, ice tray, and a two-station drink-dispensing system, which provides the operator with a choice of six different carbonated or noncarbonated beverages. The system uses an ice-bank–sweet-water bath for chilling the syrup and water, which provides for a 1-hr surge capacity of seven 6-oz drinks per minute. Six crushed fruit or syrup topping jars are also provided.

---

[1]The term "frozen custard" is often used erroneously as referring to all soft-serve products. In most areas, frozen custards are required to contain egg solids. Generally the requirements range from 2.5 to 5.0 dozen egg yolks per 90 lb of products. Custards may be served soft or hardened. The egg yolk solids content must not be less than 1.4% of the weight of the finished product.

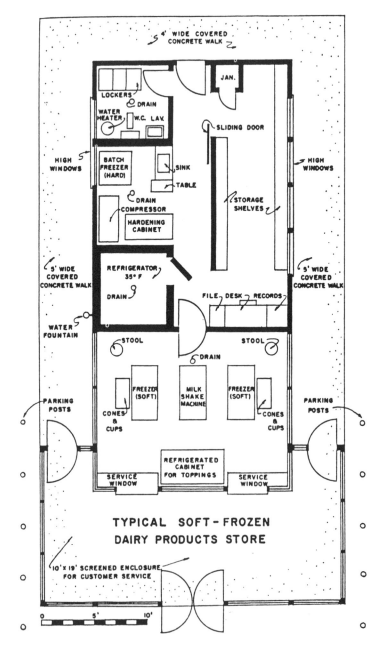

Fig. 14.1. Floor plan for a typical soft-frozen dairy products store. (Courtesy of Eugene T. McGarrahan.)

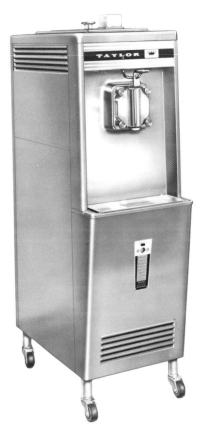

Fig. 14.2.   Taylor floor-type soft-serve freezer. (Courtesy of Taylor Freezer, Rockton, IL.)

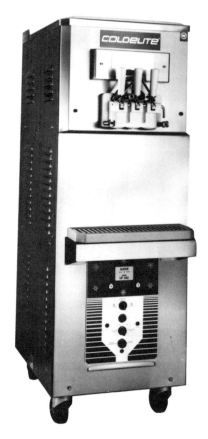

Fig. 14.3. Double-flavor soft-serve freezer. (Courtesy of Coldelite Corp. of America, South Lodi, NJ.)

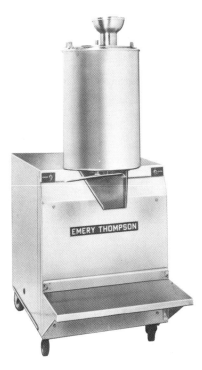

Fig. 14.4. Vertical 20-qt batch freezer with self-contained water-cooled condensing unit. Capacity, 20 gal/hr, 40–60% overrun. (Courtesy of Emery Thompson Machine Supply Company, Bronx, NY.)

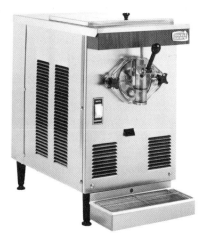

Fig. 14.5. Counter-type soft-serve freezer. Capacity, 20 qt. (Courtesy of Sani Serv, Indianapolis, IN.)

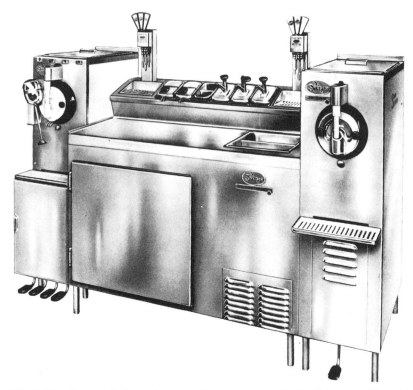

Fig. 14.6.   A complete fountain system for soft-serve products. (Courtesy of Sweeden Freezer Co.)

The machine on the right is the soft-serve freezer. This machine is rated at a continuous production capacity of 15 gal of finished product per hour, which is the equivalent of 10 2-oz (by weight) servings per minute.

CLEANING SOFT-SERVE FREEZING UNITS

The West Virginia Department of Agriculture, Consumer Protection Division, outlines the following procedure for the sanitary maintenance and cleaning of freezer units at the close of operations each day.

1.   Turn off refrigeration to freezing cylinder and turn beaters on to draw off any remaining product.
2.   Rinse freezer with 2 qt of cold tap water.
3.   Prepare 2 gal hot washing solution. Use a chlorinated detergent designed for this type of cleaning and follow the manufacturer's recommended usage for proper strength.
4.   Remove hopper cover and mix tube assembly. Fill the mix hopper with 1

gal of cleaning solution. Brush mix hopper thoroughly as solution in entering the freezer cylinder and clean mix feed tube with brush.

5. Run beaters 30 sec and draw off. Rinse with warm water.

6. Remove freezer door and disassemble all freezer parts. Brush parts, including the hopper cover and feed tube assembly, in the remaining gallon of cleaning solution.

7. Rinse all parts thoroughly. Lubricate seals and valves where necessary and reassemble in freezer.

8. Just before using the freezer, sanitize with 200 ppm chlorine solution. Drain completely but do not rinse with warm water. The freezer is ready to operate. This must be a daily clean-up operation.

SOFT-SERVE MIX COMPOSITION

The way soft-serve products are marketed makes it possible to use formulas that are considerably different from the usual formula. The principal types of mixes used in the production of soft-frozen dairy products are (1) mixes to be frozen and served in a soft form, (2) mixes to be used in the preparation of milk shakes, and (3) products to be frozen in soft-serve freezers and drawn into packages and hardened.

The composition of soft-frozen products varies according to legal standards and the type of product. Typical compositions are given in Table 14.1. The mix composition for soft frozen products may be modified to fulfill local needs and can be processed to meet specifications.

The problems involved in the preparation of soft-serve frozen products are somewhat different from those encountered in the manufacture of regular ice cream. Some of these differences include composition, freezing procedures, stability and whipping properties of the mix, and maintenance of smooth, dry, stiff characteristics of the products as drawn from the freezer.

The fat content of soft-frozen products is important. If the fat content is low (less than 4%) the product tends to be coarse, weak, and icy. If it is high (about 12%) the product may be too rich and less palatable, in addition to presenting freezing difficulties due to possible fat separation during the freezing process.

Table 14.1. Composition (%) of Soft-Serve Products

Kind of product	Fat	MSNF	Sugar	Stabilizer and emulsifier
Soft-serve products (usual range)	3–6	11–14	12–15	0.4–0.6
Soft-serve ice milk				
average	3	14	14	0.4–0.5
above average	6	11.5	13	0.4–0.5
Hardened ice milk	6	12–13	15	0.4–0.5
Ice cream				
average	12	11	15	0.3
above average	16	7–8	15	0.25
Milk shake	4.5	11	8	0.5

The MSNF content of soft-frozen products varies inversely with the fat content and may be as much as 14% for a low-fat formula. MSNF serves to provide proper firmness of body. In products with high MSNF content the lactose may separate during freezing and result in a sandy defect.

Usually the sugar content of soft frozen products is 13–15% which is somewhat lower than for regular ice cream, and the amount of corn sugar used to replace cane sugar is limited to about 25% in order to avoid too low a freezing point.

Stabilizers are used in amounts ranging from 0.2 to 0.4%. Emulsifiers are used in amounts ranging from 0.1 to 0.2% to provide smoothness, desirable whipping properties, melting resistance, and firmness. Such products as calcium sulfate used in amounts of 0.12% may be used to produce body characteristics of dryness and stiffness.

Soft-frozen products are usually drawn from the freezer at 18–20°F. Freezer design varies greatly and the automatic cycling of the ice cream in the freezer may cause major problems including fat separation, sandiness (lactose crystallization), or coarse texture.

The overrun of soft-serve products may be in the 30–50% range depending on the TS content. A higher overrun can be obtained on a product with a high TS content with the maintenance of desired body and texture characteristics.

There is variation of opinion in different areas as to the correct amount of overrun and correct serving temperature for the various soft-serve products. It is obvious that a standard of quality must be set and carefully maintained to avoid unsatisfactory products.

The standards generally used by reputable manufacturers are as follows:

Products	Overrun (%)	Serving temperature (°F)
Soft-serve	40–60	20–22
Milk shake	40–60	26–28
Sherbet	30–50	19–21
Italian ice	30–40	19–21
Hard ice cream	80–100	5–9
Super premium	10–40	5–9

Ice milk accounts for about 75% of the soft-serve volume of production, but several other products are also served soft, including frozen custards, ice cream of regular composition, milk shake base, and frozen malted milk.

Soft-Serve Ice Milk

Ice milk may range from 2 to 7% fat with a minimum of 11% total MSNF. Because of the lower fat content in the ice milk formula, a higher MSNF content is always used to provide a properly balanced mix. The following formulas are typical.

Constituents	%					
Fat	6.0	3.0	4.0	5.0	6.0	3.0
MSNF	13.0	14.0	14.0	13.0	12.5	14.0
Sugar	13.0	10.0	12.0	12.0	11.0	14.0
Corn syrup solids	—	4.0	4.5	4.0	4.0	—
Stabilizer–emulsifier	0.5	0.5	0.5	0.4	0.4	0.5
TS	32.5	31.5	35.0	34.4	33.9	31.5

Hardened Ice Milk

Production costs have been mounting steadily in recent years, a situation that has meant increased costs to consumers. To find a solution to this situation, some have turned to lower-cost formulas for soft ice milk, or to candy-covered bars, stick novelties, and other hardened products using ice milk. The MSNF does not range as high in these hardened ice milk products because storage time is involved and sandiness is less likely to occur in the lower MSNF product. When ice milk is to be used for hardened products or is to be packaged for retail sale to the consumer, the following formulas are typical:

Constituents				%		
Fat	3.0	4.0	4.0	4.0	5.0	6.0
MSNF	12.0	11.0	13.0	12.0	13.0	11.0
Sucrose	15.0	15.0	12.5	11.5	12.0	11.0
Corn syrup solids	—	—	5.0	10.0	6.0	5.0
Stabilizer–emulsifier	0.5	0.5	0.4	0.4	0.4	0.5
TS	30.5	30.5	34.9	37.9	36.4	33.5

Soft-Serve Ice Cream

Soft ice cream is very similar in composition to ice cream that is frozen and hardened. The sugar content may be 2–3% less than for regular ice cream and the drawing temperature from the freezer is 18–20°F or somewhat lower. The overrun of about 50% in soft serve is lower than for ice cream, while the amount of stabilizer–emulsifier product used and the ratio of emulsifier to stabilizer are generally greater for soft-serve ice cream. Corn sweetener solids are not used as extensively in soft-serve ice cream as in products that are hardened. Typical formulas for soft-serve ice cream are as follows:

Constituents			%		
Fat	10.0	10.0	10.0	12.0	12.0
MSNF	13.0	12.0	11.0	10.0	14.0
Sugar	13.0	13.0	12.0	12.0	13.0
Corn syrup solids	—	—	3.0	3.0	—
Stabilizer–emulsifier	0.5	—	0.4	0.4	0.3
TS	36.5	35.0	36.4	37.4	39.3

Frozen Custard

Frozen custards may be of low or high fat content, depending on state regulations. Custards are required to contain a specified quantity of egg yolk solids of not less than 1.4% of the weight of the finished custard for plain-flavored products and 1.12% for bulky-flavored products. Two typical formulas for frozen custard are given below:

Constituents	%	
Fat	5.0	10.0
MSNF	11.0	11.0
Sugar	14.0	14.0
Egg yolk solids	1.4	1.4
Stabilizer	0.5	0.4
TS	31.9	36.8

Milk Shake Mix

A milk shake mix is a product less widely manufactured and not defined in the regulations of many states. The product is of low fat content, relatively high MSNF content, and lower sugar content than ice cream. It may be frozen on a soft-serve machine that has been adjusted to accommodate the freezing of milk shakes. The best milk shakes are obtained when the overrun on the milk shake is maintained below 20%. Since a low overrun is desirable for a good milk shake, the use of an emulsifier in these products is not desirable. Legal requirements for milk shake mix are not less than 25–30% TS and not less than 3.25% milk fat. Two typical formulas follow:

Constituents	%	
Fat	3.5	4.00
MSNF	12.0	14.00
Sugar	10.0	8.00
Corn syrup solids	—	3.50
Stabilizer	0.4	0.35
TS	25.9	29.85

Milk Shake Base

Milk shake base is made from a modified milk shake mix formula. It may be frozen and placed in bulk packages and hardened in the same manner as ice cream. The percentage overrun is usually maintained at 50–60%. This product is dipped into a container to which simple syrup and milk are added in making the milk shake. The following formulas are typical:

Constituents	%		
Fat	3.5	4.0	6.0
MSNF	13.0	12.5	12.5
Sugar	12.0	13.0	13.0
Corn syrup solids	4.0	5.0	4.0
Stabilizer	0.4	0.4	0.4
TS	32.9	34.9	35.9

Malted Milk

Malted milk usually contains 4–7% fat, 10–12% MSNF, 12–13% sugar and cocoa, and malt syrup solids or a commercial malt base. The product is served in a thick, soft-frozen state. The overrun should be carefully controlled on this product also. Some typical formulas are given below:

Constituents	%			
Fat	4.0	6.0	5.00	4.00
MSNF	13.0	12.0	12.00	12.00
Sugar	10.5	10.5	10.50	10.00
Corn syrup solids	4.5	4.5	4.50	—
Malt syrup solids	—	—	0.75	0.75
Cocoa	—	—	3.00	3.00
Malt base	3.0	3.0	—	—
TS	35.0	36.0	35.75	29.75

Italian-Style Ice Cream: Ice and Gelato[2]

These products are popular in some areas. The ice is similar to an American-type ice in composition although it is usually less tart and less sweet, and is normally flavored with an extract flavoring and served in a semihard form. Gelato ice cream has a high milk fat and TS content, carries natural and abundant rich flavor, and has a very low, if any, overrun (0–10%). A variety of liqueur flavors and various fruit combinations may be used. The low overrun and high solids content gives a distinctive body and texture and desirable flavor release. The typical formula is as follows:

Constituents	%
Milk fat	18.0
MSNF	7.5
Sucrose	16.0
Egg yolk solids	4.0
TS	45.5

Soft-Serve Mellorine

These products are identified in the regulation of 14 states. Their formulation may be the same as for regular ice cream, except vegetable fat is substituted for milk fat.

The fat sources may be cottonseed–soybean blend, coconut fat, safflower oil, or other oils. The cottonseed–soybean oil blend is the most common, but the use of coconut oil results in the best product. Additional stabilizer and emulsifier may be used in the formula and some states require not less than 8400 USP units of vitamin A per gallon of 10% fat product, since vegetable fats do not contain this vitamin. The mellorine product may be hardened and marketed as such. In this case the product formula should have a reduction in the MSNF of 0.5–1.0% and a like increase in sweetener solids, with a slight reduction in the emulsifier used. Typical formulas are given below:

Constituents			%		
Vegetable fat	6.00	4.00	6.00	10.00	10.00
MSNF	13.00	13.00	12.00	11.00	13.00
Sugar	13.00	12.00	12.00	12.00	13.00
Corn syrup solids	—	5.00	4.00	4.00	—
Stabilizer	0.30	0.30	0.30	0.25	0.25
Emulsifier	0.15	0.15	0.15	0.15	0.15
Vitamins A and D	Optional				
TS	32.45	34.45	34.45	37.40	36.40

SPECIAL FORMULAS

High-Fat and High-MSNF Ice Cream

When ice cream is made and sold under the usual commercial conditions of large-scale operation, it contains between 36 and 41% TS, and is acceptable to

---

[2]The gelato product does not have a product definition or standard in the United States. Often the product offered for sale as gelato has a composition similar to ice milk but with imported flavoring material of Italian origin (see p. 78).

the largest group of consumers. Ice cream containing more than 41% TS is frequently called high-solids ice cream and seems to be preferred in certain limited or special markets. It contains a larger amount of the expensive milk fat solids than is found in ordinary commercial ice cream. A noticeable characteristic is that it does not melt down to a smooth creamy liquid. The term high-solids ice cream also may be applied to ice cream that contains less than 41% TS, but has a greater concentration of MSNF than the maximum usually prescribed.

Characteristics of High-MSNF Ice Cream

High-MSNF ice cream has been made in the western part of the United States for a long time. It is made by using such specially prepared products as soluble casein and low-lactose skim milk powder. These ingredients increase the "chewiness" and the percentage of desirable milk proteins while at the same time avoiding the lactose concentration that so often causes sandiness. It is also one way of avoiding high fat content or excessive richness. High-MSNF ice cream always contains a higher concentration of MSNF than the maximum stated earlier, but it may contain less than 41% TS provided the fat is less than 14% and no corn syrup solids are used. When balancing a high-MSNF ice cream mix, it is generally desirable to obtain part of the sugar from dextrose, which will slightly lower the freezing point so that the ice cream can be more easily and efficiently dipped from cabinets maintained at the usual temperatures. It is also possible to lower the sugar concentration by as much as 2% without sacrificing any sweetness of taste. At the same time, the MSNF concentration may be raised as much as 3 or 4%. These ice creams need slightly different processing procedures from those used for ordinary commercial ice cream. For example, the homogenizing pressures may need to be lower to avoid a curdy appearance in the melted ice cream; the capacity of the cooler may have to be increased due to the extra viscosity of the mix; and a high overrun is advisable to avoid sogginess.

High-Fat Ice Cream

High-fat ice cream contains more than 16% fat and more than 40% TS. Such ice cream, rich and smooth in texture, has long been a favorite.

High-fat[3] ice cream presents special problems because the influence of the fat on the properties of the ice cream is accentuated. The use of butter, plastic cream, or frozen cream tends to produce excessive viscosity, which interferes with cooling the mix and obtaining the proper overrun. When these products are the only source of fat they should be emulsified in fresh, sweetened skim milk or milk before the other ingredients are added. For this quality of ice cream usually only fresh cream and fresh milk are used to supply the milk

---

[3]The late Professor M.J. Mack of the Massachusetts AES did much research on high-fat ice cream, and the author wishes to credit him with much of the information given here regarding it.

solids. No additional sources, such as condensed milk, condensed skim milk, or skim milk powder, are used. Thus the resulting flavor is that of fresh cream entirely free from any MSNF flavor—an important character of this type of ice cream.

The MSNF content of these ice creams must be low, decreasing as the fat increases. For example, 7.5% MSNF with 18% fat or 7.0% MSNF with 20% fat gives good results. The low concentration of MSNF in relation to the fat content favors a crumbly body, which is a common defect of high-fat ice creams. This crumbly body may be avoided by using 16–17% sucrose (depending somewhat on the fat content), or by using dextrose (not corn syrup solids) to supply about one-fourth of the total sugar. High-fat ice cream needs a higher concentration of sugar than lower-fat ice cream in order to please the majority of consumers. This higher concentration of sugar, especially through the use of dextrose, improves the meltdown of the ice cream, which frequently is very slow and curdy. The stabilizer content must be about the same as for ice cream containing only 14% fat if smoothness is to be secured because lower homogenization pressures are used and the temperature of the ice cream when drawn from the freezer is higher. Formulas for high-fat and high-MSFN ice cream follow:

Constituents	%				
Fat	16.00	17.00	18.0	10.00	12.00
MSNF	8.50	8.00	7.5	14.00	13.50
Sugar	17.00	17.00	18.0	14.00	14.00
Egg yolk solids	0.50	0.50	0.5	—	—
Stabilizer	0.15	0.15	0.1	0.15	0.15
TS	42.15	42.65	41.1	38.15	39.65

Problems in Processing and Freezing. High-fat ice cream also presents problems in processing and freezing. Homogenization is considered essential to prevent partial churning in the freezer, especially in those freezers constructed to accomplish a drastic whipping action. However, relatively low homogenization pressures must be used, decreasing as the fat content is increased. When fresh cream and fresh milk are the only sources of milk solids, either single- or double-stage homogenization can give good results. The range of pressures in Table 14.2 is recommended as a guide.

In addition to changing the homogenization pressure, it may also be desirable to raise the freezing temperature progressively with each increase in fat content. Raising the drawing temperature avoids excessive stiffness in the

Table 14.2. Homogenization Pressures (lb/in^2) for High-Fat Ice Cream

	Type	18% fat mix	20% fat mix
Minimum	Single-stage	1500	1000
Optimum	Single-stage	2000	1500
	Double-stage	1500	1000
		500	500
Maximum	Single-stage	2500	2000

freezer and provides a more free-flowing product. High-fat ice cream may be served at serving temperatures higher than normal to avoid excessive resistance and buttery characteristics.

Different Corn Syrups

Many corn syrups are used extensively as sweeteners in ice cream. The most common method used in identifying these syrups has been by the degree of conversion used in their manufacturing process, which has been indicated as a dextrose equivalent (DE) value. As has been previously mentioned, corn syrup can be classed as low-, regular-, intermediate-, or high-conversion products. Each syrup differs in relative sweetness and influence on the properties of the finished product. It should be noted that the regular- and intermediate-conversion syrups are commonly used but the high-conversion syrup is not generally used by the ice cream industry.

Typical examples of formulas for use of the different class of syrups based on 70% sucrose and 25% corn syrup are as follows:

Constituents	Sucrose	Regular (36 DE)	Intermediate (43 DE)	High (63 DE)
Fat	10.0	10.00	10.00	10.00
MSNF	12.0	12.00	12.00	12.00
Sucrose	15.0	11.25	11.25	11.25
Corn syrup	—	8.33	7.50	5.30
Stabilizer	0.3	0.30	0.30	0.30
TS	37.3	41.88	41.05	38.85

A mix having 25% of its sucrose replaced with a 36 DE syrup shows 4.58 lb TS increase per 100 lb mix; for the 43 DE, 3.75 lb; and for the 63 DE syrup, 1.61 lb. The additional sugar solids influence the body and texture and storage preparation of the finished product.

The regular-conversion syrup has been used to supply corn syrup solids to substitute for the MSNF, but the nutritive value of the MSNF replaced is lost, including the milk protein and the milk minerals. Formulas illustrating such substitutions are as follows:

Constituents	Normal MSNF	Corn syrup solids for MSNF	Normal MSNF	Corn syrup solids for MSNF
Fat	10.00	10.00	4.0	4.0
MSNF	12.00	10.00	13.0	10.0
Sucrose	11.25	11.25	12.0	12.0
Corn syrup solids	8.33	10.33	5.0	7.0
Stabilizer	0.30	0.30	0.4	0.4
TS	41.88	41.88	34.4	33.4

Whey Solids

The results of several investigations have shown whey solids may be satisfactorily used to replace 25% of the milk solids in ice cream and ice milk and 50–100% in sherbets and novelties depending on the formula. Formulas showing the use of whey solids are as follows:

Constituents	Hardened ice cream	Soft-serve or hard ice milk	Soft-serve ice milk	Sherbet base
Fat	10.00	6.00	5.00	0.50
MSNF (total)	11.50	12.00	12.00	5.00
Dairy sweet whey solids	3.00	3.00	3.00	5.00
Other MSNF	8.50	9.00	9.00	—
Sweetener (total)	17.00	20.00	15.00	32.00
Corn syrup solids	5.00	8.00	3.00	10.00
Sucrose	12.00	12.00	12.00	22.00
Stabilizer	0.30	0.40	0.40	0.40
Emulsifier	0.12	0.15	0.12	—
TS	38.92	38.55	32.52	37.90

Diabetic and Dietetic Frozen Foods

Diabetic and dietetic frozen dairy foods are special preparations for persons on restricted diets. Diabetic frozen dairy foods are made in semblance of ice cream or ice milk using noncaloric sweeteners. Some feel the ideal fat level for diabetic frozen diary foods is 6%. The ideal butterfat content for dietetic frozen dairy foods is 3–4% and should be made free from substitute sweeteners. Sugar substitutes for diabetic frozen dairy foods include hexahydric alcohols, sucaryl (sodium and calcium), and saccharine.

The hexahydric alcohols are classified as sugar alcohols and are made commercially principally from corn sugar and are available as Sorbo (70%), Sorbitol, and Mannitol. Mannitol has 2 cal/g and Sorbo has 2.8 cal/g as compared to 4 cal/g for sugar. The hexahydric alcohols have about half the sweetening value of sucrose and they affect the freezing point and contribute to the TS as do sugars.

Sucaryl products are noncaloric sweetening agents and do not affect the freezing point. Sucaryl sodium is most often used within the rate of 0.8% as it can be added at higher concentration than sucaryl calcium within the rate of 0.5% without affecting the flavor. Sucaryl has a relative sweetness value approximately 30–50 times that of sucrose. Saccharine is a noncaloric sweetening agent. It is excessively sweet and cannot be used in amounts to affect the freezing point or TS. It has a relative sweetness of 300–500 times the sweetness of sucrose. It is used at the approximate rate of 1/4 oz per 100 lb of mix.

Diabetic base products are available commercially to build solids when substitute sweeteners are used. The following formulas have been recommended for diabetic and dietetic products:

Constituents	Diabetic product	Diabetic product	Dietetic product	Low-fat high protein
Fat	6.0	10.0	3.00	2.00
MSNF	10.5	9.0	12.00	13.50
Sucrose	—	—	13.00	13.00
Mannitol (95% TS)	8.0	8.0	—	—
Sorbo (70% TS)	8.0	8.0	—	—
Sucaryl (sodium or calcium)	0.016–0.021	—	—	—
High protein base or diabetic base	3.0	3.0	3.00	3.00
Stabilizer	0.3	0.3	0.35	0.35
TS	33.0	25.5	31.35	31.85

15
Sherbets and Ices

A sherbet is a frozen product made from sugar, water, fruit acid, color, fruit or fruit flavoring, stabilizer, and a small amount of milk solids added in the form of skim milk, whole milk, condensed milk, or ice cream mix. An ice contains the same ingredients, but with no milk solids.

Sherbets and ices are differentiated from ice cream by the following characteristics:

- A higher fruit acid content (minimum 0.35%), which produces a tart flavor.
- A much lower overrun (usually 25–45%).
- A higher sugar content (25–35%), which gives a lower melting point.
- A coarser texture.
- A greater cooling characteristic while being consumed, due to their coarser texture and lower melting point.
- An apparent lack of richness due to lower milk solids content.

An increase in the consumption of sherbets and ices has developed in recent years, as indicated by the annual U.S. production of over 85 million gallons of these products. Together they account for 6.5% of the total frozen dessert production. While sherbets and ices are in greatest demand during the summer months, they are important products throughout the year as condiments, two- or three-flavor packages, in combination with ice cream, or in fancy ice cream and specialties. An analysis of sherbet sales by flavor for the United States (Table 15.1) shows the popular flavors are orange, pineapple, raspberry, lime, and lemon.

THE COMPOSITION OF SHERBETS AND ICES

The fruit-flavoring ingredients specified for ice cream can be used as well as natural and artificial flavors for fruit sherbets. Citrus sherbets must contain a minimum of 2% fruit; berry sherbets must contain a minimum of 6% fruit; other sherbets must contain a minimum of 10% fruit.

Water ice has the same flavoring provisions as fruit sherbets. Nonfruit sherbets or ices differ from fruit sherbet and ices mainly in the flavor-characterizing ingredients. The optional characterizing ingredients include

Table 15.1. Sherbet Sales by Flavor in the United States

	United States		North Atlantic		Central Eastern		Middle Western		Southern		Western	
Flavor	Rank	%	Rank	%	Rank	%	Rank	%	Rank	%	Rank	%
Orange	1	38.62	1	37.77	1	46.03	1	42.71	2	31.22	1	38.65
Pineapple	2	22.06	3	11.41	2	20.33	2	18.91	1	34.71	2	26.75
Raspberry	3	12.30	2	27.08	5	7.53	4	9.43	5	2.63	4	7.36
Lime	4	11.44	4	9.67	3	12.54	5	7.47	3	26.40	5	4.92
Lemon	5	6.08	5	5.41	4	10.17	3	17.62	7	0.34	6	3.82
Rainbow	6	3.37	—	—	—	—	—	—	—	—	3	11.71
Strawberry	7	1.66	8	0.92	10	0.22	9	0.01	6	1.62	7	3.77
Banana	8	0.88	6	3.18	—	—	—	—	—	—	—	—
Orange–pineapple	9	0.61	13	0.08	7	0.54	8	0.17	4	2.69	15	0.04
Cranberry	10	0.60	14	0.07	9	0.39	6	3.05	8	0.32	10	0.48
Cherry	11	0.50	7	1.58	—	—	7	0.50	—	—	—	—
Grape	12	0.27	10	0.67	—	—	—	—	—	—	12	0.29
Tangerine	13	0.26	9	0.70	8	0.42	—	—	—	—	16	0.02
Raspberry salad	14	0.26	—	—	6	1.79	—	—	—	—	—	—
Lemon–lime	15	0.21	11	0.62	—	—	—	—	—	—	14	0.14
Boysenberry	16	0.19	—	—	—	—	—	—	—	—	8	0.67
Cherry mint	17	0.17	—	—	—	—	—	—	—	—	9	0.59
Hawaiian	18	0.09	—	—	—	—	—	—	—	—	11	0.31
Nectarine	19	0.08	—	—	—	—	—	—	—	—	13	0.28
Butterscotch	20	0.06	12	0.21	—	—	—	—	—	—	—	—
All others	—	0.29	—	0.68	—	0.04	—	0.13	—	0.07	—	0.20
Total	—	100.00	—	100.00	—	100.00	—	100.00	—	100.00	—	100.00

Source: IAICM (1965b).

ground spices or infusion of coffee or tea; chocolate or cocoa, including syrup; confectionery; distilled alcoholic beverages, in an amount not to exceed that required for flavoring the sherbet or ice; or any natural or artificial food flavoring (except any having a characteristic fruit or fruitlike flavor).

Researchers (Turnbow et al., 1946; Ross, 1963; Day et al., 1959) have studied the manufacture of water ices and sherbets and recommended replacing 20–25% of the sucrose with dextrose to improve the properties of the product. The use of a greater proportion of dextrose was found to cause the ice or sherbet to be too soft at hardening room and cabinet temperatures. The mixing of a high-grade gum with gelatin was recommended to prevent precipitation of the stabilizer.

It has been found that corn syrup solids in combination with sucrose improved the body and texture and prevented the development of surface crustation of the sugar. Thus, corn syrup solids have come into prominence as a component of commercial stabilizers for sherbets and ices. Carob (locust bean) products and algin stabilizers have also been used as stabilizers for these products. A sugar content of 24–32% has given satisfactory results, and formulas for ices and sherbets with combinations of sucrose and corn sugar and high-conversion corn syrup using pectin as a stabilizer are available.

Those who have studied the use of whey in sherbets have found that sherbets containing 2.6% fat and 2.4% nonfat solids with 1.9% prepared from 30% cream and whey solids were not noticeably different from sherbets made entirely with normal MSNF. A good-quality sherbet can be made that contains 4–5% whey solids. The whey sherbets possess a smooth body and texture and are more refreshing than the sherbets made with solids from milk or ice cream mix.

Investigations have been made on the use of foam spray-dried cottage cheese whey as a source of solids in sherbets. Cottage cheese whey or whey cultured with *L. bulgaricus* or *S. thermophilus* were used to replace 25, 50, 75, and 94.5% of the MSNF in orange, lemon, and raspberry sherbet. All the fresh sherbets were rated good in flavor and smooth in body and texture. The amount of citric acid required to lower the pH of orange, lemon, and raspberry sherbet to 3.7 was approximately 32, 50, and 26%, respectively, in sherbets with 94.5% of the MSNF replaced by dry acid whey.

Important factors in the manufacture of sherbets and ices include choice of stabilizer, control of kind and amount of sugar, control of acidity and pH for optimum flavor, control of composition for desirable body and texture, and maintenance of uniform natural color.

Legal standards for sherbets and ices usually require a certain minimum acidity (usually 0.35% as lactic acid) and minimum weight per gallon in the same range as for ice cream. Standards also often specify a minimum and maximum percentage of milk solids in sherbets (3–5%).

Sherbets contain a low concentration of milk solids (2–5%). Some states have established a minimum for milk solids content and in others a maximum is set for the amount of milk solids that may be contained in the sherbet. Requirements range up to a 5% minimum, while some states have a 5% maximum.

Sherbets and ices have lower melting points, coarser texture, and apparent lack of richness due to low milk solids content. The best dipping temperature ranges from $-5°$ to $+5°F$. Recent practice is to adjust the sugar composition and overrun in order to dip these products at the same temperature as ice cream.

Sugar

In general, the sugar content of these products is about double that of ice cream (25–35%). Sources of sugar include cane or beet sugar, corn sugar, corn syrup solids, invert sugar and liquid sugar. In making good sherbet it is necessary to control the sugar content and overrun. An excess of sugar results in a soft product and a deficiency results in a hard, crumbly product.

The amount of sucrose used should be the least that will give the desired sweetness in the finished ice, thus giving a higher melting point more suitable for dipping at the usual cabinet temperatures (3–8°F).

The amount of corn syrup, invert sugar, or corn sugar should be about one-third the amount of sucrose. This sugar reduces the tendency to form a surface crust, which sometimes happens when sucrose is used alone. If any appreciable amount of corn syrup solids is used in an ice it tends to keep the melting point nearer to that of ice cream, so that the product will have a firmness most suitable for dipping at the usual cabinet temperature. The amount of sugar present in the fruit added to sherbets and ices should be known. Natural sugar content is higher in some fruits than in others, and the amount of sugar added to fruit by processors may vary. By controlling the sugar content the firmness of the product can be controlled. Lack of uniformity of sherbets and ices in the past has been a serious quality defect.

The sugar contained in fruit preparations or ice cream mix, contributing to the sugar content of the sherbet or ice mix, should be given consideration in order to maintain uniform characteristics in the finished product.

Stabilizers

Most of the basic stabilizers used in ice cream may be used for sherbets and ices. The amount of basic stabilizers needed for ices and sherbets is approximately as follows: gelatin (200 Bloom) 0.45%, CMC gum 0.20%, pectin 0.18%, algin products 0.20%, locust bean gum 0.25%. Slightly less stabilizer is needed in sherbets than in ices.

Stabilization in sherbets and ices is even more important than for ice cream because of greater danger of sugar separation and body crumbliness. Stabilizers are also more important in ices than in ice cream because of the lower TS content. In the selection of a stabilizer, consideration should be given to its effect on overrun, syrup drainage, and body (crumbliness) as well as availability, convenience of use, and personal preference. Of the various stabilizers—cellulose gum, gum tragacanth, India gum, agar, gelatin, and pectin—the last two are most widely used. Best results are obtained by using a combination of two or more of these stabilizers, the ratio of combination depending on the grade and kind of stabilizers. Enough stabilizer should be used to cause a partial gelling at cold room temperatures.

Acidity of Sherbets and Ices

Citric acid is the most commonly used acid and is usually added as a 50% solution. The acid content differentiates sherbets and ices from ice cream. The amount of acid depends on the fruit used, the amount of sugar present, and the demands of the consumer. The following amounts of acids have been recommended for products depending on the sugar content: 25–30% sugar, 0.36% acid; 30–35% sugar, 0.40% acid; 35–40% sugar, 0.50% acid.

Overrun of Sherbets and Ices

Overrun also controls the firmness and dipping qualities of sherbets and ices. Overrun in sherbets is usually 30–40% while for ices it is 25–35%.

Preparation of Base Mix

This base is prepared by slowly adding the dry ingredients to at least part of the water, taking care to avoid lumpiness. Heating may be necessary to facilitate solution, especially when stabilizers like gelatin or agar are used. Pasteurization is optional, but homogenization is not practical. The prepared base is cooled before other ingredients are added. Aging is necessary only when gelatin or agar is used in the stabilizer, and then an aging period of 12–24 hr is desirable.

This base mix is now ready for the flavor and color materials. To each 80 lb of the cooled base mix enough flavor, color, and water are added to make up a total weight of 100 lb.

The flavor and color mixture is made from the following ingredients:

1. *Fruit juices.* Although the amount varies with the intensity of the flavor, it should be 15–20% of the weight of the finished ice. Avoid adding too many seeds.

2. *Flavoring.* The amount of fruit needed for flavoring varies from 3 qt to 2 gal per 10 gal of finished mix, depending on the kind of preparation and variety of fruit used. Natural extracts and artificial flavors may not produce as desirable a flavor as the fruit juices, but they are often used to fortify the flavor and thereby produce a more uniform product.

3. *Coloring.* Approved artificial food coloring aids in maintaining a uniform shade of color characteristic and suggestive of the flavor.

4. *Citric acid solution.* To obtain the desired tart flavor, a fruit acid such as citric acid or tartaric acid may be added. When fruit acids are not available, saccharic acid, phosphoric acid, or lactic acid may be used, but these do not impart an equally desirable flavor. It is a common practice to use a 50% solution (i.e., 1 lb of crystals to 1 lb of water) of either citric acid or tartaric acid. The amount of this solution generally used varies from 4 to 10 oz, depending on the acidity of the fruit juice. The titratable acidity of the finished ice should not be less than 0.35% nor more than 0.50% when expressed as lactic acid.

Additional water may be necessary to bring the total weight of this mixture up to 20 lb.

The freezing procedure in the making of ices is similar to that for ice cream. Many manufacturers prefer to use a special batch or continuous freezer since the absence of fat causes the scraper blades to become dull rapidly. The scraper blades must be sharpened more frequently since sharp blades favor more rapid freezing, smaller ice crystals, and a smoother product. The refrigerant should be at least − 10°F and should not be turned off as soon as for freezing ice cream. Frequently by using a very cold refrigerant the desired overrun and consistency for drawing can be obtained before the refrigerant is shut off. Fruit, color, citric acid, and flavor should be added at the time of freezing.

Controlling the overrun is very important in ices. A high overrun favors syrup drainage, a lack of firmness, and poor body. Therefore stabilizers that improve whipping ability are less desirable than the gum type, where it is desired to limit the overrun. Methods for controlling overrun using a batch freezer in order of preference are as follows:

1. Operate freezer with colder refrigerant and longer time before refrigerant is shut off (i.e., shorter whipping time).
2. Select the proper stabilizer.
3. Overload the freezer. Use 5-1/2 or 6 gal of mix in a 40-qt freezer.
4. Underload the freezer. Use 3-1/2 or 4 gal of mix in a 40-qt freezer.
5. Have the beater on a separate gear so that it can be made to idle while the scrapers turn.

PREPARATION OF SHERBETS

The base or stock mix described above can be used for any flavor of sherbet. This mix may be varied in order to produce a finished product with any desired body, texture, and handling characteristics. The importance and relative volume of sherbets is the same as for ices, but the dairyperson should be more interested in selling milk solids than in selling ices. One common procedure employs fresh milk or cream to furnish the total milk solids.

A base or stock mix for sherbets consists of the following:

1. Between 21 and 35 lb of sucrose (cane or beet sugar), the same as for ices.
2. Between 7 and 9 lb of glucose, invert sugar, or corn sugar, the same as for ices and for similar reasons.
3. Between 0.4 and 0.6 lb of stabilizer, the same as for ices and for the same reasons.
4. At least 35–40 lb of milk, or enough to supply 5 lb of total milk solids.
5. Enough water to make a total of 80 lb of base or stock mix.

Milk Solids Content

Milk solids should be supplied in an amount to satisfy regulations. They also enhance the body, texture, and flavor of the product, and the fat content influences the overrun. The milk solids may come from homogenized milk, condensed milk, nonfat dry milk solids, or ice cream mix. The amount of dairy products required to give approximately 5% solids in 100 lb of sherbet mix is as follows: skim milk, 55 lb; 4% milk, 45 lb; condensed skim milk (30% solids), 15.9 lb; sweetened condensed milk (27% MSNF, 42% sugar), 18.5 lb; ice cream mix (12% fat, 11% MSNF), 24 lb.

This base is prepared by slowly adding the dry ingredients to the milk and heating if necessary to obtain complete solution free from lumps. The mix need not be pasteurized provided the milk products have already been pasteurized. It should be remembered that some gum stabilizers like gum arabic will coagulate milk when heated. Therefore, when using this stabilizer the milk should be pasteurized separately. Sherbet mixes are seldom homogenized, but they must be cooled; if gelatin is used for a stabilizer, the base should be aged for 12–24 hr. Then to this 80 lb of base is added 20 lb of the mixture of fruit juices, flavoring, coloring, citric acid solution, and water as described for making ices. Since the citric acid solution may curdle the milk it is sometimes added at the freezer after some ice crystals have started to form.

Another common method employs ice cream mix to furnish the milk solids. In many ice cream factories ice cream mix is more easily available than fresh milk. Furthermore, it is already pasteurized and homogenized. Since the mix supplies some sugar and stabilizer, the sherbet base must be adjusted accordingly. The following suggestions indicate the necessary changes:

1. Between 18 and 22 lb of sucrose (cane or beet sugar).
2. Between 7 and 9 lb of corn syrup, invert sugar, or corn sugar.
3. Between 0.35 and 0.55 lb stabilizer.
4. Between 18 and 25 lb ice cream mix to furnish approximately the same amount of total milk solids as could be obtained from fresh milk.
5. Enough water to make a total weight of 80 lb of base mix.

The preparation of this base is the same as described for the first method, and the fruit mixture is added in the same manner. The freezing of sherbets is identical with the freezing of ices except that a higher overrun (35–45%) is taken. The desired body and texture characteristics may vary in different markets ranging from smooth, chewy, and heavy to medium resistant and slightly coarse. The formulas given in Tables 15.2–15.5 produce finished products of different characteristics (Day *et al.* 1959).

PREPARATION OF ICES

Ices are frequently calculated on the basis of 100-lb lots and manufacturers prepare a base or stock mix with 21–25 lb sucrose (cane or beet sugar; 7–9 lb glucose, invert sugar, or corn sugar; and 0.4–0.6 lb stabilizer. Water is added to make a total weight of 80 lb of base or stock mix. The balance of the 100 lb is flavoring and additional water. Formulas for ices are given in Table 15.6.

Table 15.2. Sherbet: Smooth, Chewy, Heavy Body and Texture[a]

Ingredients	Amount (lb)	Fat (lb)	MSNF (lb)	Sugar (lb)	TS (lb)
Cane sugar	9.0	—	—	9.00	9.00
Corn syrup solids, 42 DE (Frodex)	22.0	—	—	21.20	21.23
Ice cream mix (12% fat, 11% MSNF, 15% sugar)	17.5	2.1	1.92	2.62	6.65
Stabilizer	0.4	—	—	—	0.40
Fruit puree (5 + 1)	15.0	—	—	2.50	4.75
Water and 10-¾ oz. of 50% citric acid solution and color	36.1	—	—	—	—
Total	100.0	2.1	1.92	35.32	42.03

[a]Acidity, 0.57%; freezing point, 26.4°F.

Table 15.3. Sherbet: Medium Smooth, Medium Firm Body and Texture[a]

Ingredients	Amount (lb)	Fat (lb)	MSNF (lb)	Sugar (lb)	TS (lb)
Cane sugar	11.0	—	—	11.00	11.00
Corn syrup solids, 30 DE	10.0	—	—	9.65	9.65
Ice cream mix (12% fat, 11% MSNF, 15% sugar)	17.5	2.1	1.92	2.62	6.65
Stabilizer	0.4	—	—	—	0.40
Fruit puree (5 + 1)	15.0	—	—	2.50	4.75
Water and 10-¾ oz. of 50% citric acid solution and color	46.1	—	—	—	—
Total	100.0	2.1	1.92	25.77	32.45

[a]Acidity, 0.55%; freezing point, 28.4°F.

Table 15.4. Sherbet: Medium Coarse, Medium Firm Body and Texture[a]

Ingredients	Amount (lb)	Fat (lb)	MSNF (lb)	Sugar (lb)	TS (lb)
Cane sugar	17.0	—	—	17.00	17.00
Dextrose	7.0	—	—	6.44	6.44
Ice cream mix (12% fat, 11% MSNF, 15% sugar)	17.5	2.1	1.92	2.62	6.65
Stabilizer	0.4	—	—	—	0.40
Fruit puree (5 + 1), orange	15.0	—	—	2.50	4.25
Water and 10-¾ oz. of 50% citric acid solution and color	43.1	—	—	—	—
Total	100.0	2.1	1.92	28.56	34.74

[a]Acidity, 0.55%; freezing point, 26.4°F.

Table 15.5. Mix Formulas for Sherbet with Different Sources of Milk Solids

Ingredients (lb)	Ice cream mix	Whole milk	Condensed skim milk (30%)	Skim milk
Cane sugar	11.0	16.0	16.0	16.0
Corn sugar (Frodex)	10.0	10.0	10.0	10.0
Stabilizer	0.4	0.4	0.4	0.4
Fruit juice, color, citric solution, water	61.1	41.6	60.6	28.6
Ice cream mix	17.5	—	—	—
Whole milk	—	32.0	—	—
Condensed skim milk (30%)	—	—	13.0	—
Skim milk	—	—	—	45.0
Total	100.0	100.0	100.0	100.0

Table 15.6. Formulas for Ices

Ingredients	Amount (lb)	Amount (lb)
Cane sugar	23.0	16.0
Corn sugar	7.0	10.0
Stabilizer	0.3	0.4
Fruit juice, color, citric acid solution, water	69.7	73.6
Total	100.0	100.0

DIFFICULTIES AND DEFECTS

Control of Overrun

The overrun should be kept at 25–30% for ices and 35–45% for sherbets. This is not easy to do, especially if gelatin is used as the stabilizer, without modifying the ordinary routine of freezing. Agar, gums, or commercial stabilizers for ices are recommended largely because they retard the rate of whipping. However, many manufacturers prefer to use gelatin because it is usually on hand.

The refrigerant should be at least −10°F to freeze ices or sherbets and should be kept on until they are firm enough to draw. Usually a very cold refrigerant makes it possible to draw a low enough overrun. If not, in case of the batch freezer, the freezer must be over- or underloaded, or the beater must be on a separate gear so that it can be made to idle. Overloading the freezer is the usual procedure followed to control the overrun.

Firmness at Dipping Temperatures

Ices and sherbets should be of the same firmness at ordinary cabinet temperatures as ice cream since they usually are sold from the same cabinets. If the overrun is kept at 30–35% and the sugar content at 28–32%, the firmness will be suitable for dipping at the usual cabinet temperatures of 3–8°F.

Flavor

Sherbet and ice defects include unnatural, atypical, artificial flavor; excessive flavor, caused by addition of too much acid or flavor material; excess sweetness, resulting from a high percentage of sugar; metallic or oxidized flavor development during storage; and lack of sweetness due to the use of the improper amount or kind of sugar.

Body and Texture

Coarseness may result from insufficient solids, sugar, or stabilizer, drawing from freezer at too high temperature, or improper storage and handling. Undue coarseness may be prevented by keeping the sugar content at 28–32%; using about one-fourth of the sugar as corn sugar; using the right amount and kind of stabilizer; drawing from the freezer in a firm condition; and marketing promptly. The base should be aged for 12–24 hr and enough stabilizer should be used to cause a partial gelling at cold room temperatures.

A crumbly body indicates improper stabilizer or insufficient amount of stabilizer or sugar. The hard-body characteristic may be caused by low overrun or insufficient sugar content. A snowy body usually results from excess incorporation of air. A sticky body may be caused by use of too much stabilizer or too much sugar.

Surface crust sometimes forms on ices and sherbets. This is due to surface evaporation of moisture and can be prevented by covering with parchment paper and can cover. If about one-fourth of the sugar is corn sugar, a surface crust will not occur. With cane sugar alone as the sweetener, this trouble occurs more often. Surface encrustation sometimes appears because some of the sucrose crystallizes and liberated water freezes into ice. Use of a greater amount of stabilizer or use of corn sugar to lower the freezing point of the mix will help prevent this defect.

Other Defects

"Bleeding" is the term applied to the settling of the sugar syrup to the bottom of the can. The usual causes are excessive overrun, insufficient stabilizer, too much sugar (over 32%), and temperatures too high in the cabinet. Using more effective stabilizer or more stabilizer, reducing sugar content, and avoiding high overruns will aid in preventing this defect.

Color defects include unnaturalness, due to improper amount or kind of color, and unevenness, resulting from improperly distributed color.

Meltdown defects are that the product melts too fast, does not melt, or is curdy.

Many of the sherbet and ice products produced by ice cream manufacturers are not of the superior quality of the ice cream produced. Great strides in improving the quality of sherbet can be made by maintaining uniform composition, color, flavor, and body and texture characteristics. It is evident that standardization of quality of sherbets and ices is needed.

16
Frozen Confections, Novelties, Fancy Molded Ice Creams, and Specials

INTRODUCTION

Very early in the history of the ice cream industry, small manufacturers with imagination often emphasized the possibilities and profits to be gained in making unusual ice cream products, including quiescently frozen stick and novelty items, special flavor combination packages, cup items, and other specials and fancy molded items.[1] However, the larger manufacturers, in many instances, seem to have been a little slow in promoting this class of ice cream, due largely perhaps to the high cost of the skilled labor involved. However, recent advances in equipment for making, filling, and decorating indicate possibilities of mass production at lower costs, and plants have been established that devote the entire production to this type of products. Other plants maintain the regular production and, in addition, manufacture novelties and special products for plants that do not have sufficient volume in novelty or special products to justify investment in equipment necessary for these special products.

The factors that affect successful frozen confection production are the type of production equipment, the ingredients used in the mix, proper freezer operation, and control of production operations including correct volume, rate of freezing, sticking, extraction from molds, yield of coating, wrapping or bagging, packing, sealing cartons, and storage.

Individual Portion Control

Many of these products take the form of individual portions. The potential for the ice cream industry that exists in individual portion-controlled convenience foods has been recognized for many years. Only during the past few years have the industry changes occurred that are bringing about the increased production of such items. The success of portion-controlled products

---

[1]Provisions for the identity and labeling requirements of quiescently frozen dairy confections and quiescently frozen confections have not been made. An example of a standard of identity of these products is given in Chapter 22.

seems attributable to many factors, of which the following are generally among the most important:

1. The quality, especially the texture, of individual portions is much higher as extruded items are rapidly frozen.

2. They are convenient and easy to serve.

3. They provide the manufacturer an opportunity to use imagination in product design for merchandising advantages.

SPECIALTY EQUIPMENT

Versatile machinery that can produce ice cream novelties in nearly any shape is now available. This machinery provides an automated method for producing individual ice cream portions, slices, chocolate-coated bars, and fancy stick products. Ice cream is drawn from the freezer at 22°F, pumped through an extruder nozzle, and sliced into portions by a cutting assembly. If a stick item is desired, the stick is inserted before the extruded ice cream reaches the cutting assembly. The pieces drop onto carrier plates and pass through a freezing chamber at −43°F with rapid air circulation for fast freezing. Each piece is removed from the carrier plate as it emerges from the freezing chamber. The ice cream portions are then transferred through an enrober (if chocolate or other coating is desired) and through a chill tunnel, where the coating is set. The pieces are wrapped individually by the wrapping equipment and packed in cartons, ready for distribution.

Frozen confection equipment may be of different types or styles. There are rotary and line types of equipment, which generally use brine tanks as refrigerants, and there are extrusion types, which involve cold-air hardening. The choice of equipment is often dependent on the kind and volume of confection being manufactured. The Gram is a popular rotary piece of equipment while the Vitaline is a popular line type. Glacier and Polarmatic are popular styles of extrusion equipment.

ICE, FUDGE, AND CREAM STICK ITEMS

Quiescently Frozen Stick Items and Other Novelties

These items include water ice frozen without overrun on a stick; fudge on a stick, which has a malt flavor, contains a fudge base, may contain milk solids, and may or may not contain milkfat; and cream on a stick, which has a 2-oz ice milk or ice cream center with a quiescently frozen 2-oz outer section.

Ice Base and Ice Item Formulas

To produce an ice base that yields 38 dozen ice sticks, the following ingredients are used: water, 10 gal; cane sugar, 12 lb; corn sugar, 4 lb; stabilizer, 5 oz. The preparation is as follows:

1. Weigh stabilizer carefully and add to the 10 gal of water, agitate until suspended.
2. Add the sugar and agitate until completely dissolved.
3. Add citric acid and flavor as recommended below. Agitate thoroughly.
4. Carefully run mix into mold to within 3/16 in. of top to allow for expansion in freezing.

Table 16.1 gives formulas for producing 1000 3- and 4-oz ice items, and Table 16.2 gives a formula for producing 1000 3-oz fudge items.
The preparation of the fudge items is as follows:

1. Dissolve fudge powder in 1-1/2 gal of boiling water and mix stabilizer with sugar and dissolve in 2-1/2 gal of water.
2 Add dissolved fudge powder and suspended stabilizer mixture to ice cream mix or condensed skim milk. Agitate thoroughly.
3. Pasteurize, homogenize, and cool.
4. Fill molds carefully.

For cream-on-a-stick novelties, a special filler attachment may be used so that in one operation a freezer may be used to freeze the ice cream to 100% overrun for the center and a second freezer to freeze the ice or sherbet shell to 10–15%.

Table 16.1. Formulas for 1000 3- and 4-oz Ice Items (~24 gal of Mix)

Ingredient	Amount		Amount	
Water	20	gal	26	gal
Cane sugar	33	lb	40	lb
Corn sugar	7	lb	10	lb
Stabilizer	0.5	lb	0.7	lb
Flavor	6.5	oz	8	oz
Citric acid	22–25	oz	25–28	oz

Table 16.2. Formulas for 1000 3-oz Fudge Items (~24 gal of Mix)

Ingredient	Amount		
	Nonfat	Fat 3%	Fat 5%
Water	4 gal	10 gal	5 gal
Cane sugar	30 lb	30 lb	30 lb
Corn sugar	8 lb	8 lb	8 lb
Fudge powder	7 lb	7 lb	7 lb
Condensed skim milk (2&%)	135 lb	—	—
Ice cream mix (10%)	—	65 lb	96 lb
Stabilizer	8 oz	4 oz	4 oz
Citric acid	—	—	—

FROZEN MALTS AND ICE CREAM BARS

The frozen malt may be an ice cream or an ice milk product. Normally, 6 lb of malt per 15 gal of mix is used with an overrun of 90% on the ice cream and 80% on the ice milk product. Also included in this class are chocolate-covered bars, a novelty that consists of a sugar cone with ice cream in it with the ice cream dipped in chocolate and covered with nuts or other toppings.

The composition for coating may be as given in Table 16.3 (Erb 1942). Lecithin is added to prevent thickening on prolonged dipping. The surface of the bars should be free from moisture, which permits better adherence of the coating. Adding 5–10% coconut oil to coating increases covering ability. Other oils have melting points that are too low for satisfactory use in coatings.

Many of the more well-known novelties are controlled by patents held by commercial companies, which sell licenses to those interested. To protect these products and to ensure uniformity., the licensor insists on standard formulas and standard trademarks. (Among these novelties are Eskimo Pie, Popsicle, Fudgsicle, Creamsicle, Drumstick, and Chocolate Bar.) The licensor generally has special equipment, packages, flavoring, formulas with detailed directions, as well as advertising matter, available to those interested in making this type of product.

FANCY MOLDED ICE CREAM

Ice cream belonging to the class known as fancy molded ice cream differs from plain bulk ice cream chiefly in the form in which it is marketed. In some cases there may be a slight difference in the formula, but the principal difference is in the manner of coloring and in the size and form of the package. The difference in formula consists usually of additional stabilizer and emulsifier or more milk solids to obtain a firmer body.

The difference in packaging is one of the distinguishing features of fancy ice cream. The most common item or form is the decorated slice, which is easy to serve. The individual cup mold (enough to serve one person) is also popular. However, much ice cream is molded into the form of animals, statues, flowers, fruits, or other objects (Fig 16.1). The mold may be of individual size or it may contain a number of quarts of ice cream.

Calculated to increase sales and also to reach a different clientele, the fancy

Table 16.3. Composition for Chocolate Coatings

Ingredient	Dark coating (%)	Milk chocolate coating (%)
Sugar	28–30	28–30
Chocolate solids		
nonfat	15	12
cocoa fat	55	48
MSNF	—	10
Lecithin	0.3	0.3
Moisture	0.4	0.4

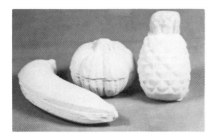

Fig. 16.1. Ice cream molded into the shape of fruits and vegetables.

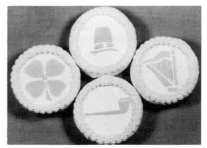

Fig. 16.2. Molds decorated for a special occasion (in this case, St. Patrick's Day).

molded ice creams are generally made for special occasions—parties, balls, banquets, and the like (Fig. 16.2). Success in this line requires no small amount of originality and artistic ingenuity, which is rewarded by a higher price and increased demand for these fancy products.

Harmony in color and flavor is even more important in fancy ice creams than in bulk. Colors and flavors should therefore be selected with great care: The color must suggest the flavor and must harmonize with it. For example, a vanilla ice cream is yellowish (creamy in color), but a strawberry ice cream is pink because that is the color imparted to the cream by the natural fresh strawberry fruit. Fruits often do not color the mix sufficiently and so it is customary to add enough coloring to remind one of the natural color of the fruit. However, it would most certainly be a bad idea to color vanilla ice cream pink or strawberry ice cream brown. Not that coloring adds or detracts from the flavor, but unless the two harmonize, there is nothing suggestive in the color.

The color, however, should not be too deep, for that suggests artificiality and cheapness. Light and dainty tints are the most pleasing to the eye. Therefore, color should be used sparingly.

Individual molds such as animals, and flowers are filled by dipping the ice cream from a bulk package, usually a 5-gal can. Large molds and center molds may also be filled in this manner. The best procedure is to fill the molds immediately after the ice cream is drawn from the freezer, while it is soft and has not had time to melt or to harden appreciably. When this is not feasible, the already hardened ice cream may be softened to the usual serving temperature (3–8°F) of retail cabinets, and then dipped into the molds. When this hardened ice cream is used, care must be taken to avoid packing too firmly because the solidly packed ice cream will be difficult to cut for eating.

DECORATING

In the past, much of the decorating of fancy ice creams was done by hand and by the use of various forms and screens. However, now in general commercial practice the decorating tool is a cone-shaped bag (the same as the bag used by pastry chefs for the same purpose) made of parchment paper into the tip of which is inserted the metal points or nozzles through which the cream is extruded and laid down on the cake surface. These points or nozzles, which come in various shapes such as cords, ribbons, leaves, roses, or stars, can be secured from dairy supply houses.

The cone-shaped bag is made by rolling the paper into a cone; just enough of the tip of the cone is cut off to allow the nozzle point to be inserted from the inside. The top flap of the cone is left to be turned down over the top after the bag has been filled. The bag is filled with the decorating medium, whipped cream, and grasped in the right hand. Using the left hand as a rest for the right wrist, the bag is squeezed enough to extrude the cream at the same time that the nozzle is moved forward over the cake to lay down the desired design. The actual process is not easy to describe but the art is easily acquired even by the novice gifted with artistic sense. The beginner should, however, seek the opportunity of watching a skilled decorator at work. Plenty of practice is needed before a perfect job can be expected. Mashed potatoes are an excellent substitute for whipped cream in obtaining this needed practice. After the decorator has acquired proficiency in handling a one-color job, a two-color job may be attempted. By carefully filling one side of the parchment bag with one color and the other side with a second color of whipped cream, a two-color effect can be produced as the cream is squeezed through the nozzle. Most decorators prefer to make up several bags, one for each of the colors they intend to use, or for the various shapes of nozzles needed for the designs.

Ice cream decorators frequently employ a small turntable on which to place the cake, pie, or brick to be decorated. This facilitates working all around the piece without disturbing its position. Such a turntable is easily made by using a block of wood 6–8 in. high for the pedestal, to which is nailed rather loosely a smooth round board for the table top. The item is placed on the turntable and is first smoothed over with a thin coating of whipped cream applied with an ordinary spatula. A 45% cream that has been aged for at least 48 hr, chilled to 40°F, then whipped to a smooth consistency (not so thick that it becomes grainy or buttery or so thin that it runs off the cake) is most satisfactory for decorating. To make it more palatable, 5% of sugar and a little vanilla or other flavoring may be added. This cream can be tinted in any desired color with flavor to harmonize, and the designs in which it can be shaped are limited only by the skill and artistic ingenuity of the decorator.

Other frostings may be used for special purposes. The thin, smooth coating to cover the surface of a mold can be made of cream, coloring, sugar, and stabilizer to give a fairly heavy batter, but not whipped. The item is quickly dipped in the batter, or the batter poured over it, and the excess allowed to drain off. Butter frosting prepared by mixing butter, sugar, color, and flavor can also be effective.

A variety of special effects is also possible. The "fuzzy" coloring effect on peaches can be obtained by chilling the molded cream on dry ice and then spraying it with colored water from an atomizer. A shiny glazed surface is obtained by chilling the molded cream on dry ice and then briefly dipping it in water, which may or may not be colored. Silhouette effects can be created by stencils, as described below.

Decorated Slices

The decorated slice is perhaps the most popular of the decorated pieces. There are many special designs available (Ess-Dee Craft Industries 1968). Special colored whipped cream is spread over the stencil design with a spatula and the stencil is quickly removed before it freezes to either the ice cream or the whipped cream design. When the stencil is removed the sharp colored outline of the pattern will remain. The decorated pieces are hardened in the hardening room and placed in appropriate packages for protection.

FANCY EXTRUDED ICE CREAM

Versatile extrusion equipment is available that can produce ice cream portions in nearly any shape and flavor combination (see Fig 16.3).

To be able to produce ice cream shapes by extrusion, the ice cream must be frozen to a certain stiffness so that it retains its form between the time it is extruded until it enters a hardening tunnel. Extruded ice cream is drawn from the freezer at 20–22°F.

The external contour of the slice may be almost any desired shape and is determined by the shape of the extrusion nozzle, subject to certain limitations. Complex extrusions utilizing more than one flavor or color can be produced from multiflavor extrusion nozzles supplied by more than one continuous freezer barrel. By placing different extrusion devices inside each other, faces with eyes, nose, and mouth can be formed, as well as other intricate designs (see Fig. 16.4).

Ice cream can be extruded both vertically and horizontally. In both cases, the principle is the same. As the stiff, extruded ice cream flows through the extrusion nozzle, portions of appropriate size are cut off by an electrically heated wire. In vertical extrusion, the flat portion of the ice cream slice falls precisely onto a continuous row of stainless steel supporting plates fastened to a conveyor chain, which carries the portions into the hardening tunnel for rapid freezing. The temperature in the hardening tunnel is usually in the range of −45 to −50°F. Horizontally extruded "log" products are placed lengthwise onto the conveyor plates. They are usually longer than they are high. They, too, may have external contours of nearly any shape and multiple flavors.

A 10% butterfat mix with 85–100% overrun is the most commonly used. However, a wide range of fat content (both butter and vegetable fats) can be extruded, given a proper balance of emulsifiers and stabilizers. Furthermore, in recent years, highly stabilized water ices have become popular as extruded items. Product quality, especially texture, is excellent due to the rapid freezing process.

Extruded product capabilities include single flavor, multiflavored, decorated, chocolate-coated, and drycoated sticked and stickless slices; coated and uncoated ice cream sandwiches; single-portion and large horizontally extruded fancy decorated logs; and bite-size chocolate-coated miniatures. Additionally,

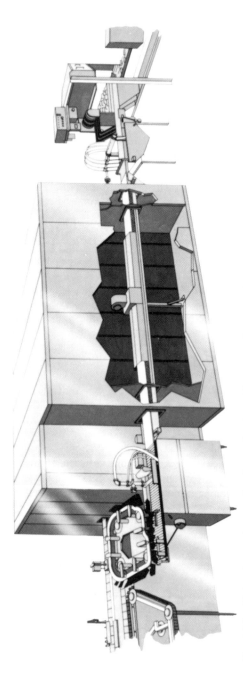

Fig. 16.3. Extrusion equipment for the production of frozen confections. This particular setup includes vertical and horizontal slice cutters, rosette decorator, syrup dispenser, automatic product transfer, enrober, coating hardening belt, top decorating station, and tray loader. (Courtesy of Glacier Industries Inc., Austin TX.)

regular and boat-shaped cones can be produced with the addition of cone-filling equipment.

Recently, production volume has been greatly increased. Extrusion equipment that produces 300 5-oz chocolate coated stickless slices (six slices per plate) per hour is now available (Fig. 16.5).

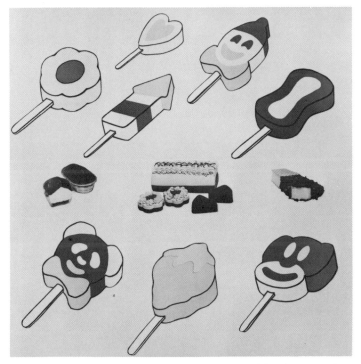

Fig. 16.4. Some of the products that can be produced by the extrusion process. (Courtesy of Glacier Industries Inc., Austin TX.)

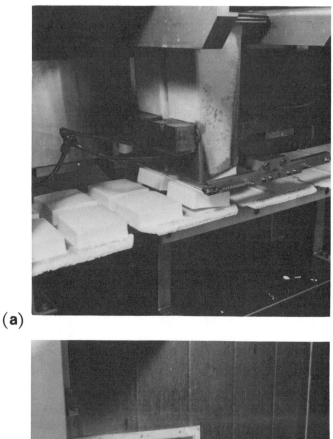

(a)

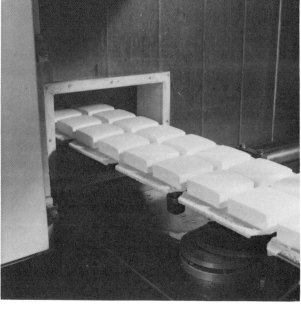

(b)

Fig. 16.5. The Glacier 600-E enlarged tunnel for the high-volume production of slices. (a) Extrusion from double nozzle, two slices/cut, four slices/plate. (b) Slices entering freezing tunnel. (c) Organized rake-off of frozen slices in dual lanes from

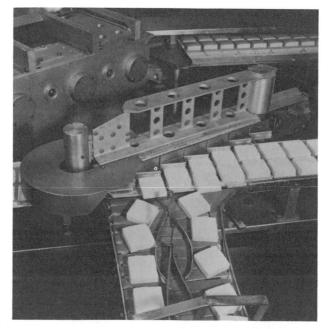

(c)

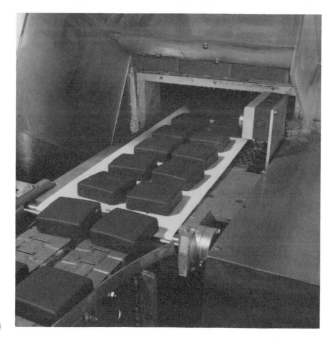

(d)

product plates prior to chocolate enrobing. (d) Coated slices emerging from side cooling chamber on coating hardening belt. (Courtesy of Glacier Industries Inc., Austin TX.)

OTHER SPECIAL PRODUCTS

Fancy Centers with the Continuous Freezer

The continuous freezer fitted with special discharge outlets makes it possible to produce many combinations including fancy centers for different type packages (Fig. 16.6) with both speed and economy. The sundae-type product provides many different variations. Split flavor nozzles will produce designs of different flavors of ice cream or ice cream and sherbet. Many square designs, which may appeal to customers, can be effected with such a nozzle.

Ice Cream Cakes and Pies

These products can be made with freezer attachments designed for filling the cake or pie plate (Fig. 16.7). The cake is usually inserted into a cardboard package to support the form of the cake during handling and delivery.

Ice cream pies can be modified by using fruit-flavored gelatin instead of the filling of preserved fruits or fruit ice cream ordinarily used. The fruit gelatin used in ice cream pies is similar to that used in modified aufait ice cream (see below). The pie crusts are about 1/2 in. in thickness and may be made by hardening vanilla ice cream between two pie plates. Closed or open pies may be made.

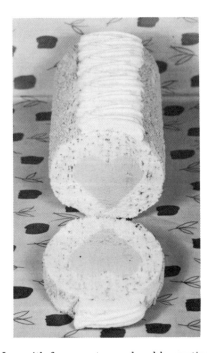

Fig. 16.6. Log with fancy center produced by continuous freezer.

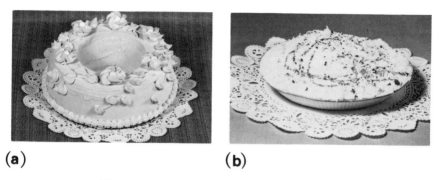

(a)   **(b)**

Fig. 16.7. (a) Ice cream cake, (b) ice cream pie.

The modified ice cream cake is made by placing alternate layers of ice cream and fruit-flavored gelatin in cake pans. The gel is the same as that used in modified ice cream pies. It is desirable to have the gel filling for ice cream pies and cakes and modified aufait slightly weaker than that used for gelatin cubes. The pies and cakes can be decorated with whipped cream.

Frozen Malted Milks

Frosted malteds are increasing in popularity during the winter as well as summer, according to recent reports (IAICM 1984). In some places the consumption of this product has increased substantially. Frosted malteds are made of a mix similar to that of malted milk shakes, and are frozen in a freezer as is ice cream. The partially frozen mix is held in the freezer and drawn into cones or paper cups when the customer's order is taken. In consistency it resembles soft ice cream ready to be drawn from the freezer.

Spumoni

This is a fancy ice cream generally made in cup-shaped form in pint or quart size. The outside layer is usually made of vanilla ice cream. In the bottom of this shell is placed macaroon or chocolate mousse and this is topped with tutti-frutti mousse. In serving, it is cut in wedge-shaped pieces like cake (Fig. 16.8).

Combinations

Various new combinations of fruits can be appealing flavors for ice cream specials. As examples, pineapple combinations such as grape–pineapple, mint–pineapple, orange–pineapple, pineapple–marshmallow prisms, glacé cherry mix, or pineapple, nuts, raisins and cherries. Caramel flavor combinations offer other attractive specials as well as do candies and candy–nut combinations such as buttercrunch, butterscotch, peppermint, lemon drops, butter toffee, maple pecan, and pecan crunch.

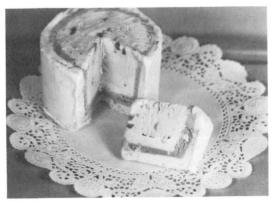

Fig. 16.8. Spumoni.

Aufait Ice Cream

Aufait ice cream usually consists of a layer of fruit between two layers of ice cream.

Variegated Ice Cream

Variegated or rainbow ice cream is made by carefully mixing (marble fashion) several different colors as the product is packaged. The variegated ice cream, sundae products, and other colorful products packaged in transparent plastic containers have additional consumer appeal.

Freeze-Dried Ice Cream

In the freeze-drying process more than 99% of the moisture is removed. The composition of freeze-dried ice cream is the same as the ice cream mix from which it is made in all constituents except water. It is important that the ice cream contain overrun in order to obtain a better product structurally. The length of freezing time depends upon the thickness of the ice cream; for a product thickness of 1/4–3/4 in., freezing time is 4–6 hr. Freeze-dried ice cream can be used as centers for candy and other confections.

An ice cream mix with a composition of 12% fat, 11% MSNF, 15% sugar, and 0.3% stabilizer would result in a freeze-dried product of approximately 19.3% fat, 17.7% MSNF, 25.1% sugar, and 0.48% stabilizer.

THE USES OF SPECIAL FLAVORS
AND OTHER NOVELTIES

The ice cream manufacturer should make more of an attempt to look at things from the consumer's viewpoint. Manufacturers should encourage consumer desires for new flavors and styles of products by developing new ideas, new specials, for different seasons and occasions, to keep interest from lagging. Any progressive ice cream manufacturer or retailer can offer the consumer some variety in ice cream specials. Although it is not ordinarily considered wise for the small concern to carry too many kinds of ice cream at one time, a definite plan for specials on a weekly basis or for festive occasions is good business.

Many manufacturers in different parts of the United States have taken advantage of new flavor appeals to increase their local business. Thus, coffee and maple have become popular sellers in New England and Canada, prune is successful in California, and ginger is popular among some ethnic groups. Many ice creams contain fruits and nuts that can be featured at appropriate times of the year.

Fall and winter have traditionally been the sluggish periods for the ice cream business. However, there is ample evidence to indicate that if special flavors are pushed when they are in season, and if fancy ice creams and novelties are developed and offered as they synchronize with the various holidays and seasons, business can be materially increased, even in these off-seasons. Although catering to this type of demand requires energy and imagination, ice cream makers can make use of the suggestions that follow to help their particular local businesses:

- Wedding and showers: Decorated cake; individual molds (slipper, bell, dove, bride and groom, tulip, heart, cupid, ring, etc.)
- Baby showers: Decorated cake with emblems such as stork and baby; individuals of the same designs
- Bridge parties: Decorated cake; individual molds of ace of hearts, clubs, spades, and diamonds; sometimes a stencil with similar designs can be used satisfactorily on sliced bricks
- Birthdays: Decorated cake, with "Happy Birthday" and/or name and numerals; individual molds with the stenciled numerals
- Children's parties; Individual molds of animals, toys, etc.
- Athletic functions: Ice cream cake in the form of a football, basketball, soccerball; individual forms showing athlete or ball
- New Year's Eve: Decorated cake with the baby New Year or a bell; brick with a bell center
- Lincoln's Birthday: Decorated cake with bust of Lincoln, flag, or other patriotic decorations; individual molds or sliced brick with the same decorations
- Washington's Birthday: Decorated cake; hatchet, flag, cherry tree, Washington bust either in cake or individual form
- Valentine's Day: Heart and cupid decorations on cake; heart center or cupid center bricks and individual molds of same design
- St. Patrick's Day: Shamrock cake or shamrock center brick; individual molds, carrying out the shamrock idea (see Fig. 16.2)
- Easter: Cake decorated with egg or lily; individuals in the shape of lilies, eggs, or rabbits; the same designs in the center of slices, large (2-qt, for example) rabbit
- Mother's Day: Whipped-cream decorations with appropriate wording; individual molds of assorted flowers
- Memorial Day: Special decorated cakes
- July 4: Individual designs (flags, shield, cannon, liberty bell, etc.); red, white, and blue bricks; cakes with patriotic decorations
- Halloween: Individual pumpkin, witch, corn cob, black cat, owl molds; cakes with these for decorations
- Thanksgiving: Decorated cakes showing turkey, horn of plenty, pumpkin, or other symbols suggestive of Thanksgiving; individual molds of the same kind

- Christmas: Decorated cakes with appropriate wording or designs; individual molds in the form of bells, stockings, Christmas trees, Santa Claus; bricks with Christmas tree centers

17
Defects, Scoring and Grading

Quality and price are two major factors in determining not only the volume of current business but also the future of the entire ice cream industry. Since quality is so vital in establishing price, it is necessary to understand the causes and remedies of defects in quality. Defects result from faults in flavor, body and texture, melting characteristics, color and package, bacterial content, or composition. The common defects in ice cream cause diminished consumer good will, sales, and income to the manufacturer. In their efforts to improve quality, manufacturers assume an ideal of perfection for each of these characteristics. This ideal standard is embodied in a score card, which is used to measure the degree of perfection by deducting from a perfect score for the various defects of the ice cream. This score card, which is discussed later, assigns points as follows: flavor, 45 points; body and texture, 30 points; bacteria, 15 points; color and package, 5 points; melting quality, 5 points.

The scoring of ice creams, sherbets, and ices presents some difficulties not encountered in scoring other dairy products. In the first place, the ideal flavor is far more variable than the ideal flavor for other dairy products, since it depends not only on the flavoring matrial used but also on the presence of other substances that blend with and modify the added flavoring material. Consequently, the ideal standard is a blend of the ideal flavor in dairy products and the ideal flavor in the added flavoring material. The ideal product should be packaged in an attractive container, possess a typical, pleasant, and desirable flavor, have a close, smooth, uniform body and texture, have desirable melting properties, possess a uniform natural color, and have a low bacterial count.

FLAVOR DEFECTS

Sources of flavor defects are

- Dairy products of poor quality: with common old ingredients, oxidized, acid, cooked, or unclean off-flavors
- Sweetness: excessive or deficient
- Flavoring: excess, deficient, or atypical
- Blend: may not be pleasing
- Serving conditions: too hard or too soft.

Flavor Characteristics

The qualities imparted by the flavoring material may be designated as high, low, delicate, harsh, and unnatural.

High flavor is characterized by the presence of large amounts of the flavoring material. In some cases an excess of flavoring material will impart a sharp or bitter flavor to the ice cream. A poor quality of flavoring may have the same effect; hence it is quite important to determine, if possible, whether the bitter flavor is due to poor quality or to excessive flavoring material, although both are undesirable defects.

Low flavor refers to an insufficient amount of flavoring material, that is, there is not enough to make the flavor easily recognized. It may be due to insufficient or weak flavoring material, to some other substance obscuring the flavor, or to the ice cream mix being cooked after the volatile flavoring material is added. However, low flavor should not be confused with delicate flavor.

Delicate flavors, are, as a rule, the most pleasing and desirable and most easily blended, and they do not cause one to get tired of them quickly. Natural flavors, such as fruit and nut flavors, are delicate and pleasing to taste but they are also readily dissipated by careless handling.

Harsh flavors are sharp and lingering, such as ginger, onion, and vinegar. A good illustration of this defect in ice cream is obtained when quite large quantities of lemon or orange extract are used, giving a flavor entirely due to the lemon or orange oil. Harsh flavors are usually due to the use of inferior flavoring substances, but in some cases may result from the use of too much flavoring extract. Inferior and artificial extracts lack the fine, delicate qualities of the high-grade extracts and frequently give a very pronounced, but not pleasing, flavor to the ice cream.

Unnatural flavors are considered defects, but to an extent that will depend upon the source of that flavor. For example, because of its acidity lemon juice is sometimes added to reinforce certain fruit flavors. However, should any of the oil from the rind of the lemon find access to the mixture, it is likely to impart a lemon flavor where it is not wanted. In such a case, the resulting blended fruit flavor would be "unnatural" but not of a particularly undesirable sort. Similarly, a pronounced vanillin flavor in vanilla ice cream, caramel flavor in maple ice cream colored with caramel, and synthetic flavors that are not perfect imitations of the true flavors are considered unnatural. Flavors due to poor cream, poor gelatin, fermented syrups, overripe or unsound fruit, and rancid nuts are also considered unnatural flavors.

Fruit and fruit juices may impart undesirable flavors if the fruit is unsound or the juice fermented. The naturally delicate flavor imparted by sound fruit may be quite easily distinguished from the artificial flavors. An artificial flavor, being somewhat unnatural, is not regarded as highly as a natural flavor.

Nut flavors are judged in the same way as fruit flavors. The way in which the nuts have been prepared also is important: whether the nuts have been blanched, finely chopped, and evenly distributed through the ice cream.

Syrups and sugar may be used in excess, making the mixture too sweet. When an insufficient amount is used, the ice cream has a flat flavor. Sometimes a sour or yeasty flavor may be imparted by the use of a syrup that has begun to ferment.

The flavors imparted by the dairy products are the most important from a hygienic standpoint. The flavor given to ice cream by good, pure dairy products is rich, creamy, and delicate. Flavor defects are usually described as "cooked" and "feed" (when due to normal feeds) are not of a particularly undesirable sort. Lower scores are given for flavors due to the use of tainted dairy products. These flavors may be grouped under such terms as "feed" (due to weeds, etc.), "high acid," "old ingredient" (yeasty, cheesy, musty, bitter, etc.), "oxidized," "rancid," "salty" (when due to salty cream), and "unclean."

Defects Caused by Chemical Changes

Flavor defects described as "storage" (stale) and "oxidized" (resembling cardboard or tallow) sometimes develop in ice cream as a result of chemical changes and are particularly objectionable. An especially unpleasant flavor, suggesting a stale and unclean flavor, may be absorbed from the air of the hardening room when moisture-soaked wood is exposed through lack of paint or cracked paint. This absorbed flavor defect is usually most noticeable in the whipped cream decorations of specialties being hardened without wrapping.

Lack of fine flavor is a minor flavor defect and may be corrected by using fresh dairy products and true flavoring materials.

Acid flavor is caused by the presence of an excessive amount of lactic acid. It can be remedied by using fresh dairy products; prompt, efficient cooling of the mix; or avoiding prolonged storage of the mix at high storage temperatures.

Bitter flavor results from the use of inferior products and may be prevented by using true extracts; avoiding use of dairy products stored for long periods at low temperatures, as certain types of bacteria produce bitter flavor under these conditions; or using products free from off-flavors.

Cooked flavor is caused by overheating the mix or using overheated concentrated dairy products. This defect can be prevented by carefully controlling the pasteurization process, or using concentrated products free of cooked flavor.

Flat flavor is a result of the use of insufficient flavor, sugar, or milk solids, and can be remedied by increasing the amount of these materials.

Unnatural flavor indicates the presence of a flavor not typical to ice cream. This condition may be remedied by using high-quality flavoring products, or using high-quality dairy and nondairy products.

Metallic flavor is caused by copper contamination and in some cases may be the result of bacterial action. It may be prevented by avoiding copper contamination of the mix during processing, or avoiding the use of products having a metallic flavor.

Salty flavor may be due to the use of more than 0.1% salt in the mix, or too high MSNF content of the mix.

Old ingredient flavor may be prevented by using only clean fresh dairy products.

Oxidized flavor is also sometimes called tallowy or cardboard. It may be avoided by using fresh dairy products; using only stainless steel equipment; using antioxidants; or pasteurizing the mix at high temperatures (170°F).

BODY AND TEXTURE

Body and Texture Characteristics

Body may be said to be the quality that gives weight and substance to the product and enables it to stand up well. Thus it refers to consistency ("chewiness") or firmness and to the melting character of ice cream. The ideal body is produced by the correct proportion of milk solids (both butterfat and MSNF) together with the proper overrun, and melts fairly rapidly at room temperature to a smooth liquid similar in appearance and consistency to sweet cream containing about 40% fat. It results from the proper combination of composition and processing, each being somewhat limited by the other.

Texture refers to the grain or to the finer structure of the product, and depends upon the size, shape, and arrangement of the small particles. Ice cream having an ideal texture will be very smooth, the solid particles being too small to be detected in the mouth.

The body and texture characteristics are closely associated and are important in influencing consumer acceptance of ice cream and related products. The internal structure factors that influence body and texture include the size, shape, and distribution of ice crystals; the size, shape, and distribution of air cells; and the amount and distribution of unfrozen material. The microtographs in Fig. 17.1 show ice cream samples having different body and texture characteristics.

Body and Texture Defects

Sources of common body and texture defects are improper composition of mix, improper processing methods, and improper storage conditions. Composition affects body and texture in general through an increase or decrease in TS of the mix. Body defects are commonly described as crumbly, soggy, and weak, while the common texture defects are called coarse, icy, fluffy, sandy, and buttery.

A "crumbly" body lacks cohesion and pulls or breaks apart very easily—a common defect of sherbets and ices where it is less serious than in ice cream. It is frequently associated with a low TS content, insufficient stabilization, excessive overrun, low homogenization pressure, large air cells, and imperfect homogenization. Factors (such as improper salt balance, enzymatic improvers, and certain gum stabilizers) that limit the hydration of the proteins are also thought to cause crumbliness. It is similar to the defect sometimes referred to as "dry" body, which results from excessive use of emulsifiers, egg yolk solids, certain types of vegetable stabilizers, excessive homogenization pressure, or the addition of dry milk solids at the freezer. Crumbly body may be remedied by increasing the solids content, increasing the stabilizer, or decreasing the overrun.

A "soggy" body is dense and may be somewhat "wet" in appearance. In some

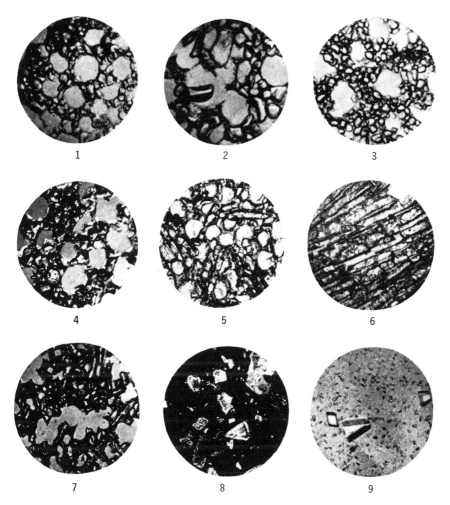

Fig. 17.1. Micrographs of ice cream showing body and texture characteristics. (1) Close, smooth; (2) coarse, open; (3) short, fluffy; (4) soggy; (5) coarse, icy, due to temperature fluctuations; (6) coarse, icy, flaky, due to slow freezing without agitation; (7) coarse, icy, surface heat shock; (8) lactose crystals from sandy ice cream; (9) lactose crystals.

market areas this defect is not too objectionable. It is due to a low overrun (especially if the TS content is high), a high concentration of sugars that lower the freezing point, hand packaging after hardening the ice cream, or excessive concentration of stabilizer. It is frequently confused with defects described as "gummy," "doughy," "sticky," and "gluey." Excessive stabilization or a high TS content produces a "chewy" or "gummy" body, while syrups and certain types of gum (pectin, oatgum, etc.) favor a "pasty," "sticky," or "gluey" body. Sogginess and its related defects contribute to a high melting resistance.

A "weak" body lacks firmness or chewiness and is invariably accompanied by rapid melting. It should not be confused with "fluffy" or "snowy" texture and excessive overrun. A weak body is particularly undesirable from the consumer's viewpoint and should receive a very low score. The defect is due to a low TS content combined with insufficient stabilization, and results, therefore, in a thin mix—a mix of weak consistency.

"Buttery" texture refers to lumps of butterfat large enough to be easily detected in the mouth. When a lump of butterfat is chewed, the sensation is different from that obtained from ice crystals or from lactose crystals. This defect is due to churning (usually during the freezing process), which results from incomplete homogenization, high fat content, mix entering the freezer at too high a temperature, and slow freezing.

"Coarse" or icy texture indicates that the ice crystals are large or not uniform in size, or that the air cells are too large. The coarseness due to large air cells should not be confused with high overrun obtained by small air cells. This is the most common texture defect and is affected by many factors. For example, large air cells may be due to the type of freezer used, or to a mix of low whipping ability. Large ice crystals are favored by insufficient stabilizer, slow freezing in the freezer, slow freezing in the hardening room (such as happens after partial melting before entering, and refreezing in the hardening room or when storage temperatures fluctuate and slightly softened ice cream is rehardened), and insufficient hydration of the protein (lack of aging, high acidity, poor salt balance, etc.). "Coarse and icy" also includes the presence of ice pellets, which are caused by droplets of water getting into the ice cream, frequently from the retailer's scoops. Coarse texture may be controlled by avoiding low solids in mixes, sufficient stabilizer, lower drawing temperatures at the freezer, fast hardening, avoiding heat shocking, and short storage.

"Fluffy" texture is readily detected by the presence of large air cells and an open texture. It is due to the incorporation of an excessive amount of air. This defect may be expected when the TS content is not more than one-third of the overrun. When the air cells are large and the amount of air is excessive, the texture is sometimes described as "snowy" or "flaky." Such a condition might be more properly noted as both "fluffy" and "coarse." It may be corrected by decreasing the overrun, increasing the TS, or decreasing the amount of emulsifier.

"Sandy" texture is a roughness like sand in melted ice cream that is noted not only when rubbed against the roof of the mouth but also when chewed. Sandy texture jeopardizes the marketability of the ice cream. It is due entirely to fairly large lactose crystals, which are slow to dissolve. Conditions favoring the development of a sandy texture include a high lactose content (usually expressed as high MSNF content), high and perhaps fluctuating temperatures (as in retail cabinets), high temperature when drawn from freezer, low viscosity of the unfrozen liquid phase, and perhaps the presence of substances that initiate crystal formation. This defect may be controlled by reducing the MSNF content of the mix, acid standardization, replacing part of the cane sugar content with dextrose, or maintaining uniformly low storage temperature.

Factors Affecting Texture

The factors affecting texture are (1) mix composition, (2) ingredients used, (3) physical and chemical characteristics of mix, (4) methods of processing, (5) method of freezing, (6) rate of hardening, and (7) storage conditions.

Increased TS content of the mix as resulting from increasing the percentage of any of the mix constituents may produce a smoother texture because there is less water to be frozen, the increased concentration of mix causes mechanical obstruction to crystal growth and air incorporation during the freezing process, and the freezing point may be lowered.

Fat content influences texture by its ability to reduce ice crystal size through mechanical obstruction, and to produce a lubricating effect causing a smooth sensation in mouth. The effect on ice crystal size is as follows:

Fat content (%)	Ice crystal size (μm)
10	82.6 × 60.8
16	47.2 × 38.0

MSNF affects texture by reducing freezing point, increasing the amount of unfrozen material, mechanically obstructing ice crystal and air cell formation, and holding a portion of the water as water of hydration (Table 17.1). Increased MSNF shows a pronounced effect upon the texture, resulting in smaller ice crystals, smaller air cells, and a reduced thickness of the air cell walls. The occurrence of smaller air cells with increased amounts of MSNF is significant in that MSNF is probably the constituent in the mix with the greatest influence in the air cell size. These factors also influence the body characteristics.

Increasing the sugar content causes a smoother texture because the freezing point is lowered and the amount of unfrozen material is increased, and sugar holds a portion of the water.[1]

Sugar content (%)	Ice crystal size (μm)
12	67.5 × 51.0
18	48.8 × 35.5

Added increments of corn sugar may decrease ice crystal size because of lowering the freezing point of the mix. The unfrozen material is increased and the body characteristics may show improvement.

The percentage overrun is an important factor in influencing body and texture of ice cream. The influence of overrun on ice crystal and air cell size and distribution is shown in Table 17.2.

The effect of 1% increase of mix components in decreasing ice crystal size is shown in Table 17.3. It seems that after the texture reaches a certain degree of

---

[1]Neutralization of mix or ingredients is not permitted in any case.

Table 17.1. Effect of MSNF on the Internal Structure of Ice Cream[a]

MSNF content of ice cream (%)	Average ice crystal size (μm)	Average air cell size (μm)	Cell wall thickness (μm)	Texture observations
9	55.8	176.6	165.4	Slightly coarse
11	52.3	188.4	148.7	Medium smooth
13	39.4	158.0	116.0	Smooth
15	32.2	103.2	124.0	Very smooth

[a]Arbuckle (1940).

Table 17.2. Effects of Overrun

Overrun (%)	Ice crystal size (μm)	Air cell diameter (μm)	Unfrozen material (μm)
85	62.7 × 51.2	165.2	11.2
100	53.9 × 47.3	142.3	10.0
115	50.4 × 44.1	109.0	8.5
130	49.8 × 43.1	104.0	7.0

Table 17.3. Effects of Component Increase on Crystal Size

	Reduction (μm)
Fat, 1%	4.5
MSNF, 1%	4.3
Fat, 0.5%; MSNF, 0.5%	5.8
Sugar, 1% in 11% MSNF	2.8
Sugar, 1% in 13% MSNF	2.4
Overrun, 10%	1.6

closeness, further changes of components of the mix have little influence upon ice crystal size.

The acidity of the mix influences texture characteristics, as shown in Table 17.4.

Special products such as sodium caseinate, calcium sulfate, and delactosed milk solids have various effects on body and texture. Sodium caseinate improves whipping properties and affects air cell and ice crystal distributions. Calcium sulfate produces a dry stiff ice cream and has little effect on smoothness.

Mix processing procedures most effective in influencing body and textures are pasteurization, homogenization, and aging. Pasteurization temperatures may range from 150 to 300°F. The effect of higher temperatures on mix components is to produce a smoother product. Effective homogenization results in smooth ice cream; excessive pressure may produce adverse results. Aging or storing of mix 2–4 hr allows stabilizer and other mix constituents to become oriented.

Table 17.4. Effect of Acidity on Crystal Size

Acidity (%)	pH	Ice crystal size (μm)
0.24	6.5	50.7 × 42.5
0.18	6.8	42.5 × 37.4
0.12	7.5	49.2 × 44.3

Table 17.5. Effect of Emulsifiers on Texture[a]

Product	Ice crystal diameter (μm)	Air cell diameter (μm)	Comments
Gelatin	38	188	Very slightly coarse
plus lecithinated products	32	156	Medium smooth
plus mono- and diglycerides	36	151	Medium smooth
plus fatty acid esters	31	122	Smooth
plus polyoxyalkylene derivatives	35	135	Smooth

[a]Arbuckle (1950).

The viscosity or thickness of the mix has little relationship to the body and texture characteristics of the finished ice cream.

Stabilizers are effective in producing a smooth texture through their ability to combine with a portion of the water of the mix. This results in mechanical obstruction to ice crystal formation and smaller ice crystals. Stabilizers also prolong whipping time, which provides for a more uniform distribution of internal structure components.

Emulsifiers produce smooth stiff ice cream with smaller ice crystals and more evenly distributed and somewhat smaller air cells (Table 17.5). Egg yolk solids produce similar but usually not as pronounced effects.

The rates of freezing and hardening affect texture. Fast freezing produces small ice crystals.

Such factors as container size, air circulation, hardening room temperature, and use of air blast in tunnel influence the rate of hardening, and the resulting texture of the product. Uniform hardening room temperature is extremely important in maintaining uniformity of texture. A temperature as high as −5°F will produce good results if fluctuations are avoided. Partial melting and rehardening should always be avoided.

Lactose crystallization in the finished product results in a sandy texture defect. Rapid turnover of the product and the use of delactosed milk solids and mineralized solids have been proposed to prevent this.

The effect of stabilizers in the fruit on the texture characteristics of strawberry ice cream is shown in Table 17.6. Fruit particle size used in ice cream is also important. It is difficult to get smoothness in large fruit portions. Particles that are too small result in good texture but poor flavor appeal.

Table 17.6. Effects of Fruit Stabilizers on Texture

Kind of berry preparation used	Observations
Frozen berries stabilized by fruit picker	Smooth, berries firm, ice crystals not detectable
Frozen berries thawed and stabilized (by the ice cream plant)	Slightly coarse, berries tend toward coarseness
Frozen strawberries not stabilized	Medium coarse, berries icy

It is quite essential to avoid the presence of undissolved particles of any of the mix constituents if a desirable body and texture is maintained. The importance of body and texture should never be overlooked in the production of ice cream that will have maximum consumer acceptance.

MELTING QUALITY DEFECTS

Desirable melting qualities are shown when the melted ice cream is very similar in characteristic to that of the original mix.

The melting appearance of ice cream is sometimes distinctly foamy. This should be considered a defect and is due particularly to large air cells and large amounts of egg solids. Emulsifiers or excess gelatin in low-solids mixes, as well as a heavy mix consistency, are likely to augment the condition.

"Curdy" meltdown includes not only the finely divided particles of protein in watery liquid, but also a dull, finely wrinkled, scumlike surface on the melted ice cream. This defect leads the consumer to assume that inferior ingredients were used. Actually it is the result of protein destabilization, which may be caused by one or a combination of the following: excess acidity, low concentration of citrates and phosphates in proportion to the calcium and magnesium content, melting and refreezing even in the freezer, the use of enzymatic improvers, the use of certain stabilizers, excessive homogenization pressures, long storage at low temperatures, and shrinkage of the ice cream.

Curdled meltdown indicates high acidity in the mix or any other factor that might cause instability of milk protein. The condition may be corrected by using fresh dairy products, avoiding the use of any product that might disturb the natural salt balance of the mix, or avoiding high-acid mixes.

"Does not melt" includes not only ice cream that retains its shape when warmed but also the various degrees of slow melting to a liquid. It frequently accompanies body defects such as "soggy," "gummy," "doughy," and "sticky." The conditions causing these body defects also contribute to high melting resistance. Other factors producing this melting defect include a high fat content, drawing at a low temperature from continuous freezers, high freezing point, and excessive viscosity resulting from slow cooling, the use of calcium neutralizers, or certain types of stabilizer.

Slow melting indicates overstabilization or improper processing of the mix. The condition can be corrected by reducing the amount of stabilizer or emulsifier, using fresh dairy products, or homogenizing at proper temperature and pressure.

Whey leakage occurs during the melting of ice cream when the mix is of poor quality or if the mix is improperly balanced or stabilized. This defect can be remedied by using high-quality dairy products, balancing the constituent of the mix carefully, or using a more effective stabilizer.

Foamy meltdown is caused by the incorporation of too much air in the ice cream. The foamy defect may be corrected by reducing the overrun or reducing the amount of emulsifier or egg product used.

COLOR AND PACKAGE DEFECTS

Coloring and packaging help present the tempting appearance essential in ice cream. Therefore, good workmanship as evidenced by delicate, appropriate colors, uniformity of colors, not only the uniformity of layers but also the clearness of object outlines in molded ice creams, and the cleanliness and neatness of packages should receive consideration. The ideal color is characteristic of the flavor, true in shade, and neither too pale nor too intense. For example, vanilla ice cream should be the color of cream produced on early pasture.

Uniform, natural color is desirable in ice cream. Excessive color is the result of adding too much artificial color to the mix. An uneven color results if the color is not properly added and also if care is not exercised when changing flavors. An unnatural color is caused by carelessness in adding the color, improper use of color, or use of foreign materials.

Unnatural color describes defects due to insufficient (pale) color, excess (intense) color, and colors that are not characteristic (true in shade) of the flavor. Examples of defective shades are the tannish brown of caramel instead of the reddish brown of chocolate, or egg yellow for annatto color in vanilla ice cream, or a dull, grayish appearance (due to lack of acidity) in cranberry ice cream.

Other defects such as uneven color, no parchment lining of cans, rusty cans, and unclean cans are too obvious to need discussion here.

COMPOSITION AND BACTERIAL DEFECTS

Standards for composition and bacterial content are now adopted by nearly all communities, so that the public may be assured of a safe, healthful product. These standards represent the lowest quality (i.e., the least expensive) permissible for market, and should not be interpreted as either optimum or ideal. As yet there is no widely accepted procedure for scoring variations in either bacterial content or composition except to require compliance with local legal standards.

"Sediment" designates insoluble foreign material. It proves extreme carelessness and therefore is very objectionable. It may enter as part of the ingredients, when the ingredients are carelessly produced or stored (as in open containers), or it may be due to carelessness while manufacturing.

The disadvantages of strainers and filters for removing foreign materials are it is almost impossible to sanitize these utensils after they are assembled for use, they encourage the operator to use contaminated ingredients, erroneously thinking that strainers and filters will remove bacterial contamination, and they tend to encourage carelessness on the part of the operator. However, in commercial practice they have some advantages, such as preventing serious damage to expensive equipment by bolts, wrenches, rings, buttons, etc., dropping into vats or ice cream hopper either accidentally or through carelessness of employees; and catching such other foreign substances as should not, but sometimes do, get into the milk, cream, or ice cream mix.

However, foreign substances such as buttons, hairpins, and jewelry sometimes gain access to the hardened ice cream after it leaves the factory, when lids are removed while handling cans for storage in retail cabinets or for dispensing the ice cream over the counter. Hence precautions against these mishaps should be taken at every step from the factory to the consumer.

"Pancake" (a taffylike deposit at the bottom of the package) is similar to the bleeding defect in ices and sherbets. When hardened, these so-called pancakes are very coarse and unpalatable. Conditions favoring this defect are storage at too high a temperature, near the melting point of the ice cream; draining the freezer too completely, i.e., collecting unfrozen mix; and a weak body due to an improper balance of the mix constituents, such as a high sugar content, low concentration of stabilizer, and low TS content. Although not specifically mentioned on the score card, this defect is serious and greatly reduces the score.

"Shrinkage" adequately describes a particularly vexatious defect. After well-filled packages are hardened, the volume of the ice cream shrinks, leaving a space either at the top or side of the package, which then appears "not full." It is probably a special type of the "weak" body defect combined with a texture defect (therefore closely associated with whipping ability) and becomes apparent with certain temperature changes or types of package (see Fig. 17.2).

Although it has been widely studied, and many factors have been suggested as causes, shrinkage is still difficult to produce at will; in fact, frequently it occurs in only a portion of the packages frozen under similar conditions from the same batch of mix. Conditions accepted as probable causes include:

- Neutralization of the mix or some of the ingredients used
- Containers that are porous to air, such as paper not properly waxed on the side in contact with the ice cream
- Abnormally low temperatures either when freezing, drawing from the freezer, hardening in tunnels, or hardening by dry ice before storage
- Conditions favoring bleeding or pancakes
- Excessive overrun as in fluffy texture (though the product may not appear fluffy the air content may be greater than can be contained at conditions to which the product is exposed)
- Excessive smoothness (the texture is too fine grained) possibly results from an unusual combination of conditions (such as too rapid freezing) that favor the formation of small-sized particles, and conditions arising from a combination of emulsifiers, as yet not too well understood, but which seem to favor very small air cells
- Texture that favors curdy meltdown, i.e., partially destabilized protein.

Shrinkage might be expected in ice cream receiving severe criticism for weak body.

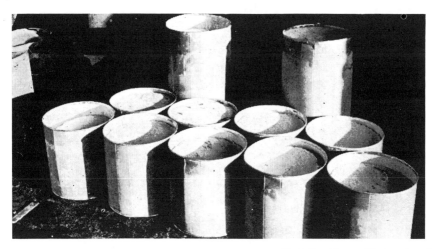

Fig. 17.2. Shrinkage defect in ice cream. (Courtesy of D. J. Hankinson, University of Massachusetts.)

THE SCORE CARD

Ice cream as yet is not sold on the basis of score. However, the score card (Fig. 17.3) is a convenient tool or guide with which to measure the degree of perfection of any given ice cream. The ideal or standard as indicated by the highest score on the score card serves as the measuring stick by which to compare or judge the ice cream. Some practice in the use of the score card should be valuable in improving the quality of ice cream. The reliability of the score depends partly upon the judge's conception of the ideal standard and partly upon an ability to recognize very slight defects. The degree of perfection or score may or may not agree with the acceptability of the ice cream in a certain market area, although there is usually a rather close agreement.

The Use of the Score Card

The purpose of scoring ice cream is to emphasize the degree of perfection and the opportunity for improvement. Figure 17.4 is a summary of the relative significance of the defects described in previous paragraphs of this chapter and a guide to scoring them.

A defect is considered "slight" when recognizable by the connoisseur but not detected by most consumers; (2) "definite" when detectable by many consumers; (3) "pronounced" when detectable by most consumers. Usually the defects are scored to the nearest half point, and a product with a score below the normal range should generally be considered unsalable.

There are several ways scoring can be done:

Write scores opposite the rating for perfect score. Check criticisms in the space opposite the defects noted and in the proper sample column.

Perfect Score	Criticisms	Sample Number			
		1	2	3	4
FLAVOR: 45	CONTESTANT SCORE ▶				
	GRADE ___ SCORE / CRITICISM				
	Cooked				
	Lacks flavoring				
NO CRITICISM: 10	Too high flavor				
	Unnatural flavor				
	High acid				
	Lacks fine flavor				
	Lacks freshness				
	Metallic				
NORMAL RANGE: 1–10	Old ingredient				
	Oxidized				
	Rancid				
	Salty				
	Storage				
	Lacks sweetness				
	Syrup flavor				
	Too sweet				
	Whey				
BODY AND TEXTURE: 30	CONTESTANT SCORE ▶				
	GRADE ___ SCORE / CRITICISM				
NO CRITICISM: 5	Coarse/icy				
	Crumbly				
	Fluffy				
NORMAL RANGE: 1–5	Gummy				
	Sandy				
	Soggy				
	Weak				
COLOR: 5	ALLOWED PERFECT IN CONTEST ▶				
MELTING QUALITY: 5	ALLOWED PERFECT IN CONTEST				
BACTERIA: 15	ALLOWED PERFECT IN CONTEST				
TOTAL: 100	TOTAL SCORE OF EACH SAMPLE ▶				
	TOTAL GRADE PER SAMPLE				

Fig. 17.3. The official ice cream score card. Scores are written opposite the defects, and averaged for entry in the "contestant score."

Guide for Scoring Flavor of Ice Cream

No flavor criticism: 10 Normal range: 1–10	Intensity of defect					
	Slight		Definite		Pronounced	
Cooked	9	(39.5)	7	(38)	5	(36)
	7	(37.5)	6	(36)	3	(33)
Lacks flavoring	9	(39)	8	(38)	7	(37)
Too high flavor	9	(39)	8	(38)	7	(36)
Unnatural flavor	8	(37)	6	(35)	4	(33)
High acid	4	(34)	2	(31)	*	—
Lacks fine flavor	9	(39.5)	8	(38)	7	(37)
Lacks freshness	8	(38)	7	(37)	6	(36)
Metallic	6	(36)	4	(34)	2	(32)
Old ingredient	6	(36)	4	(34)	2	(32)
Oxidized	6	(36)	4	(34)	1	(31)
Rancid	4	(34)	2	(31)	*	—
Salty	8	(38)	7	(37)	5	(35)
Storage	7	(37)	6	(36)	4	(34)
Lacks sweetness	9	(39)	8	(38)	7	(37)
Syrup flavor	9	(39)	7	(37)	5	(35)
Too sweet	9	(39)	8	(38)	7	(37)
Whey	9	(39)	7	(37)	5	(35)

Guide for Scoring Body and Texture of Ice Cream

No body and texture criticism: 5 Normal range: 1–5	Intensity of defect					
	Slight		Definite		Pronounced	
Coarse/icy	4	(29.5)	2	(27)	1	(25)
Crumbly	4	(29)	3	(27)	2	(26)
Fluffy	3	(28)	2	(27)	1	(26)
Gummy	4	(29)	2	(27)	1	(26)
Sandy	2	(26)	1	(25)	*	—
Soggy	4	(29)	3	(28)	2	(27)
Weak	4	(29)	2	(27)	1	(26)

Guide to Converting Criticism Range to Point Score

Quality class	Flavor score range	Body and texture score range
Excellent	10 (40)	5 (30)
Good	8–9 (38–39.5)	3–4 (28–29.5)
Fair	6–7 (36–37.5)	2 (26–27.5)
Poor	5 or less (35.5 or less)	1 or less (25.5 or less)

Fig. 17.4. The use of the score card—a guide.

1. By putting the characteristic into a quality class (excellent, good, fair poor) and then assigning the appropriate point rating.
2. By judging the characteristic by intensity (slight, definite, pronounced) and then scoring accordingly.
3. By rating the characteristic from 1 to 10 and then finding the appropriate score.
4. By assigning a point rating to the characteristic.

After each characteristic has received a point score, the scores in both groups are averaged, and the average is entered as a contestant score under the correct sample.

Sensory Rating and Evaluation of Ice Cream Quality

Dethmers *et al.* (1981) presented a comprehensive sensory evaluation guide for testing food products and stated that sensory evaluation has been defined as a scientific discipline used to evoke, measure, analyze, and interpret reactions to those characteristics of foods and materials as they are perceived by the senses of sight, smell, taste, touch, and hearing. The most commonly occurring industrial applications of testing methodology and objectives and types of tests are set forth.

Ice cream is probably among the most variable and complex foods to evaluate by sensory analysis. Scoring may be done by an individual, by a panel of judges, or by a profile of panelists. The latter has many advantages as the members discuss their findings on each sample and make a common judgment. Group perception is generally more comprehensive and meaningful.

The Clinic

The carefully conducted clinic is a very valuable way for manufacturers to evaluate the characteristics of their products. The following steps can be taken to organize a clinic:

1. Select a competent taste panel to judge the finished products.
2. Choose a regular time, at least once a month, when the products are to be judged.
3. Have an employee who is not a member of the judging panel pick up samples from retail outlets, if possible the oldest samples available.
4. Have an employee pick up sample packages of your competitor's product of the same flavor as your own from retail outlets. Sample packages collected from stores must be held cold during transport to the clinic site.
5. All samples should be tempered to 5–10°F.
6. All samples are placed in paper bags, and the bags taped around the top so as to hide the identity of each sample.
7. Number all samples and maintain a key to their identity.
8. Place all samples in numerical order.

The steps in the examination of the ice cream samples are as follows:

1. Dip out a small portion for meltdown observation,.
2. Each member should use two spoons: one for dipping, one for tasting.
3. Numerical scoring is not necessary; score by quality class: excellent, good, fair, poor, or without criticism.
4. Criticism should give an insight as to what is wrong so that immediate steps can be taken to correct the defect.
5. Tabulate results and comments in a manner in which they will be most

useful to those responsible for correcting defects. Insist that corrections are made immediately.

6. Recall products that do not meet salable standards.

The most common defects encountered in clinics are

1. Flavor: cooked, old ingredients, unnatural, oxidized, syrup, whey.
2. Body: weak, soggy, short.
3. Texture: coarse/icy.
4. Meltdown: does not melt, flaky, curdy, wheys off.
5. Color: unnatural, too high, lacking.
6. Fruit and nut distribution: uneven, lacking.

Fundamentals of Ice Cream Judging

Judging ice cream is performed by use of the senses of sight, taste, touch, and to a lesser degree smell.

1. The judge should learn to recognize and evaluate visible defects, such as color, body and texture, appearance, flavor, and particle distribution.

2. Flavor is a combination of both taste and aroma. An individual can detect four basic taste sensations: bitter, acid, salty, and sweet. These are detected by the taste buds in the mouth on certain areas of the tongue: sweet, top central section of the tongue; acid, side halfway back of tongue; bitter, base of tongue; salty, tip and sides of tongue.

Many of the flavors in ice cream, other than those listed above, must be identified by taste. This is accomplished by tasting the product and permitting the volatile flavor of the product in the mouth to pass over the taste buds and the olfactory organs in the back of the nostrils. One then becomes familiar and experienced with a flavor and gains the ability to recognize it by memory whenever it occurs. Some flavors or combinations of flavors occur that may be difficult to identify.

3. Body and texture are determined by the senses of sight and touch. Melting quality may be observed by allowing a portion of ice cream to remain at room temperature for about 30 min.

The sequence of observations is as follows:

1. Examine condition and appearance in container.
2. Note color, flavor, and candy, fruit, and nut distribution.
3. Take portion for judging: note the way the product cuts and feels.
4. Place portion in mouth and examine for body and texture.
5. While moving sample about mouth to ascertain body and texture, observe the flavor.
6. Make decisions, evaluations, and expectorate.
7. Repeat above sequence to assure correct evaluation.

The scoring of ice cream is difficult because the flavor is quite variable as it is dependent on several aspects: the flavor in the dairy products, the flavor of the added flavoring material, and the sweetening agent.

Color defects may be excessive, uneven, unnatural, due to careless adding of color, processing methods, different freezers, lack of uniformity in flavoring materials.

Melting quality defects may include curdiness, foamy, does not melt, and whey leakage. The causes may be lack of aging the mix, high-acid ingredients, excess stabilizer and emulsifier, too high overrun, improper homogenizing temperature or pressure, poor-quality ingredients.

Tasting Technique

- Dairy product judges generally rinse their mouths out with water after tasting a decidedly off-flavor product or return to a good or excellent sample to prevent the off-flavor from carrying over to the next sample.
- The amount of product tasted may range from 10 to 30 ml.
- It is the consensus that there is much merit in retasting products during scoring.
- The time interval of 2–5 min between samples has been used to allow all the organs to return to normal taste conditions. A comparatively brief time is required to sense a flavor, as little as 5–10 sec.
- The judging panel of five or six judges may be expected to operate with a narrower range in score. A larger number of judges does not necessarily result in a more accurate judging.

Contrary to general opinion there is no limit to the number of samples an experienced taster can taste in one day.

Suggested Fundamental Rules for Judging

1. Be in physical and mental condition for scoring.
2. Know the score card and ideals established for the product.
3. Know product defects and defect intensities allowed.
4. Have samples properly tempered.
5. Always secure a representative sample to be judged.
6. Use a sufficiently large sample for examination.
7. Fix an ideal in mind. Compare to this ideal.
8. Observe the sequence in flavors.
9. Observe the body and texture characteristics.
10. Concentrate on the sample being examined to the exclusion of everything else.
11. Do not be too critical.
12. Be honest with yourself. Do not be influenced by comments of others.
13. Check your own scoring occasionally.
14. Avoid facial expressions or remarks that may influence other judges of the group.
15. Clean your mouth occasionally by rinsing with water or an excellent sample.
16. Never eat strong-flavored foods just before judging.
17. Avoid excessive fatigue.
18. Recognize that practice and experience are helpful in improving ability.

Table 17.7. Guide to Market Rating of Ice Cream, Sherbet, and Ices

Rating	Flavor score		Body and texture score		Sum of score on color, meltdown, bacteria	Total score
	Range	Common criticism	Range	Common criticism		
Excellent	40	None	29.5–30	None	25	93–95
Good	38–39.5	Cooked	28–29.0	Slight coarse	23–24.5	90–92.5
		Salty		Slight weak		
		Lacks fine flavor		Slight fluffy		
		Lacks flavoring		Slight gummy		
		Lacks freshness		Slight soggy		
		Too high flavor				
		Too sweet				
Fair	35–37.5	Cooked	26–27.5	Definite coarse	21–22.5	87–89.5
		Old ingredient		Definite weak		
		Syrup flavor		Definite fluffy		
		Too high flavor		Definite gummy		
		Storage		Definite soggy		
		Salty		Slight sandy		
		Metallic				
		Oxidized				
Poor	31–34	Oxidized	25–25.5	Pronounced coarse	19–20.5	Less than 87
		Old ingredient		Pronounced weak		
		Storage		Pronounced fluffy		
		Rancid		Pronounced gummy		
				Pronounced soggy		
				Pronounced sandy		

MARKET GRADES

Market grades or classes have not as yet been accepted in the ice cream industry in spite of the fact that many consumers would welcome a system of market grades. The fluid milk or market milk industry has a widely accepted system of market grades in which the methods of producing and handling the milk receive more emphasis than does the score, i.e., its degree of perfection. These market grades of milk are closely associated with the relative value of the milk not only to the consumer but also as determined by the cost of production and distribution. Similarly the market grades of butter are closely associated with the score, even though the distinction between the grades is based primarily upon the relative value of the butter to the consumer. A similiar system of market grades based primarily upon the relative value to the consumer might be beneficial to the ice cream industry.

Table 17.7 suggests a possible system of market ratings together with the approximate correlation to the ice cream score. It should be recognized that the score primarily measures differences in degree of perfection, which may not represent significant differences in value to the consumer—the latter differences being the primary distinction in market rating. Therefore, a market rating will include a range of scores all of which will represent the same market value to the consumer.

18
Sanitation and Quality Control

A high-quality ice cream can be made only from good mix ingredients properly balanced to produce a desirable composition, along with proper processing, freezing, hardening, and distribution, under proper sanitary conditions. All of these factors are important and must be carefully controlled if the most acceptable product is to be produced. It must be remembered that product inferiority constitutes one of the greatest menaces to the success and progress of the ice cream industry. The consumer has learned to depend upon ice cream as a safe, enjoyable, energy-giving, nourishing, and refreshing food. Consumer interest in the quality of ice cream is one of the industry's greatest assets.

Although the quality of ice cream is usually judged by the flavor, body and texture, melting quality, package, color, and keeping quality characteristics, it is the bacterial content that plays an important role in determining sanitary quality.

The usual methods of measuring sanitary quality include the sediment test, the standard plate count for bacteria, the coliform test, and the usual tests for proper pasteurization. The combined tests will help indicate whether there has been contamination with pathogenic (disease-producing) bacteria and careless methods of handling. However, they do not measure toxic (poisonous) materials resulting from certain types of spoilage or from the use of ingredients containing them. There are also some unsanitary practices, such as straining out foreign materials or contamination with undesirable soluble materials, that are not easily detected. The hygienic quality of poor ingredients cannot be entirely corrected even though pasteurization does destroy whatever pathogenic bacteria are present. Therefore, the need for conscientious, constant detailed attention is apparent.

Factors of ultimate importance to the ice cream manufacturer in producing a finished product of high sanitary quality include the following: (1) clean, healthy employees who are quality minded; (2) quality ingredients; (3) proper processing methods; (4) proper plant sanitation; (5) good equipment; and (6) proper distribution methods.

Almost as important as the quality of the finished product are clean, healthy employees who are industrious and quality minded, of good character and integrity, with a knowledge of the business and an appreciation for laboratory facilities and quality control.

The highest quality ice cream can be made only from good, clean, fresh raw materials. The extensive use of dairy products of questionable quality or products held for long storage periods may result in a finished product of less desirable quality. Standards are given in Table 18.1.

Plant sanitation is essential in order to comply with legal requirements and to produce a product free from objectionable bacteria. Effective bacterial control promotes health protection, product popularity, quality, and less spoilage loss. A high count may be due to any one or more of the following: (1) high count in raw products, (2) ineffective processing methods, (3) ineffective sanitizing methods, (4) carelessness, or (5) prolonged storage of mix.

The types of microorganisms important in the sanitary quality of dairy products include bacteria, yeast, and molds. Bacteria are unicellular microscopic organisms belonging to the plant kingdom, classed as coccus, which are spherical shaped; bacillus, which are rod-shaped; or spirillum, which are spiral shaped. They reproduce by fission or division. Yeast are unicellular, but are larger than bacteria. They reproduce by budding. Molds are multicellular branched fungi, which produce visible surface growth.

Factors affecting microorganism growth are (1) temperature, (2) light, (3) chemicals, (4) food materials, (5) oxygen, and (6) moisture. The types of fermentation that may be produced by these organisms are acid, gas, sweet curdling, proteolytic, and color.

Mix ingredients that usually have low bacterial counts are butter, milk, sugar, vanilla, preserved fruits, dry MSNF, and stabilizers or emulsifiers. Products that may have higher counts or be a source of off-flavor are cream, bulk condensed milk, fresh or frozen fruits, raw nuts and, sometimes, liquid color.

Processing methods or equipment may be responsible for wide variations in bacterial counts. Proper pasteurization will give effective bacterial reduction, but the homogenization process may increase the count as a result of breaking up bacterial clumps or because the machine has not been properly cleaned. The cooler, freezer, and especially the packaging machine may also increase the count. Prolonged storage in the storage tank may be an important cause of a high count. Maintenance of all equipment in good repair, free from dented surfaces and leaks, will help avoid high counts due to equipment.

Table 18.1. Recommended Microbial Standards for Ice Cream[a,b]

Ingredient	Raw state	Processed state
Milk	<200,000	50,000
Cream	<400,000	50,000
Egg products	<200,000	<100[c]
Flavor and color materials	<10,000	<100[c]

[a]Numbers are given in plate count per gram of ingredient.
[b]Coliform microorganisms are not to exceed 10 per gram in any product.
[c]Mold and yeast count per gram of ingredient.

SANITARY EQUIPMENT

Washing and Rinsing

The importance of thorough washing and rinsing cannot be overestimated in making equipment hygienic. Either sterilizing or sanitizing is very difficult, if not impossible, when the equipment is not thoroughly cleaned. Thorough washing also offers an excellent opportunity to inspect the equipment for wear, loss of tinned surface, rust, pitting, etc. The first step in washing any piece of equipment is rinsing with lukewarm (80–110°F) water to remove milk remnants. Soaking may be necessary when the milk film has been allowed to dry. Rinsing should be followed by vigorous scrubbing with a stiff-bristled brush and hot (115–120°F) water containing a washing powder (cleaning agent). Extra effort should be applied to corners and any other places that are difficult to reach. This scrubbing is essential for removing the film that remains after the visible milk, fat, or foreign material has been removed. A stream of washing solution under pressure can be as effective as a brush. The outside of the equipment also should receive the same careful washing treatment. When the surface has been scrubbed to a high polish with washing solution, it should be rinsed again with clean, warm water (100–110°F) to remove the thin film of washing solution. When this process is carefully done, the equipment will have a bacteria count not exceeding that of the final rinse water. Cleaning in place (CIP) of ice cream processing equipment is becoming more popular. The success of the CIP procedure depends upon the following:

- The effectiveness of the CIP installation.
- The temperature and velocity of cleaning solution.
- The use of proper detergent solutions and adequate circulation time.
- The proper adaptability of the processing equipment to CIP.

The steps that should be taken in the CIP procedure are as follows:

1. Rinse system with water (100°F or less) until rinse water runs clear. This rinse should be directed to sewer.
2. Use centrifugal pump to circulate cleaning solution containing sufficient acid (phosphoric and hydroxyacetic) to give 0.15–0.6% acidity, at 150–160°F, and 5–7.5 ft/sec velocity for 20–30 min.
3. Rapidly drain and rinse system with water at 145°F for 5–7 min.
4. Flush for 20–30 min with 150–160°F water containing 1–1.25 lb alkali detergent for each 10 gal of water.
5. Rinse with cold water until equipment is cool.

Washing powders (cleaning agents) should contain no soap because this ingredient leaves a surface film that is difficult to rinse away. Free alkalis, as sodium hydroxide and caustic, should not be used on metallic surfaces if corrosion is to be prevented. Sodium metasilicate, sodium carbonate (washing soda), and trisodium phosphate are satisfactory types of cleaning agents. The effectiveness of these materials is improved by a small amount of so-called wetting agents (i.e., materials like sulfonated alcohols sold under various trade names). Water containing appreciable amounts of calcium or magnesium is described as "hard" water. The use of such water is a contributing cause of a deposit know as "milk-stone" on the surface of the equipment. This can be avoided by adding a water-softening agent (such as pyrophosphate or metasilicate) to the washing compound, but these are not necessary when soft water is used. A very satisfactory cleaning agent for use in hard water may be prepared by thoroughly mixing 100 lb of trisodium phosphate with 20 lb of tetrasodium pyrophosphate and 2 lb of Syntex beads. Where soft water is available, excellent results are obtained from a mixture of 40 lb of trisodium phosphate, 60 lb of sodium carbonate, and 2 lb of Syntex beads. Preparing these mixtures is somewhat troublesome even though it frequently is more economical. There are many similar mixtures available under trade names, and these may give equally good results.

Sterilizing the equipment should follow the washing and rinsing process. Ideally, sterilizing will kill all organisms on the equipment—a goal that is desirable and not impractical. However, most commercial workers and many milk sanitarians are satisfied with merely preventing "public health hazards" and therefore substitute sanitizing for sterilizing.

Sanitizing kills all pathogenic organisms but may leave a few bacteria ("reasonably small number" or "insignificant number"). It is a less expensive, less exacting, and less time-consuming process than sterilizing, although the same two groups of agents are used. For example, heat (as hot water) at 170°F for 10 min will sanitize, while heat (as steam under 15-lb/in^2 pressure) at 240°F for 15 min will sterilize.

Sanitizing Agents

The recommended sanitizing agents together with their advantages and the precautions to be observed in using them may be outlined as follows:

1. Heat is the most reliable agent, especially when both temperature and time are carefully controlled. Its main advantages are its penetrating ability and the fact that it facilitates drying of the equipment.

(a) Dry heat at 240°F for 5 min sanitizes.
(b) Steam under pressure (15 lb/in^2 at 240°F) for 5 min sanitizes.
(c) Steam at zero pressure (212°F) for 10 min sanitizes.
(d) Hot ("boiling") water (180–212°F) for 10 min sanitizes.

Lower temperatures or shorter times at that temperature will not properly sanitize or leave the equipment dry.

2. Chemical agents are effective only under four conditions: (a) When the surface is entirely clean, (b) when the surface is in intimate contact with the chemical, (c) when there is sufficient concentration of the active constituent of the chemical, and (d) when there is sufficient time of contact with the surface. The first three requirements are difficult to satisfy. Many mechanical washers do not clean the surface sufficiently for chemical sanitizing agents. Furthermore, pipe lines may appear to be completely filled with sanitizing solution and yet contain air pockets that will prevent complete sanitization. This is especially true of fittings, joints, and pumps. Also, vat covers may not come in

contact with the chemical agent. The concentration of the solution will change if the chemical agent is not properly stored, if it is used repeatedly, or if it is used for too many pieces of equipment.

Temperatures of 110°F or more usually cause rapid loss of concentration, and therefore volatile chemical sanitizing agents should be used and stored at lower temperatures. Since low temperatures are used, the equipment is seldom left dry. This is a serious objection, for moisture even without the chemical will favor corrosion of the equipment. However, this low-temperature sanitizing has three advantages: (1) It permits sanitizing immediately before the equipment is to be used, when hot equipment would be injurious to the quality of the milk. (2) It avoids excessive strain on equipment, which occurs by expansion and contraction when high temperatures are used. This is particularly important in freezers and equipment having stuffing boxes, as in pumps. (3) It encourages the flushing out of equipment immediately before use, thereby removing any possible dust that may have entered the cans or equipment.

Chemical Sanitizing Agents

Only three types of chemical sanitizing agents have sufficiently pleasing odors to permit their use; all others have odors that are objectionable in dairy products. There are many trade-named products containing one of these three types as the active ingredient.

1. Hypochlorites, usually sodium hypochlorite, are rapid in action, lose strength easily, and are rather corrosive on equipment. Sanitizing solution should contain not less than 50 parts (many recommend as much as 200) of available chlorine per million parts of solution (50 ppm). The solution should be in contact with the surface for at least 15 sec.

Sodium hypochlorite is prepared by the electrical decomposition of salt in a slightly alkaline solution and many preparations are available under trade names. It may also be prepared in a stone crock as follows: To 4 lb of "chloride of lime" add 5 gal of water, and to this add 1-1/2 lb of washing soda. Thoroughly mix with a wooden paddle and allow to stand until the lime settles to the bottom. Then drain off the clear solution into a bottle. Use 1/2 pint of this solution to 2 gal of water for a sanitizing solution.

2. Chloramines are available under many trade names. Chlorine is the active ingredient in the hypochlorites. These are less rapid in action, lose strength less rapidly, and are less corrosive than the hypochlorites. Sanitizing solutions should contain not less that 50 ppm of chlorine (many recommend as much as 200 ppm). The solution should be in contact with the surface for at least one minute.

3. Quaternary ammonium compounds (QACs) have been found to be effective sanitizers. The following is quoted from Henderson (1971):

> Products containing n-alkyl (C_8–C_{18}) dimethyl benzyl ammonium chlorides, n-alkyl (C_{14}–C_{18}) dimethyl benzyl ammonium chlorides, and n-alkyl (C_{12}–C_{18}) dimethyl ethylbenzyl ammonium chlorides are effective in waters ranging from 550 to 1100 ppm hardness without added sequestering agents (U.S. Public Health Service 1965). Certain other compounds, such as sodium tripolyphosphate, require a sequestering agent to reduce the hardness.

The bactericidal effectiveness of specific quaternary ammonium compounds varies and is influenced by the chemical nature and concentration of the active agent, temperature of application, pH, exposure time, and interfering substances in natural waters (Elliker 1964). The removal of calcium or magnesium will assist in the effectiveness of the QAC. When the solutions are properly formulated, they are effective at 200 ppm or more, at pH levels of 5.0 or higher, and at 75°F or higher for an exposure time of 30 sec.

The quaternary ammonium compounds are odorless, nontoxic, noncorrosive to dairy equipment, and do not irritate the hands or the udders of cows. They are effective in hot water and are less affected by pH than are the hypochlorites and the iodine compounds. They combine with protein and, hence, like the halogens are effective only on clean surfaces. Soaps, phospholipids, calcium, and magnesium decrease their effectiveness.

A special application of the quaternary compounds is due to their ability, as a wetting agent, to spread on a cleaned surface, thus creating a bacteriostatic film that will inhibit bacterial growth after sanitizing the equipment. The equipment should be thoroughly drained, however, since solution residues can influence flavor and as little as 3 ppm can inhibit the growth of starter bacteria.

Iodophors are a combination of iodine with a nonionic wetting agent. This sanitizer has been developed in recent years and as a result is not used as extensively as other sanitizers. Iodophors are used at the rate of 12.5–100 ppm in sanitizing solutions at a pH ≤ 5 at temperatures ≤ 120°F for best results.

Wetting agents are synthetic organic compounds which improve the wetting of particles and penetration of washing solutions. These agents are of the anionic, nonionic, and cationic types. The cationic type is not used extensively because of expense.

Drying is the last process in sanitization. It should be accomplished by heat and ventilation, never by the use of a cloth or towel of any kind. While sanitization is not complete without drying, the drying process may be omitted when the equipment is to be immediately refilled with a dairy product. Drying is essential to reduce deterioration and corrosion. It also inhibits the growth of organisms that may find access to the properly cleaned, rinsed, and sterilized surface. Drying should also be accompanied by ventilation insofar as this is possible without recontamination. Resanitizing with a chemical agent immediately before the dried equipment is put into use again is advisable.

SANITARY SURROUNDINGS

Equipment can be kept more uniformly hygienic in sanitary surroundings, i.e., in rooms having hygienic construction and kept sanitary by hygienic personnel. All rooms, even toilets and locker rooms, of the factory should be kept sanitary by the same method described for producing hygienic equipment.

Hygienic construction is probably more important than hygienic methods, since it encourages hygienic practices, especially at an economical cost. The essential factors in hygienic construction are very similar for utensils, equipment, work rooms, buildings and surroundings:

1.   Surfaces should be smooth and free from scratches and grooves. This is particularly essential for surfaces coming in contact with the product, such as

the inside of utensils and equipment. Floors of work rooms are the only exception, and these should be slightly rough (like the commonly known "wood finish" on concrete) to prevent accidents by slipping on the wet floor.

2. Surfaces should be sloping and free from depressions that do not drain quickly and completely. This is desirable not only in equipment but also for all floors, window sills, ledges, shelves, etc.

3. Corners should be rounded and large enough to permit scrubbing with a brush. Sharp corners and crevices must be avoided in surfaces that come in contact with dairy products. In walls, floors, the outer surface of equipment, etc., sharp corners and crevices are objectionable because they are difficult to get completely clean.

4. All surfaces should be easily accessible for scrubbing. Pipe fittings should be tees, never elbows, and easily dismantled to permit visual inspection for cleanliness. Coils in vats should not interfere with scrubbing the entire surface of the coil and the vat. Equipment should be mounted on the floor to avoid leaving corners and floor space under the equipment that cannot be scrubbed daily.

5. Materials used in construction should be impervious to moisture and free from objectionable odors. Certain woods and paints have odors that are easily absorbed by dairy products. Some metals tend to dissolve in the product and to cause undesirable flavors, which are frequently described as "cardboard," "tallowy," or "metallic." This injurious effect can be avoided by covering the metal with a film or coating of tin. When such tinned equipment is used it should be frequently inspected for small spots where the tin coating has been removed by scratching or wear. Most modern equipment is made from stainless steel, which has no injurious effect on the flavor of dairy products.

6. Light is essential for proper cleaning. It should be available especially during cleaning operations without interfering with the operation (i.e., the operator should not have to stand in the light and cast a shadow on the surface being scrubbed).

7. Ventilation with fresh, clean air is essential. All equipment, utensils, rooms, cupboards, etc., should be constructed to permit thorough ventilation without contamination. This not only avoids undesirable odors but reduces the objectionable moisture in the atmosphere.

8. Rodents and insects should have no place to collect or hide. Dark, moist, and unclean places attract rodents, ants, roaches, flies, etc. Removal of all such places eliminates the pests. Sprays, poisons, screens, and traps should be used only as a temporary measure, preferably not at all. Neither the pest nor the usual "control measures" belong in a respectable dairy, and either one is evidence of careless methods.

9. Segregation of operations is necessary in the construction of buildings. There should be separate rooms for unpasteurized or raw products to avoid contamination of equipment and possible mixing of unpasteurized with pasteurized products; for products with pronounced odors that may be easily absorbed by other products; for wash rooms, for cans, bottles, etc.; for boilers, engines, refrigeration compressors, etc.; for all storage rooms whether refrigerated or not; and for rest rooms (toilets) and locker rooms.

10. Special facilities are necessary in the construction of buildings and

work rooms. Conveniently located facilities for obtaining an ample supply of both hot and cold water are most essential. The supply of both hot and cold water should be unrestricted if cleanliness is expected. Mixing outlets, permitting adjustment of temperature, should be located for convenience in applying an ample supply of water to all parts of every room. Floor drains in each room are equally essential. They should be located so as to drain the floor completely and not leave even shallow puddles. When possible it is desirable to locate them at the sides or at least out of the traffic lanes, but they must be easily accessible for cleaning when they become clogged; for this reason they are often located in the center of the room. A most important special feature of each room is a lavatory, i.e., a small basin for washing hands. This lavatory should be equipped with a mixing faucet for hot and cold water, soap or cleaning agents, a cold-water drinking fountain, and single-service (paper) towels. Thus personal cleanliness is encouraged, and the improper use of equipment (such as sinks for washing utensils, drinking from a hose, contamination by handling equipment with dirty hands) is avoided.

Hygienic personnel is probably the most important factor not only in obtaining but also in maintaining healthful quality in the product. Every person associated with dairy products should be hygienic minded and constantly observant of sanitary details. This applies to mechanics, electricians, janitors, stenographers, truck drivers, etc., as well as to persons actually operating equipment for processing the dairy product. The three characteristics of hygienic personnel are as follows:

1. Hygienic conscience, or a subconscious desire to employ only healthful practices and habits as well as a determined conscious effort to correct errors in hygienic behavior.
2. Physical health, especially freedom from contagious diseases. Medical examination for contagious diseases (particularly typhoid, which supports "carriers") should be required once a year. Rigid isolation should be practiced even in the event of less fatal contagious diseases such as common colds.
3. Hygienic habits including innumerable personal details such as the following:

    (a) Hands and nails should be clean. The hands should be washed before touching dairy products or clean utensils, especially after touching unsterile cans, shaking hands with anyone, coughing against the hand, wiping the nose, scratching, visits to the toilet, etc.

    (b) Unsanitary practices such as coughing in or near the equipment or spitting on the floor should be avoided.

    (c) A net or cap should be worn to prevent loose hair from contaminating the product or equipment.

    (d) Clothes should not be worn longer than one full day between launderings, and should be changed more often when they become untidy. Clothes worn on the streets or outside the work-room should not be worn while handling the product. Footwear used while cleaning larger vats that must be entered should not be worn elsewhere, even on the floor of that room.

(e) Wounds or sores should be bandaged to prevent any possible contact with the equipment or product. Wet equipment may make contact by soaking through the bandage. When this cannot be avoided the person should not touch the equipment or product.

The recontamination problem is very complex because the product is exposed to so much equipment, some of which is difficult to sanitize, and the product is exposed to human contact. Hygienic ingredients can be reasonably assured by obtaining bacterial counts on all products used in the ice cream. Bacterial counts and coliform tests on samples of ice cream taken at various places between the pasteurizer and the retailer aid in discovering recontamination. Wherever possible human contact should be eliminated. Where it cannot be avoided, the health of the workers should be supervised and they should be compelled to practice hygienic habits. Some sanitarians believe that:

1. Every employee should be required to have a complete medical examination by a competent physician and submit the necessary samples of blood, feces, and urine for laboratory examination, together with any other test necessary, at the time employed and semiannually thereafter. If the Board of Health does not require such an examination, employers should require it for their own protection.

2. Supplementing the above examination and as an added protection, all employees coming in direct contact with food, milk, or other dairy products should be examined regularly by a nurse, foreperson, or some other competent person for evidence of contagious diseases. By means of education and intelligent application, many causes of potential or actual disease may be found in this way.

3. Whether this system or any other is used in trying to find persons suffering from contagious disease, employees must not be penalized by being discharged or temporarily laid off without due compensation.

4. Only persons who are inherently clean should be employed in the food or dairy industry. All new employees should be watched carefully until they have been so classified.

QUALITY CONTROL PROCEDURES FOR FINISHED PRODUCTS

Finished product quality control procedures are extremely important in the production of a good product. Comply with all composition standards for all products by testing biweekly. Fat content should not vary more than 0.2% and TS not more than 1%.

Weekly bacteriological analyses should be made for all regular flavors and the results should comply with Health Department standards.

Weekly examinations should be made for quality of each product manufactured. These examinations should include flavor, body and texture, color, and appearance.

Packages should be clean, neat, and properly labeled.

Weight control of packages is important. Usually 1-gal units should weigh within 4 oz, 2-1/2 gal units within 5 oz, and 5-gal units within 8 oz of the standard desired.

Routine checks on processing procedures including mix preparation, homogenization, flavoring and coloring materials, freezing, packaging, storage, and distribution play an important role in producing the best product. The rate of turnover of products in the hardening room should be as rapid as possible. The maximum time should not exceed 6 weeks.

Spillage, broken packages, and overaged products should be kept at a minimum and this material should be discarded rather than used as a rerun.

Products showing defects in periodic examinations may be given prompt corrective attention. In this manner, products may be maintained at the desired standards.

19
Refrigeration

Refrigeration is the removal of heat from a substance and therefore is concerned with heat exchange (i.e., heat transfer). The excess heat in the substance being cooled (refrigerated) is transferred to a cooler substance, which becomes heated. Therefore "refrigeration" is the reverse of "heating," both occurring simultaneously and being dependent upon the same principles and factors of heat exchange. However, the ice cream industry uses the term "refrigeration" to mean cooling to temperatures between 40 and −30°F.

METHODS OF REFRIGERATION

The Ice and Salt Method

Natural ice, in very early times, was harvested from ponds and stored to be used for refrigeration. Since ice melts at 32°F, lower temperatures could be obtained only by mixing ice and salt. This method, now called "the ice and salt" method, is still used when only a small amount of refrigeration is required. Under usual conditions it is not practical to obtain temperatures below 0°F by this method, although theoretically −6°F is possible when using 1 lb of salt to 3 lb of ice.

The lowest temperature obtained by this method depends upon the proportion of ice and salt, the rate at which heat is supplied, the density of the brine, the original temperature of ice and salt before mixing, and the size of both the ice and salt particles. Smaller lumps of ice and more concentrated brine favor rapid cooling and are used when the rate of heat transfer is high.

Mechanical Refrigeration

Mechanical refrigeration is now almost universally used and has the advantages of requiring less labor, being less cumbersome, yielding lower temperatures, and more uniform temperature control. It is also faster, cleaner, and drier. It is based on the principle that a liquid absorbs heat when it vaporizes, as in the case of water changing into steam; the vapor can be collected, cooled to a liquid state, and used again. The particular liquid, called the refrigerant, to be used in a mechanical refrigeration system depends on many factors, the more important of which are (1) the boiling point of the liquid, (2) pressure characteristics (the pressures under which it can be used), (3) the latent heat of vaporization (amount of heat absorbed when the refrigerant vaporizes), (4) the ease with which a leak is detected, (5) its corrosive action on metals used in the system, and (6) its toxicity.

TYPES OF REFRIGERANTS COMMONLY USED

Of the many and various refrigerants, only two have been found sufficiently satisfactory to be widely used in the ice cream industry: ammonia, which has been used a long time, and Freon-12, a representative nontoxic refrigerant used in ice cream cabinets, in small installations (home refrigerators, counter freezers, etc.), and where very low temperatures are not required.

The most important advantages of ammonia are (1) it absorbs a large amount of heat when vaporizing, (2) operating pressures are reasonably convenient, (3) leaks are easily detected, (4) its toxicity is not great in low concentrations though its odor is very pungent, and it has a very pronounced irritating effect on mucous membranes and wet skin, and (5) it usually operates at pressures above atmospheric, thereby keeping foreign gases and liquids out of the system.

Its main disadvantages are (1) it is very corrosive to brass and other copper alloys (since only iron and steel can be used in the system, the equipment is rather bulky), (2) the relatively large volume of gas requires large compressors, (3) mechanical automatic operation is difficult to obtain, (4) maintenance of temperature within a narrow range is difficult (the last two of these disadvantages are due to the large amount of heat absorbed during vaporization but are not significant in many installations), and (5) for some installations the objectionable odor from even minor leaks becomes very important.

Freon-12 (dichlorodifluoromethane) is one of the many Freon refrigerants. The advantages of these refrigerants are (1) they require lower operating pressures, (2) their odor is neither objectionable nor toxic, (3) they are not injurious to food materials, (4) they are not corrosive to most metals, although alloys containing magnesium must be avoided, (5) smaller and more compact refrigeration systems can be used, because of the lower pressures, as well as copper alloys (hermetically sealed units are becoming popular), (6) they are carriers for oil, thus facilitating the lubrication of compressors, (7) mechanical automatic operation is fairly simple, and (8) more uniform temperatures can be maintained.

The main disadvantages of Freon refrigerants are (1) they must be free of moisture, (2) leaks are not easily detected (a special Halide torch that gives a pink flame in the presence of Freon can be used to detect leaks), (3) the system must be tighter than for ammonia to avoid leaks (small leaks are not noticeable and the refrigerant may be lost just when it is most needed), and (4) they are less satisfactory than ammonia for very low temperatures.

PRINCIPLES OF MECHANICAL REFRIGERATION

The mechanical refrigeration system has only three essential parts: (1) the compressor, (2) the high-pressure side, and (3) the low-pressure side (see Fig. 19.1). The compressor consists of one or two cylinders, usually surrounded by a water-jacket for cooling, and containing pistons, similar to those of a gasoline engine, operated by a crankshaft that runs in oil in the crankcase. The compressor is usually belt-driven from a motor, engine, or other source of power. The purpose of the compressor is to concentrate the vapor. It takes the vapor from the low-pressure side in large volume at low pressure and low temperature, and discharges it into the high-pressure side. Thus the compressor occupies a position dividing the two sides. The high-pressure side extends from the compressor to the expansion valve and includes the condenser and receiver. The hot vapor leaving the compressor passes through the condenser, i.e., coils of pipe cooled by water or air. This cooling in the condenser changes the vapor into a liquid at about room temperature and still under a high pressure, the liquid being collected in a tank (the receiver). This liquid refrigerant passes on to the expansion valve, which is the other position dividing the high and low sides. The low-pressure side extends from the expansion valve to the compressor. The expansion valve is usually an ordinary needle valve permitting fine adjustment and may be operated manually. It derives its name from the fact that the liquid refrigerant passes through the valve and then expands into a vapor. The liquid refrigerant is under high pressure at room temperature before passing through the valve, and under low pressure at low temperature as it leaves the expansion valve to go through the expansion coils, i.e., coils of pipes located where refrigeration is to be produced, and leading back to the compressor. In this way the refrigerant is used repeatedly, being compressed, condensed, and expanded. The refrigerant never wears out, but slight leaks invariably occur, making it necessary to replenish the supply. The refrigeration or cooling is obtained by means of the expansion coils since in these coils the liquid refrigerant absorbs heat while vaporizing. The pressure in these expansion coils determines the lowest temperature obtainable, and this pressure is often called the suction pressure or back pressure of the system. The expansion coils may be located in the hardening room, in a tank of water or brine, in the ice cream freezer, etc., to give refrigeration in that particular place.

A large amount of heat is absorbed as the liquid changes to a vapor, and a smaller amount of heat is absorbed by the vapor when it expands further. This heat absorbed in the expansion coils is carried in the vapor to the compressor and on to the condenser, where it is transferred from the hot refrigerant vapor to the cooling water or air around the condenser coils. Sometimes this cooling water is used only once and wasted; in other places it is more economical to reuse this water. In these cases the water is pumped to the top of a cooling tower (usually on the roof) and allowed to trickle down over the tower, being cooled by partial evaporation in the process. This proves very economical where the cost of water is high. In some Freon systems the condenser is air-cooled, usually by a fan blowing air around condenser coils that have fins to facilitate radiation of the heat.

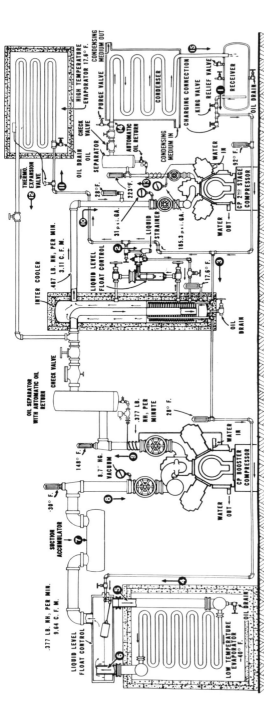

Fig. 19.1. An example of a mechanical refrigeration system. (Courtesy of Crepaco, Inc.)

1. Liquid refrigerant leaving receiver.
2. Liquid refrigerant passing through float control to intercooler.
3. Liquid refrigerant passing liquid cooling coil in intercooler.
4. Subcooled liquid refrigerant passing through float control to low-temperature evaporator.
5. Liquid refrigerant from accumulator circulating through low-temperature evaporator.
6. Refrigerant liquid and vapor mixture circulating from evaporator to accumulator.
7. Excess liquid not evaporated in the evaporator but carried as entrained liquid in the suction gas is separated from the suction gas at the accumulator. The liquid can be returned to any portion of the system, which is designed to handle liquid NH_3 (usually required where there is more than one evaporator.)

8. Low-pressure refrigerant vapor entering booster compressor.
9. Hot intermediate-pressure refrigerant vapor leaving compressor to oil separator and intercooler.
10. Cold intermediate-pressure refrigerant vapor leaving intercooler and entering second-stage compressor.
11. Liquid refrigerant passing through expansion valve to high-temperature evaporator (optional).
12. Intermediate-pressure refrigerant vapor leaving high-temperature evaporator and entering second-stage compressor (optional).
13. High-pressure refrigerant vapor leaving second-stage compressor and entering and entering oil separator.
14. High-pressure refrigerant vapor leaving oil separator and entering condenser.
15. Liquid refrigerant returning to receiver.

Although the principle involved in the mechanical refrigeration system is rather simple, the construction and installation is too complicated for a brief discussion. Usually it is more economical to obtain the services of a refrigeration engineer to supervise the planning and installation of the system.

OPERATING PRECAUTIONS

Some precautions to observe in operating refrigeration systems are as follows:

1. When opening valves on refrigerant lines, open them slowly.
2. Keep the suction pressure as high as possible. It must be sufficiently low to give the desired temperature. The pressure on the low side should correspond to an ammonia boiling point 10°F lower than the temperature of the brine (or other medium surrounding the expansion coils) for maximum efficiency. A lower back pressure than this reduces the refrigeration capacity. There is a temperature drop of about 10°F between the brine and the ammonia due to the wall of the expansion coil. This is the same principle as in a milk cooler. The cooling medium must always be cooler than the temperature to which it is desired to cool the milk. Table 19.1 shows the boiling point of ammonia at different gauge pressures.

To illustrate, if a minimum brine temperature of $-10°F$ is wanted, the pressure on the low-pressure gauge should be that at which ammonia will boil at $-20°F$ or 3.45 lb/in^2. Table 19.1 shows that it is not necessary to carry a vacuum on the low side unless extremely low temperatures are desired. Head pressures (pressures on the high side) are determined by the temperature of the refrigerant in the condenser.

3. Keep the head pressure as low as possible to save power. The head pressure depends on (a) size of the condenser, (b) temperature of water used for cooling the condenser, (c) amount or volume of water flowing through the condenser, (d) impurities in the refrigerant (mainly oil and air), and (e) cleanliness of the condenser outside as well as inside.

Table 19.1. The Relation of Gauge Pressure to Boiling Point of Ammonia

Gauge pressure (lb/in^2)	Boiling point of ammonia (°F)	Minimum brine temperature (°F)
1.17	−25	−15
3.45	−20	−10
5.99	−15	−5
8.77	−10	−0
10.93	−5	5
15.37	−0	10
19.17	5	15
23.55	10	20
27.93	15	25
32.95	20	30
38.43	25	35
44.41	30	40

4.   Avoid operating the compressor at zero suction pressure or under vacuum, since this favors oil passing out of the compressor into the condenser.

5.   Avoid frost on the compressor. The suction pipe at the compressor should carry frost up to the compressor when operating most efficiently.

6.   Inspect and drain all oil traps regularly. Some oil always passes along with the refrigerant and collects at low spots in the system. Valves at these points permit the oil to be drained out, thereby improving the efficiency of the heat transfer. Worn piston rings favor oil passing into the refrigerant.

7.   Keep air out of the system. Air and some other gases do not condense into a liquid, but collect at high spots in the system. Valves at these points permit the removal of the air. Air decreases the efficiency of the condenser, causing excessive head pressures. Usually the air is removed at the high point of the condenser; this operation is called purging.

8.   Keep the expansion coils as free from frost as possible. This is especially important in hardening rooms, since frost and ice beyond a certain thickness reduce the rate of heat transfer.

DEFROSTING METHODS

The common methods of defrosting are as follows:

1.   Brushing the coils with a stiff or wire bristled brush: This is not very effective as it may leave a thin layer of ice which gradually increases in thickness.

2.   Scrubbing with hot water: A wet, messy, disagreeable operation leaving much moisture in the room and warming up the entire hardening room. However, it is nearly always used when the expansion coils are in a separate cabinet through which the hardening room air is circulated.

3.   Passing hot liquid refrigerant through the coils: This requires extra valves and pipes in the installation, but does not raise the temperature of the room much. The frost and ice are easily removed from the quickly heated coils before the ice melts.

4.   Passing hot refrigerant vapor or gas through the coils: This is similar to the use of hot liquid refrigerant.

5.   Using a brine drip or spray over the coils: A trough containing calcium chloride crystals is placed above the coil so that as the crystals absorb moisture the brine drips down over the coil to collect in a pail at the bottom.

METHODS OF COOLING

Brine

The brine method of cooling (sometimes called the brine system) represents the first application of mechanical refrigeration. The expansion coils of the mechanical refrigeration system are immersed in a large tank of brine (a calcium chloride solution) to cool the brine. Then the brine is pumped through pipes to the freezer (or other place where refrigeration is desired) and back to the brine tank to be cooled again. This method involves additional investment in brine tank, brine solution, pumps, pipes, etc. It is less efficient since the heat removed for refrigeration must be transferred to the brine and then to the mechanical refrigeration system. Other disadvantages are the corrosiveness of the brine, the difficulty in obtaining very low temperatures, and the more bulky installation. The most important advantages are that it permits storing up of refrigeration and can be used where ammonia leaks would be dangerous. Although it has been largely replaced in modern factories, it continues to find application in certain operations such as making ice cream novelties and in making artificial ice.

The care of brine systems is important and may be summarized as follows:

1. Test the brine every month for concentration, alkalinity, and ammonia.

2. Keep the concentration of the brine high enough to give a freezing point at least 10° lower than the lowest temperature to which it will be cooled (see Table 19.1). Otherwise, brine will freeze onto the expansion coil, and this ice will act as insulation preventing the heat in the brine from penetrating the expansion coil.

3. Adjust the alkalinity by adding a solution of sodium hydroxide (caustic soda) or of lime until the brine is neutral to litmus or phenolphthalein. If the brine is acid to litmus it is too corrosive.

4. Use only one metal, preferably a pure grade of cast iron, in contact with the brine. Two different metals favor corrosive action.

5. Immerse a bar or strip of zinc in the brine to decrease the corrosion when two different metals favor corrosive action.

6. Add a solution of sodium dichromate and caustic soda to reduce corrosion; however, this will cause irritation of the skin. Care must therefore be used in handling the dichromate, as well as the brine containing it. To make the solution, thoroughly dissolve, by stirring, a mixture of 5 lb commercial dichromate and 1.4 lb caustic soda in 1 gal of water. This amount will be sufficient to treat 375 gal of brine the first time. Once a year it will be necessary to add from one-fourth to one-half the original amount.

7. Avoid air coming in contact with the brine since air makes the brine acid and more corrosive. Keep the brine tank covered, and avoid bubbling air through the brine or spraying the brine.

8. Avoid ammonia leaks from the expansion coils, which cause the brine to become more alkaline. They can be detected by boiling a sample of brine in a narrow-necked flask and testing the vapors with red litmus paper. If the red litmus paper turns blue, the steam from the boiling brine contains ammonia.

Direct Expansion

The direct-expansion method of cooling has replaced the brine method in many installations, since it represents increased efficiency and a saving in investment. In this method the brine pipes in the freezer (or other place where refrigeration is desired) are replaced by the expansion coils of the mechanical refrigeration system. These expansion coils may or may not contain much liquid refrigerant in addition to the refrigerant vapor.

Flooded System

The flooded system or method of cooling is a special case of the direct expansion method in which the liquid refrigerant collects in the expansion coils nearly filling the coils. The compressor draws off the vapor as the absorbed heat vaporizes the liquid. Thus in the operation of this flooded system the liquid refrigerant under high pressure and room temperature passes through a valve (usually controlled by a float) to the expansion coils, where it is a liquid under a lower pressure and lower temperature. As heat is transferred to the liquid refrigerant, evaporation takes place; the vapor from this evaporation is constantly removed by the compressor and the liquid level maintained by the float.

The important advantages of the flooded system are (1) it is more efficient, since heat is more readily transferred between liquids than between vapors, gas, or liquid to gas, (2) less cooling surface or coil surface is needed, (3) there is less fluctuation in temperature. The fact that float valves occasionally stick causing liquid refrigerant to enter and damage the compressor is the main disadvantage.

TERMS USED IN REFRIGERATION

1. *BTU*:   British thermal unit, or the amount of heat required to raise the temperature of 1 lb of water through 1°F when water has its greatest density (at about 39°F). Roughly the amount of heat required to raise the temperature of 1 lb of water from 39 to 40°F.

2. *Latent heat of vaporization*:   The amount of heat (in BTU) required to change 1 lb of liquid into 1 lb of vapor without changing the temperature or pressure.

3. *Latent heat of fusion*:   The amount of heat (in BTU) required to change 1 lb of liquid into a solid without changing the temperature or pressure.

4. *Ton of refrigeration*:   288,000 BTU per 24 hr, or the amount of heat required to melt 1 ton of ice per day at 32°F without changing the temperature or pressure. Other convenient ton of refrigeration equivalents are 12,000 BTU/hr and 200 BTU/min.

5. *Ton refrigeration machine*:   A compressor or machine that will produce 1 ton of refrigeration during 24 hr of continuous operation under a particular set of conditions. (For example, 5°F suction vapor and 86°F condenser.)

Refrigeration compressors are frequently rated in tons of refrigeration at a certain suction pressure and this numerical figure is approximately one-half the horsepower rating of the motor driving the compressor. However, many engineers find it more satisfactory to list the size of compressor in terms of piston diameter and length of piston stroke, since the following factors affect the size of motor and capacity of a compressor:

1.   The refrigerant used: Compressors are made for a particular refrigerant.
2.   The diameter of the cylinder: This influences the volume of refrigerant vapor that can be handled at one stroke.

3. The length of the piston stroke, which also determines the volume of refrigerant vapor handled at one stroke.
4. The speed, which determines the volume of refrigerant vapor handled per minute, hour, or day.
5. The suction pressure or pressure on the low-pressure side, which determines the weight of refrigerant vapor per volume handled by the cylinders.
6. Volumetric efficiency of machine, i.e., the ratio between the piston displacement and the actual amount of gas delivered.

The first four of these factors are usually constant in a particular installation, but the capacity of the compressor decreases rapidly with a decrease in the suction pressure. Also it should be remembered that the pressure on the high-pressure side has almost no influence on the capacity of the compressor, although it does greatly affect the power consumption of the motor.

20
Laboratory Testing

Proper laboratory control is important for efficient operation and for maintaining uniform quality of ice cream. It consists of both chemical and bacteriological analyses of the ingredients used, of the finished product, and of other samples taken in an attempt to remedy undesirable conditions. Sometimes arrangements are made with a competent commercial laboratory to make these analyses on the basis of a fixed price per sample or per month. However, it is generally desirable and economical to have at least the most essential routine testing done in the plant by plant personnel.

Some of the tests described here can be done in a small laboratory. The simplest and least expensive equipment is required, and the operator needs only a small amount of specialized training.

TAKING AND PREPARING SAMPLES FOR TESTING

Taking the Samples

Whether the sample to be tested is milk, cream, butter, or ice cream, it is equally important that it be taken in such a manner as to make absolutely sure that it is a fair and representative sample of the product to be tested. Otherwise time and money are wasted in carrying out the test. Therefore, a considerable portion of the product to be tested should be carefully and thoroughly mixed before the sample is taken.

Preparing the Samples

Plain Products. Let the sample soften at room temperature. Because melted fat tends to separate and rise to the surface, it is not advisable to soften the sample by heating in a water bath or over a flame. Mix thoroughly by stirring with spoon or egg beater, or by pouring back and forth between beakers.

Frozen Desserts Containing Insoluble Particles. Use malted-milk mixer capable of comminuting product to a fine, uniform pulp.

Use enough sample (4–8 oz) to fill mixer cup one-quarter to one-half full. Melt at room temperature or in incubator set at 37°C in a closed container (a Mason jar is suitable), transfer entire sample to mixer cup, and mix until insoluble particles are finely divided (2–5 min for fruit ice creams and up to 7 min for nut and certain candy ice creams). Transfer the mixed sample to a suitable container for convenience in weighing.

FLAVOR AND AROMA TEST

This is perhaps the most essential routine test. It is one of the best and most accurate measures of quality. The aroma (or odor) is best observed in a place where there are no strong odors, and when the observation is made immediately after the sample bottle is opened. The flavor is obtained by taking a small portion (about a teaspoonful) into the mouth, allowing it to warm and then carefully rolling it to the back of the mouth without swallowing any of it. After the flavor has been observed, the portion is delivered into a sink or garbage receptacle instead of being swallowed. Then the next sample may be tested. Care is necessary to avoid contaminating the product.

BABCOCK TEST FOR FAT IN MILK

Preparing the Sample. Cool milk to a temperature of 60–70°F and mix thoroughly by vigorous shaking.

Apparatus and Reagents. Standard Babcock test equipment; commercial sulfuric acid (sp.gr. 1.82–1.83).

Procedure
1. Using a 17.6-ml pipette, transfer 18 g of the sample to the milk test bottle, being sure to drain the pipette completely by blowing out the last drop.
2. Add 17.5 ml of sulfuric acid, at the same temperature as above, pouring it down the side of the neck of the bottle in such a way as to wash any traces of milk into the bulb.
3. Mix the milk and acid thoroughly, first by a rotary motion and finally by vigorous shaking, until all traces of curd have disappeared.
4. Transfer the bottle to the tester; counterbalance it; and after the proper speed has been attained, whirl for 5 min.
5. Add soft water, at 140°F or above, until the bottle is filled to the neck.
6. Whirl the tester again, this time for 2 min.
7. Add hot water until the fat is brought well within the scale on the bottle neck.
8. Whirl again, this time for 1 min.
9. Transfer the bottle to a water bath maintained at a temperature of 130–140°F, and immerse it to the level of the top of the fat column, allowing it to remain for 5 min.
10. Remove bottle from the bath and wipe it dry.

11.   With a pair of dividers measure the fat column, in terms of percentage by weight, from its lower surface to the highest point of the upper meniscus.

At the time of measurement, the fat column should be translucent, of a golden yellow or amber color, and free from visible suspended particles. All tests in which the fat column is milky or shows the presence of curd or of charred matter, or in which the reading is indistinct or uncertain should be rejected and the test repeated.

BABCOCK TEST FOR FAT IN CREAM

Preparing the Sample.   In collecting the sample of cream, the same general procedure is followed as in sampling milk. The cream to be tested should be warmed to a temperature of 100–110°F just before it is mixed. After the cream is warmed it should be thoroughly mixed and all lumps broken up. Precaution should be taken to avoid overheating or allowing the sample to stand too long at 110°F which would cause it to "oil off."

Apparatus and Reagents.   Standard Babcock test equipment; commercial sulfuric acid; liquid petrolatum (Glymol, e.g.).

Procedure.   Use the cream test scales and weigh 9 g of prepared sample into a 9-g cream test bottle, or 18 g into an 18-g bottle. Proceed by one of the following methods.

Method 1
1.   After the cream has been weighed into the test bottle, add 8–12 ml of sulfuric acid in the case of the 9-g bottle, or 14–17 ml in the case of the 18-g bottle; or add acid until the mixture of cream and acid, after shaking, has assumed a chocolate-brown color.
2.   Shake the bottle with a rotary motion until all lumps have completely disappeared.
3.   Add 5–10 ml of soft water at a temperature of 140°F or above.
4.   Transfer the bottle to the tester, counterbalance, and after the proper speed has been attained whirl for 5 min.
5.   Add hot water until the fat column is brought well within the graduated scale on the bottle neck and whirl 1 min longer.
6.   Transfer the bottle to the water bath as in the testing for fat in milk, immerse the bottle to the level of the fat column, and allow it to remain for 5 min.
7.   Place 2 or 3 drops of Glymol on the surface of the fat column, allowing the Glymol to run down the side of the neck in order to keep it from splashing and getting beneath the fat column.
8.   Remove the bottle from the bath and wipe dry.
9.   With a pair of dividers measure the fat column from its lowest surface to the line of division between the fat column and the Glymol.

Method 2 (for use only with the 9-g bottle)
1. After the cream has been weighed into the test bottle add 9 ml of soft water and mix thoroughly.
2. Add 17.5 ml of sulfuric acid and shake with a rotary motion until all lumps have completely disappeared.
3. Transfer the bottle to the tester, counterbalance, and after the proper speed has been attained whirl for 5 min.
4. Fill the bottle to the neck with hot water and whirl again for 2 min.
5. Add hot water until the fat column is well within the graduated scale on the bottle neck and whirl 1 min longer.
6. Transfer to the water bath and continue as in Method 1.

As in the test for fat in milk, the fat column, at the time of reading, should be translucent, of a golden yellow or amber color, and free from visible suspended particles. All tests in which the fat column is milky or shows the presence of curd or charred matter, or in which the reading is indistinct or uncertain, should be rejected and the test repeated.

Precaution. Avoid overheating the sample or allowing it to stand for too long at 110°F, which would cause it to "oil off."

MODIFIED BABCOCK TESTS FOR ICE CREAM

The original Babcock test is not satisfactory for testing ice cream because the strong sulfuric acid used reacts with the sugar in the product and charred material is formed to such an extent that it is next to impossible to obtain an accurate test. The ice cream mix is homogenized, which also makes the fat more difficult to separate. It has been necessary then to develop modifications of the Babcock test for testing ice cream. Numerous modified tests have been recommended. The most popular modifications are the Pennsylvania, Minnesota, Nebraska, Illinois, and Glacial acetic–sulfuric acid tests. The Pennsylvania and Minnesota tests have probably gained the greatest acceptance; however, all of the above tests check within ±0.3° of the other extraction method.

The main use of the modified tests is to serve as a guide as to whether the mix complies with the legal composition standard or to the composition standard the manufacturer wishes to meet.

In general, the modified Babcock tests that employ sulfuric acid of a reduced strength require a base such as ammonium hydroxide to aid in digesting the protein present, and alcohol and/or ether to aid in freeing the butterfat. The modified tests that employ alkaline reagents also require an alcohol or ether to help dissolve and free the fat.

Pennsylvania Test

This method, which uses a diluted sulfuric acid to complete the digestion after ammonium hydroxide and alcohol have been added to the sample, gives clear fat columns and ranks high from the standpoint of accuracy.

Preparing the Sample. Melt the ice cream at room temperature and, if necessary, heat to eliminate the foam. Warm ice cream mix to approximately 70°F. Reduce large particles in fruit and nut ice cream to a finely divided state.

Apparatus and Reagents. Standard Babcock test equipment, including ice cream test bottles; ammonium hydroxide (28–29% NH_3); normal butyl alcohol (bp 117°C); diluted commercial sulfuric acid (1.72–1.74, prepared by adding 3.5 parts, by volume of commercial sulfuric acid to one part of water in a heat-resisting container); Glymol.

Procedure
1. Weigh 9 g of the representative sample into a 9-g 20% ice cream test bottle, keeping the fruit or nut ice cream thoroughly mixed.
2. Add 2 ml of ammonium hydroxide (preferably from a burette) and mix for approximately 30 sec.
3. Add 3 ml of butyl alcohol and mix for approximately 1 min (samples containing chocolate require additional mixing).
4. Add 17.5 ml of the diluted sulfuric acid and mix thoroughly until digestion is completed.
5. Centrifuge the bottles for 5 min.
6. Add water (130–140°F) to bring the contents to within 1/4 in. of the base of the neck of the bottle and centrifuge for 2 min.
7. Add enough water (130–140°F) to keep the fat within the graduated portion of the neck of the bottle until read and centrifuge 1 min.
8. Place the bottles in a water bath at 130°F for 5 min.
9. Allow a few drops of glymol to run down the inside of the neck of the bottle just before reading.
10. Measure the length of the fat column from the bottom of the lower meniscus to the sharp line of demarcation between the glymol and the fat.

Precautions
1. The small amount of sample that adheres to the inside of the neck of the bottle should be washed into the bottle by the reagent; otherwise it may collect at the base of the fat column and make the correct reading of the fat column difficult.
2. Use care in transferring ammonium hydroxide—add to test bottle from burette.
3. Be sure chemicals are of proper purity and strength.
4. Use care in preparation of dilute acid.
5. Use precautions observed in testing milk by the Babcock test.

Minnesota Test

This is an alkaline test. It requires four chemicals that are available at chemical supply houses, or the ready mixed reagent can be obtained.

Preparing the Sample. Prepare the sample in the same way as for the Pennsylvania test.

Apparatus and Reagents. Standard Babcock test equipment, including ice cream test bottles; Minnesota reagent (prepared by mixing 645 g sodium salicylate, 355 g potassium carbonate, 160 g sodium hydrozide; add 3 qt water; after solution is complete add 1 qt isopropyl alcohol); Glymol.

Procedure

1. Weigh 9 g of the well-mixed melted ice cream into 20% ice cream test bottles. (An 8%, 18-g milk test bottle may be used, but the fat reading must be multiplied by 2.)

2. Add 15 ml of the Minnesota reagent and shake thoroughly.

3. Digest in water bath at 180°F or above until the fat layer at the surface is clear and well-defined. (Do not shake the tests vigorously and no more than is absolutely necessary to cause complete digestion. The digestion period usually requires about 12–15 min.)

4. Centrifuge for 30 sec.

5. Add hot water (135–140°F) to bring the fat within reading scale of bottle.

6. Centrifuge 30 sec.

7. Place bottles in a water bath at 133–137°F for 5 min.

8. Read test in same manner as for cream, using Glymol.

Precautions

1. The same precautions observed for testing milk by the Babcock test.

2. Store reagent in glass-stoppered bottle to prevent evaporation and absorption of CO_2 but use caution to prevent glass stopper from sticking in bottle.

3. Store reagent in cool place.

4. Use proper water bath temperatures and times.

5. Mix samples frequently during heating period.

6. Use care to prevent the alcohol from boiling out of test bottle during this period.

THE BABCOCK TEST FOR FAT IN BUTTER

Preparing the Sample. All that has been said about the need for care in sampling milk applies even more strongly to the sampling of butter, because the sample must be taken so as to represent the composition of the whole batch to be tested. A butter trier is used to take the samples (or "plugs" as they are called) from various places in the butter container and from top to bottom. The sample may be prepared in several different ways but the following method is quite generally used: As they are taken, place the plugs in a clean, dry, tightly stoppered sample jar. Warm only enough to soften the butter so that it can be stirred easily. Using an electric food mixer of the doublebeater type, with shafts attached to a metal screw cover to fit the sample jar, insert the beaters into the jar, screw the cover down tightly, and mix the contents at high speed for about 3 min. Rotate the jar until all portions of the contents are incorporated in the mixture. Remove the beater and proceed with test.

Apparatus and Reagents. Standard Babcock test equipment, including a 90% butter test bottle; commercial sulfuric acid; Glymol.

Procedure

1. Weigh 9 g of the prepared sample into the 90% butter test bottle. (Fat clinging to the neck of the bottle may be melted by holding the bottle neck under the warm water tap till the fat melts and runs into the bottle.
2. Add about 9 ml of the sulfuric acid and mix thoroughly by gently rotating the bottle.
3. Centrifuge and complete the test as described for testing cream.

The Babcock test is not quite as accurate for butter as for cream. It is generally thought to read about 0.5% too high. The operator with more experience may wish to use more accurate tests such as the Kohman or the Mojonnier.

Precaution If for any reason the testing is not done within a few hours, or if the sample has been allowed to become so warm that it melts, remix the sample just before the test is to be performed.

MOJONNIER ANALYSIS FOR FAT AND TOTAL SOLIDS IN ICE CREAM

Preparing the Sample. Prepare the ice cream sample in the same way as for the Babcock tests.

Apparatus. Balance; fat dishes, solid dishes; tongs; dish contact maker; extraction flasks; pipets 1, 2, and 5; cooling desiccator; hot plate.

Reagents. Distilled water, free from residue; ammonia, chemically pure, about 26° Baumé, sp. gr. 0.8164 at 60°F; ethyl ether, not more than 4% water, free from residue, sp. gr. 0.713–0.716 at 77°F; bp, 95°F; petroleum ether, free from residue, sp. gr. 0.638–0.660 at 70°F; bp 120–140°F; alcohol, 95% sp. gr. 0.8164.

Procedure for Fat

1. Prepare a representative sample and mix thoroughly by pouring from one container to another.
2. Weigh a 5 g sample into a properly labeled extraction flask.
3. Add 5–6 ml of water.
4. Add 1.5 ml of ammonia and mix thoroughly.
5. Add 10 ml of alcohol, insert cork, and shake for 30 sec, keeping finger over cork.
6. Add 25 ml of ethyl ether, insert cork, and shake for 30 sec.
7. Add 25 ml of petroleum ether, insert cork, and shake for 30 sec.
8. Centrifuge 30, taking 30 sec.
9. Pour off the ether mixture containing the extracted fat into previously tared and weighed fat dishes. Avoid getting any of the residue into the dish.

10. Add 5 ml of alcohol to the flask.

11. Add 25 ml each of ethyl and petroleum ether, insert cork, and shake for 30 sec after each reagent.

12. Centrifuge 30 turns, taking 30 sec.

13. Pour off the other mixture into the same fat dishes used in the first extraction.

14. Evaporate the ether from the fat dishes on an electric hot plate at 135°F.

15. Place dishes in vacuum oven at 135°F for 5 min with not less than 20 in. of vacuum.

16. Cool dishes in the cooling desiccator for 7 min.

17. Weigh dishes and fat rapidly and record weight of fat to the fourth decimal place.

18. The percentage of fat is calculated by dividing weight of fat by weight of sample, and multiplying by 100.

Procedure for Solids

1. Mix the sample thoroughly by pouring several times from one container to another.

2. Weigh a 1-g sample into a solids dish that has been previously heated for 5 min in a solids oven at 212°F and then cooled for 5 min in a solids cooling desiccator.

3. Record the weight of the dish and the sample to the fourth decimal place with cover on the dish.

4. Add 1 ml water.

5. Tilt the dish in order to spread the mix in a thin film over the entire bottom of the dish.

6. Place the dish on the hot plate at 350°F and heat until the residue begins to turn a light brown. Use the contact maker to ensure uniform evaporation.

7. Place the dish into the solids vacuum oven at 212°F and heat for 10 min under not less than 20 in. vacuum.

8. Cool for 5 min in the cooling desiccator.

9. Weigh the dish and solids. Record the weight.

10. The percentage of TS is calculated by dividing weight of solids by weight of sample, and multiplying by 100.

OTHER METHODS OF FAT DETERMINATION
Roese–Gottlieb Method

Preparing the Sample. Standard.

Apparatus and Reagents. Mojonnier fat extraction flask (or Röhrig or similar type); free-flowing pipet; ammonium hydroxide; alcohol.

Procedure

1. Accurately weigh 4–5 g of thoroughly mixed sample directly into flask.

2.   Dilute with water to about 10 ml, work charge into lower chamber, and mix by shaking.

3.   Add 2 ml of ammonium hydroxide, mix thoroughly, and heat in water bath for 20 min at 60°C with occasional shaking.

4.   Cool, add 10 ml alcohol, and mix well.

5.   Add 25 ml ether (all ether must be peroxide-free), stopper with cork or stopper (synthetic rubber) unaffected by usual fat solvents, and shake very vigorously for 1 min.

6.   Add 25 ml petroleum ether (redistilled slowly at 65°C) and repeat vigorous shaking.

7.   Centrifuge Mojonnier flask at 600 rpm or let it (or Rohrig tube) stand until upper liquid is practically clear.

8.   Decant ether solution into suitable flask or metal dish.

9.   Wash lip and stopper of extraction flask or tube with mixture of equal parts of both solvents and add washings to weighing flask or dish.

10.   Repeat extraction of liquid remaining in flask or tube twice, using 15 ml of each solvent each time.

11.   Evaporate solvents completely on hot plate or steam bath at temperature that does not cause spattering or bumping.

12.   Dry fat in oven at temperature of boiling water to constant weight.

13.   Weigh cooled flask or dish, using as counterpoise duplicate container handled similarly, and avoid wiping either immediately before weighing.

14.   Remove fat completely from container with warm petroleum ether, dry, and weigh as before.

The loss in weight is then the weight of the fat. Correct the weight of the fat by a blank determination of the regents used.

Separation of Fat from Ice Cream

Preparing the Sample.   Standard.

Apparatus and Reagents.   No. 20 sieve; separator; ammonium hydroxide; alcohol; petroleum ether; anhydrated Na_2SO_4.

Procedure

1.   Melt sample and screen out any large pieces of fruit or nuts with sieve.

2.   Place 300 ml of melted sample in 1-liter separator, add 100 ml of water and 50 ml of ammonium hydroxide, and shake well.

3.   Add 200 ml of alcohol and shake for 1 min.

4.   Add 200 ml of petroleum ether and shake for 1 min.

5.   Let stand until emulsion breaks, and drain and discard lower layer.

6.   Add 25 g of anhydrated Na_2SO_4, shake, and decant thru rapid folded paper.

7.   Evaporate ether and alcohol, and let fat dry at 55°F overnight.

8.   The separated fats can then be used for the various determination and values desired.

TOTAL SOLIDS—OFFICIAL[1]

Into a round flat-bottomed dish not less than 5 cm in diameter, quickly weigh 1–2 g of sample. (Sample may be weighed by means of short, bent, 2-ml measuring pipet.) Heat on steam bath 30 min, then in air oven at 212°F for 3.5 hr. Cool in desiccator and weigh quickly to avoid absorption of moisture.

THE ACIDITY TEST FOR MILK

Preparing the Sample. Samples for this test should be taken and prepared in the same manner as for fat tests.

Apparatus and Reagents. 17.6-ml pipet as for the Babcock test; 9-ml pipet; white porcelain cup; glass stirring rod; buret graduated to read to 0.1 ml; alkali solution (0.1*N*); indicator (1.0% phenolphthalein).

Procedure
1. Using the 17.6-ml pipet, transfer 18 g of the sample to the white cup.
2. Add 3–5 drops of indicator.
3. Fill the buret with alkali solution, making sure that no air bubbles remain in the tip of the buret when it is filled to the 0 mark.
4. Slowly titrate the milk with the alkali solution until a faint pink color appears. (This color should persist for about 30 sec.)
5. Read to the nearest 0.1 ml the amount of alkali solution used.
6. Divide the amount of alkali used by 20 to get the percentage of acidity in the milk.

THE ACIDITY TEST FOR CREAM AND PLAIN ICE CREAM MIX

Preparing the Sample. Proceed as for testing acidity in milk.

Apparatus and Reagents. The same as for testing acidity in milk.

Procedure
1. Using the 9-ml pipet, transfer 9 g of sample to the white cup.
2. Add 9 ml of distilled water, and 3–5 drops of indicator.
3. Titrate with the alkali solution as described for milk.
4. Read the amount of alkali solution used.
5. Obtain the percentage of acidity by dividing the amount used by 10.

---

[1]Official means here that this is a method of analysis of the Association of Official Agricultural Chemists (AOAC).

THE ALCOHOL COAGULATION TEST
FOR PROTEIN STABILITY

This is a simple test to indicate the protein stability of an ice cream mix.

Preparing the Sample. Standard

Apparatus and Reagents. Alcohol (95%); test tubes.

Procedure
1. Place 5 ml of mix in a test tube.
2. Add distilled water and then alcohol in various proportions, starting with 9 ml water and 1 ml alcohol, then 8 ml water and 2 ml alcohol in the next test tube, etc. (The total volume of alcohol plus water should always equal 10 ml.)
3. Starting with the tube with the least alcohol, mix by closing the tube with the thumb and slowly inverting three times.
4. Continue from tube to tube until a slight precipitate can be seen on the wall of the test tube as the mix drains away.
5. Record the amount of alcohol (to the nearest 0.1 ml) necessary to form the slight precipitate.

Protein stability to alcohol is assessed according to how much alcohol is required to form the precipitate: 2–3 ml, poor; 4–5, fair; 6–7, good; over 7, excellent. Those mixes with poor stability may have problems in processing and handling, and there may be deterioration in the finished product.

DETERMINATION OF PROTEIN IN
ICE MILK AND ICE CREAM

A formol titration procedure appears to have application as a quality control test for rapidly checking the total protein content of frozen desserts.

Preparing the Sample. Standard.

Apparatus and Reagents. 100-ml beaker; pH meter; NaOH (0.03N); saturated potassium oxalate.

Procedure
1. Weigh 20-g sample into a 100-ml beaker.
2. Add 0.8 ml of saturated potassium oxalate and mix for about 1 min.
3. Titrate with standard 0.03N NaOH to an endpoint of pH 8.5 using a pH meter.
4. Add 4 ml of 40% formaldehyde and titrate back to the endpoint of pH 8.5.
5. Run a blank using 20 ml of water instead of 20 g of frozen dessert.
6. The net formol titration is the amount of NaOH (minus the blank) required to titrate the sample after the formaldehyde is added.

7. The percentage of protein is given by NaOH (ml) × (normality of NaOH) × 9.04 − 0.14

WEIGHT PER UNIT VOLUME OF PACKAGED ICE CREAM

Apparatus and Reagents
1. Overflow can: Use a No. 10, or 1-gal can (see Fig. 20.1). Upper edge of opening of spout should be above lower bend.
2. Iron bar: slightly longer than diameter of can, equipped with a bridge of tinned metal, may be used to submerge sample in kerosene of known density at 20/4° and cooled to 5–10°C (40–50°F) before use.
3. Balance: Capacity 1 kg, sensitive to 1 g.
4. Cylinders or beakers: 500–1000 ml, graduated.

Procedure. Obtain packaged samples (pints preferred) from freezing compartment or cold room and immediately place in insulated container. Surround package with slabs or pieces of dry ice until frozen solid.

Place overflow can on level table so that overflow discharges into sink. Fill can with the cooled kerosene until it overflows through spout. When overflow ceases, place tared 500-ml graduated cylinder (or beaker) under spout.

Remove frozen brick from dry ice, quickly remove from carton, and weigh to accuracy of 1–2 g. Slowly immerse brick in kerosene, finally submerging it completely by holding it under surface with small spatula, or bridge described above, until overflow ceases. Weigh displaced kerosene to accuracy of 1–2 g, and subtract tare weight of cylinder or beaker to ascertain net weight of kerosene displaced. Divide net weight of kerosene by its specific gravity to obtain its volume. The weight per unit volume will then be found from the relationship.

$$8.345 W/V \quad \text{lb/gal}$$

where W is the weight of the ice cream and V the volume of the displaced kerosene.

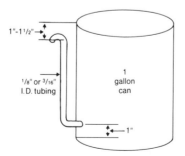

Fig. 20.1. Overflow can.

If the ice cream is packed so that it is difficult to remove from the carton, then determine the gross weight of carton and contents by opening the ends or sides of the carton enough to avoid formation of entrapped air bubbles, and submerging the entire carton and contents in the kerosene. After overflow ceases and the displaced kerosene has been weighed, remove contents from carton, dry the empty carton, and weigh it. Transfer the kerosene to a 100- or 200-ml graduated cylinder, filling to the halfway mark, and record the volume of the carton by slipping it into the cylinder until it is completely immersed in the kerosene. The increase in volume is the volume occupied by the carton. Correct for the weight and volume of carton in the formula above, weight in lb/gallon.

A graduated cylinder may be used instead of a beaker to catch the overflow. The volume reading may be used as a check against calculated volume of the kerosene. Volume calculated by weight is more accurate.

STABILITY TO HEAT SHOCK

Use a portion (1/2 gal) of ice cream in a container. Temper and store the container of ice cream at $-4°F$. After storage transfer it to a temperature-controlled area at 68°F for 1.5 hr and then return it to refrigerated storage. The next day (or 24 hr later) transfer the sample to the temperature-controlled area for another 1/2-hr shock. Repeat this treatment each day for 6 days. Then return the sample to the refrigerated storage and evaluate it after 24 hr. Product stability is assessed as poor, fair, or good based on appearance, coarseness of texture, degree of product breakdown, and conversion to serum.

MELTDOWN TEST AND SHAPE RETENTION

A rectangular block of ice cream (pint) that has been stored at $-4°F$ is placed on a wire gauze (10 wires/in.) in an atmosphere maintained at 60°F. Make arrangements to collect the liquid drained from the gauze. The time for collection of the first 10 ml of liquid is noted. The volume of liquid collected in each subsequent 10-min period is measured and the slope of the graph obtained by plotting the volume collected against time is recorded as the meltdown milliliters per hour. After the sample is melted (up to 4 hr) the residue is examined and the degree of shape retention and appearance is assessed as bad, poor, fair, good, or excellent.

A graduated cylinder is suitable for measuring the melted liquid. In case of excess foam, it may be desirable to record the weight of the residue at the intervals. Photographs of the residue may be taken as a record.

MICROSCOPIC EXAMINATION OF
ICE CREAM TEXTURE

The ice cream is hardened at $-15°F$ for 48 hr before texture measurements are made. All apparatus including a microscope, lamp, slides, cover glasses, sectioning knife, immersion liquid, tweezers, and lens paper are tempered at hardening-room temperature. Representative freehand sections several microns in thickness are made. These sections are then embedded in a few drops of an immersion liquid with a refractive index of 1.42 on a microscope slide. The section is covered with a cover glass and examined with the microscope using a magnification of approximately 100×. Measurements of ice crystal size, air cell size, distance between cells, and unfrozen material are made. An average number of measurements is taken on each item by means of an eyepiece micrometer. Examination of duplicate packages, sections, and fields contributes to accuracy.

FARRALL HOMOGENIZATION INDEX

Make a dilution of ice cream mix to be tested by using standard medicine dropper for measuring 3 drops of mix to 10 ml water solution of glycerine (1/3 glycerine). Add diluted product to special slide, cover with cover glass, and let set for 5 min. Count the number of each size fat globule over 2 μm in diameter in each of five fields.

Size ranges of fat globules are grouped as 2–2.5, 2.5–3, 3–4, 4–5, 5–6, 6–7, and 7–8 with a K value for each group of 1.4, 2.6, 5.4, 11.4, 21.0, 34.0, and 53.0, respectively. To obtain the index, the number of globules counted in each group is multiplied by the K value of each group and the values obtained are added. For example, if an examination of five fields showed two globules 2–2.5 in size, one globule 2.5–3, and one globule 3–4, the homogenization index would be 10.8, the sum of 2×1.4, 1×2.6, and 1×5.4.

VISCOSITY MEASUREMENTS

Pipet Method

In the pipet method, a measuring pipet of 50–100 ml capacity, marked at an arbitrary place below the bulb, is used to make the comparison. The sample to be tested is tempered to a standard temperature in the range 60–70°F. The pipet is tempered by putting water at 60–70°F into the pipet. The time in seconds required to discharge the sample to the lower mark is determined for water and then for the sample being tested for comparison purposes. Comparisons are made of the flowtime of mixes of the same composition on different days and on different mixes.

Borden Flow Meter Method

This instrument is available from the Borden Co., Columbus, Ohio. The tube-out type is available in different sizes to handle products of greatly different viscosities. The instrument and ice cream mix to be tested are tempered to 65–70°F. The sample is mixed gently, then placed in the instrument, and the excess is allowed to flow out the overflow tube. The time (in seconds) that a continuous stream of mix flows from the instrument is recorded as flow time and can be used for comparison purposes.

Surface Tension Measurements

The drop method can be used for comparison purposes: A tube of uniform bore is used and the number of drops of the sample falling per unit time is compared with that of water.

The tensiometer, employing a platinum ring, is a more accurate method of measuring surface tension. The ring is connected to a sensitive balance and the force (in dynes) required to draw the ring from the liquid is measured. The surface tension of water is 72–73 dynes while the value for ice cream mix is typically 50 dynes.

TESTING GELATIN

The Dahlberg Test

Sometimes called the test tube test, this serves as a guide in determining the amount of gelatin needed in the mix, and in comparing the stabilizing ability of different gelatins when used in ice cream.

Apparatus. Butter moisture scales, or scales of equal accuracy; set of weights, 1–100 g; 250-ml beaker (for weighing skim milk); 1-liter Erlenmeyer flask; 24 test tubes, 12–14 mm diameter; test tube rack; 2 pipets, capacity 10 ml in 0.1-ml graduations.

Reagents. Gelatin sample; at least 1 qt of fresh skim milk.

Procedure
1. Weigh and put into the flask exactly 495 g fresh skim milk, below 80°F.
2. Weigh exactly 5 g gelatin, and add it to the skim milk in the flask, thus obtaining a 1.0% gelatin solution.
3. Allow to soak for 30 min.
4. Using a water bath, heat the gelatin solution to 145°F and hold at this temperature for 15 min, keeping the flask stoppered to prevent evaporation while heating.
5. Cool the solution to room temperature.
6. Put at least 10 clean, dry test tubes in a rack, and number them.
7. Using one pipet for the gelatin–skim milk solution, and another for the fresh skim milk, prepare the series of solutions shown in Table 20.1.
8. Mix each tube by inverting it, and then set the tubes in ice water for 18–20 hr.
9. Then examine each tube in turn by placing a thumb over the top of the tube and quickly inverting the tube, holding the inverted tube still for 30 sec.
10. Do not allow the hand to warm the tube; record the number of the tube in which the solution just fails to break when inverted for 30 sec.

Table 20.1. The Dahlberg Test for Gelatin Strength

Tube no.[a]	Gelatin–skim milk (ml)	Skim milk (ml)	Factor
1	10.0	0	1.00
2	9.5	0.5	0.95
3	9.0	1.0	0.90
4	8.5	1.5	0.85
5	8.0	2.0	0.80
6	7.5	2.5	0.75
7	7.0	3.0	0.70
8	6.5	3.5	0.65
9	6.0	4.0	0.60
10	5.5	4.5	0.55
11	5.0	5.0	0.50
12	4.5	5.5	0.45

[a]Additional tubes may be needed for some gelatins.

The factor (the percentage gelatin in the tube) corresponding to this tube is used to calculate the amount of this sample of gelatin needed in an ice cream mix as follows:

$$gelation \ (\%) \ = \ factor \ \times \ \frac{100 \ - \ TS \ (\%)}{100 \ - \ serum \ solids \ in \ skim \ milk \ (\%)}$$

For example, the skim milk used in the gelatin test contained 8.7% serum solids. When the tubes were inverted for 30 sec the solutions in tubes 10 and 11 broke and ran down, but the solution in tube 9 failed to break. The factor corresponding to tube 9 is 0.60. Therefore,

$$gelatin \ (\%) \ = \ 0.60 \ \times \ \frac{100 \ - \ 36.09}{100 \ - \ 8.7} = 0.42\%$$

which is the percentage of gelatin to use in this ice cream mix provided no other ingredients used act as a stabilizer.

When using the Dahlberg test to compare different gelatins, the following conditions must be kept uniform for all gelatins: (1) the quality, i.e., acidity, of the skim milk; (2) the soaking time, heating time, and temperature in making the solutions; and (3) the temperature and time of the ice water bath.

This test is not satisfactory for gum-type stabilizers. In fact, there is, as yet, no really accurate test of stabilizing ability for either the gelatin- or the gum-type stabilizer.

TESTS FOR AMMONIA LEAKS

Apparatus and Reagents. Clean tumbler; piece of glass large enough to cover it, ammonia test papers purchased from refrigeration companies (similar papers may be prepared from heavy white paper strips, about 1×5 in.); these are dipped in phenolphthalein solution, the indicator solution used for acidity tests; if dried and stored for future use, these test papers must be moistened with distilled water when used).

Procedure

1. Pass a strip of the test paper along the ammonia pipes, valves, or compressor head suspected of leaks.

2. If there is a leak, the phenolophthalein-treated paper will turn pink where it comes in contact with the escaping ammonia.

3. Ammonia leaking into the brine or the cooling water may be detected as follows: Fill a tumbler half-full of the suspected brine or cooling water and add about 1/8 teaspoonful of dry caustic soda or lye, whichever is available.

4. Cover with the piece of glass.

5. Insert right under the cover, but not in the solution, a small strip of the phenolphthalein-treated paper.

6. If paper becomes pink after a few minutes, ammonia has been escaping into the brine or cooling water.

OTHER LABORATORY PROCEDURES

Mix density, acidity, viscosity, surface tension, interfacial tension, and freezing point determination are discussed in Chapter 4.

Rheological methods involving body and texture measurements and gas chromatography in establishing body and texture and flavor profiles are based on sophisticated instrumentation. Instrument operation procedures must be referred to in adapting them to the analysis of ice cream. Deb (1983) has conducted extensive investigation and done rheological studies in adapting advanced technological methods to the evaluation of flavors, body and texture, and rheological properties of ice cream.

The advent of chromatography and its application to carbohydrate analysis has provided a quantitative determination for sugars in ice cream. The following sugars have been resolved on a single chromatographic strip: fructose, glucose, galactose, sucrose, maltose, lactose, and higher sugars.

Bruhn *et al.* (1980) used the dye-bending method of determining protein and analyzed 24 samples of vanilla ice cream and ice milk. They concluded that when the Kjeldahl protein results were corrected for the nonprotein nitrogen present, the resulting protein values averaged 0.20% lower than dye-binding values. The results indicated the dye-binding method was sufficiently accurate for monitoring protein concentration in the frozen desserts studied.

Douglas and Tobias (1982) reported on a procedure for determining casein and whey protein in ice cream by measuring its phosphorus:nitrogen ratio. They stated that this procedure can also be used to demonstrate whether or not ice cream has been adulterated with other proteins.

Water activity A_W, the amount of water in the total water content, is usually defined as the percentage of relative humidity generated in equilibrium with the product sample in a closed system at constant temperature. Moisture content is often defined as the percentage by weight of the water content to the weight of the sample. The active part of the moisture content (free) water in relation to the total including (bound) water has gained attention in the food-processing industry. A water activity specification has been included in FDA regulations (FDA 1979).

Water activity influences change in color, flavor, and aroma, spoilage (food poisoning), loss of vitamins, and consistency (body and texture).

Water activity is important in the control of bacteriological, chemical, and physical food stability. It is not possible for most bacteria to grow or have a minimum A_W value of 0.90 or less. The oxidization of fats decreases at A_W values below 0.2. Body and texture are affected at A_W values of 0.5–0.6. The A_W value of frozen fruit, ripple sauce, and the ice cream mix may be important to consider.

OTHER TESTS USED IN A
QUALITY CONTROL PROGRAM

Other chemical and bacteriological tests require more elaborate equipment and skilled operators. However, their use is important in any well-organized quality control program. Among these tests are the Mojonnier test for fat and total solids; the phosphatase test for detecting improper pasteurization; the coliform test, used as a measure of the sanitary handling of dairy products; the sediment test, used to detect the presence of insoluble foreign matter that does not properly belong in dairy products; tests for antibiotic and pesticide residues.

Directions for these and other analytical tests can be found in Standard Methods for the Examination of Dairy Products published by the American Public Health Association, New York; and in Official and Tentative Methods of Analysis published by the Association of Official Agricultural Chemists, Washington, D.C.

21
Sales Outlets

In recent years the merchandising of ice cream has become highly competitive, and profit margins have been greatly reduced. Marketing methods have also changed extensively. Ice cream manufacturers have been required to adapt to these changes to be assured of dependable markets for their products. The supermarket has become a dominant factor in ice cream distribution to the consumer along with an increase in volume of 1/2-gal packages and other prepackaged items. Less bulk ice cream is being sold in drug stores and more through special confectionery stores and institutional outlets. There are several types of markets available to the ice cream manufacturer: (1) wholesale to drug stores, specialty confectionery stores, dairy stores, supermarkets, and food service establishments; (2) retail directly to customers through the manufacturer's special ice cream stores, dairy bars, or ice cream parlors; (3) wholesale to other manufacturers by developing a specialized operation for novelties, special formulations, or packaging.

WHOLESALING

If this type of marketing is chosen, the supermarket, drug store, and dairy store offer good outlets for the packaged products. The dairy bar, drug store, ice cream parlor, and food service institutions provide good outlets for bulk ice cream. There is a current trend for the food distribution companies to manufacture ice cream for their supermarkets, and some manufacturers establish dairy or confectionery stores to retail to their customers. The development of a large, effective specialty operation for manufacturing packaged ice cream or ice cream novelties for wholesale distribution over a wide territory is also a trend.

RETAILING

Retailing by the manufacturer has been facilitated in recent years by the availability of large shopping centers and by improved transportation and packaging along with the increased competition and reduced profit margins in some areas of wholesale operations. The dairy store, confectionery store, and dairy bar are important retail outlets.

MERCHANDISING

Baumer and Jacobson (1969) submitted an economic and marketing report on frozen desserts which included studies on demand elasticity, consumption patterns, competition among ice cream and related products, and competition from other desserts and snacks. They concluded that ice cream consumption responds readily to price changes—that price increase comes close to decreasing consumption by a proportional amount. Demand analysis suggested that an industry average price increase of 10% would result in approximately an 8% consumption drop; a 10% increase in the price of private label ice cream and ice milk might be expected to result in a 17% decline in sales of these products.

Price changes may be expected to result in greater changes in ice cream consumption as increased volumes are mass merchandised through large retail outlets and as the availability of substitutes increases, particularly in the snack market.

Consumption patterns for ice cream have remained about constant during recent years, but ice milk and mellorine have shown large sales growth. Ice milk sales now represent more than 20% of industry sales.

Baumer and Jacobson stated that because ice cream, ice milk, and mellorine are readily substituted for each other by consumers, there is competition among these products, and changes in price relationship can have great sales impact. They concluded that while ice cream has generally been thought of as a dessert, it has taken on increased importance as a snack food in the past few years; that about 50% of the ice cream and related products are being consumed as snacks and 45% as desserts; and that price competition from other desserts and snack goods will likely become more intense in the future.

Supermarket package sales accounted for 59%; institutional bulk pack sales for 19%; and novelties for 22% of the total sales of ice cream in the study.

A study of consumer use of frozen desserts (Traugott 1965) indicated that 60–70% of purchases of ice cream were in supermarkets, 9% in drug stores, 18% in ice cream stores, and 10% in other categories.

Potter (1966) stated that food service establishments have a wide variety of products and flavors to choose from in the frozen dessert industry and that careful attention should be given to the purchase of these products. He claims that the use of product specifications is essential to ensure that the proper product is being purchased.

Tracy and McGarrahan (1957) discussed the planning and operation of the dairy products store. IAICM (1968) has set forth the aspects of proper merchandising of ice cream.

DRIVE-IN STORE

The main requirement for the drive-in store (second only to the store itself, of course is plenty of parking space for customers' cars. If possible, the site chosen should have a pleasing background and a good view, and the parking area should be kept neat and tidy. Since it has been estimated that about 75% of ice cream business is in repeat orders, obviously the drive-in store should be on the edge of a residential area, preferably near and in view of a well-traveled highway.

The store itself should be attractive, well-lighted, well-arranged, and convenient for service. It should be kept clean and sanitary in every detail.

The manager of such a store (of any food store, in fact) should make it a first rule to become familiar with state and local community health regulations and insist that all employees and persons delivering food products to the establishment comply with such regulations.

THE SODA FOUNTAIN[1]

Soda fountain service is a profitable addition to many of the types of food outlets. However, this kind of business should be ventured into only if there is sufficient capital to do a good and attractive job of installation, and only if the management understands the soda fountain business and is sufficiently interested to become familiar with the many phases of this kind of merchandising.

If properly rightly equipped and managed, and staffed with perfectly trained personnel there is no doubt that the soda fountain can be a great help in selling ice cream. Keep in mind, however, that service must be given in an accommodating, eye-appealing, and taste-tempting manner. The ice cream dispenser and the soda fountain itself should have a neat, well-cared-for appearance. About everything connected with the fountain and its environment there must be an intangible atmosphere that suggests wholesomeness, cleanliness, and sanitation (see Fig. 21.1).

General Housekeeping

Both the inside and the outside of the fountain need regular cleaning and upkeep. For sanitary reasons, the inside must be kept scrupulously clean. Keeping it clean both inside and outside also retards corrosion of the metal linings and thus prolongs the life of the fountain. Keep in mind, too, that a spotless general appearance has definite customer appeal and generally pays off handsomely in additional profits.

Glass or Paper Dishes?

At the fountain, either glass or paper cups and serving dishes may be used. Many people perfer glassware, but if it is used great care must be taken to

---

[1]The soda fountain , which at one time was known as "ice cream parlour," is being increasingly called "ice cream shop" in some parts of the country. However, no matter what it is called, the soda fountain is characterized by sit-down service of a wide (and—for children as well as adults—wonderful) variety of ice cream products and concoctions.

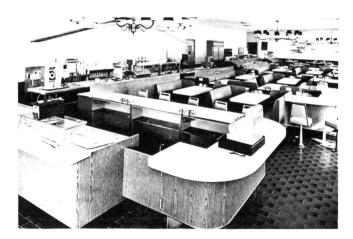

Fig. 21.1. Food service establishments, like this restaurant, find a soda fountain installation offers opportunities to increase sales volume. This one includes a wall fountain, liberal storage facilities, a storage and display case, and an efficient arrangement for customer servicing. (Courtesy of Grand Rapids Cabinet Co.)

prevent breakage and to keep dishes sanitary. With glass there is also the danger that chips of glass may fall into the open ice cream cans, and cleaning dirty dishes is always extra work. When paper cups and dishes are used, good housekeeping is made easier, serving can be more sanitary, there is no danger of broken glass, and no expensive delay for dishwashing.

PERSONNEL

Soda fountain success depends upon the selection and training of the right type of personnel for giving good service. This applies equally well to dairy bar or dairy store personnel. The men and women behind the counter should be schooled to follow a well-planned routine regarding the best form of greeting and approach to customers in taking the order, in serving the food, in making suggestions for increasing the order, in presenting the customer's bill or check, and in cleaning the counter before the next customer is served. In short, the good dispenser, or salesperson, will cultivate cheerfulness, meet customers with a smile, be dignified and quiet, give quick, accurate, and gracious service, and be dependable and honest.

Health Habits

The public is becoming more and more health conscious. Therefore, persons handling and serving food should be trained to live up to definite and rigid health standards. Hair should be well groomed; employees with long hair should cover their hair; teeth should be well cared for, hands and fingernails clean and trim, uniforms clean and neat, and shoes clean and polished. Soap and water should be easily accessible and used as freely as commonsense sanitary regulations dictate.

Keep Hands Clean

"Hands," someone has said, "are the tools of the food worker," essential in many operations in filling orders. The following rules about cleanliness of the hands must be observed by all operators: Keep them clean. Always assume they may carry germs. Wash them before handling tableware and food. Wash them after each visit to the lavatory; after coughing, sneezing, or combing the hair; and after handling refuse or waste of any kind. Always be sure they are clean before they touch food.

TRAINING FOR FOUNTAIN SERVICE

Quite likely the retailer's principal interest in the soda fountain is to increase profits. To do this more and more customers are needed. In order to attract customers and have them come back for repeat orders, the ice cream must be of high quality, good cream and good flavoring substances must be used in making it, and an equally good quality of syrups and toppings must be used to combine with the ice cream at the fountain. Generally it is best to buy and use only the best and most palatable materials for toppings and syrups and then be familiar with how and when to use them most effectively. Therefore, it would pay the retailer to train workers to sell more ice cream and thereby make larger profits. If the staff of store and fountain is to function well, training for the job is necessary for all employees. The work expected of them should be carefully explained and ably demonstrated to them.

The dispensers, the people in charge of the fountain, should have some special training in soda fountain work until they have thoroughly mastered the know-how of what and how to serve. They should be familiar with the best methods of preparing toppings and of blending fruits, nuts, and toppings with simple syrups. They should also know how to dip ice cream most economically, and know the most attractive ways in which the variously colored and flavored ice creams should be served.

Employees as Sales Representatives

The men and women employed for fountain service are the principal contact retailers have with the public who buy their products. It is really a waste of money to advertise, build and equip a fine building, and manufacture or buy high-quality ice cream if the employees who represent the establishment create an unfavorable impression on the public—the consumer who is counted upon to buy this delicious product.

Choosing a Manager

The manager must be honest, conscientious, able to handle personnel, to work with them and yet be their leader; must be efficient and have some administrative ability; must have enough originality to be able to develop new sales ideas; and finally must be loyal to the proprietor or organization.

All that has been said about employees' training, ability, and qualifications has been said simply to emphasize the fact that these employees really reflect the business and managerial ability of the proprietor. A good manager will make a business prosper. If a business is too large to handle personally, much will depend on the store or fountain manager chosen to help run the business.

The management that has thus thoroughly trained its representatives, i.e., its employees, for their respective jobs, should be well on the way toward a profitable business.

How to Dip Ice Cream

While it may seem like an easy thing to do, it really takes practice and planning to dip ice cream properly. To lower the ice cream surface evenly in the can, to cut from the highest surface of the ice cream, and to keep the can stationary while dipping the ice cream for the cone require skill that comes only with practice. Experienced fountain operators have found that it is best to press the ball of ice cream gently on the side of the cone with the outside of the dipperbowl, pressing just enough to make it stick but not enough to spoil its shape or to break the cone. The dispenser should learn early at what temperature ice cream will dip or cut easily and still not be so soft as to spoil the texture and cause shrinkage. This feel for dipping comes only by practice (see Figs. 21.2 and 21.3).

The dipped package usually refers to carry-out packages filled by the retailer, who dips the hardened ice cream from a bulk package in the cabinet and presses it into the new container.

It is common knowledge that the volume of ice cream after dipping is less than the volume before dipping. This decrease in volume is due to air being compressed or expelled from the ice cream with a corresponding loss in overrun. The retailer cannot sell the same volume of ice cream received from the manufacturer, but sustains what is known as a dipping loss. Several factors may affect dipping losses, among which are overrun, dipping temperature, and composition. These factors were studied in detail by Bierman (1926): his findings still offer valuable information.

The percentage overrun is important in determining the number of quarts or servings that the ice cream dealer can dip from a container of ice cream. Table 21.1 shows the effect of overrun on dipping losses.

The most uniform weight quarts were dipped from ice cream containing 80–100% overrun. The percentage dipping loss increases as the overrun of the ice cream increases. A dealer who observes this fact will be in a better position to establish proper dispensing procedures.

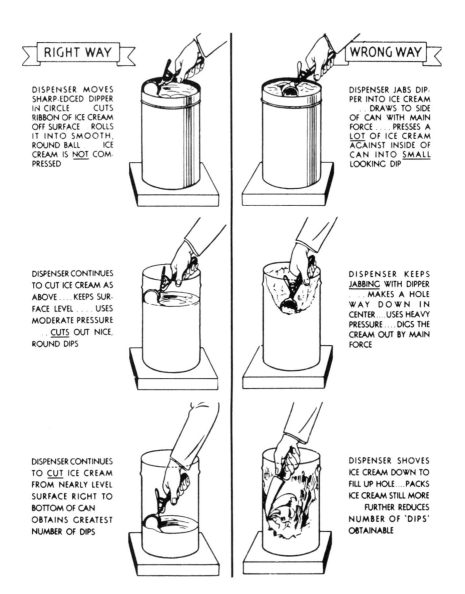

RIGHT WAY

DISPENSER MOVES SHARP-EDGED DIPPER IN CIRCLE CUTS RIBBON OF ICE CREAM OFF SURFACE ROLLS IT INTO SMOOTH, ROUND BALL ICE CREAM IS NOT COMPRESSED

DISPENSER CONTINUES TO CUT ICE CREAM AS ABOVE....KEEPS SURFACE LEVEL....USES MODERATE PRESSURE ..CUTS OUT NICE, ROUND DIPS

DISPENSER CONTINUES TO CUT ICE CREAM FROM NEARLY LEVEL SURFACE RIGHT TO BOTTOM OF CAN OBTAINS GREATEST NUMBER OF DIPS

WRONG WAY

DISPENSER JABS DIPPER INTO ICE CREAM . DRAWS TO SIDE OF CAN WITH MAIN FORCE.... PRESSES A LOT OF ICE CREAM AGAINST INSIDE OF CAN INTO SMALL LOOKING DIP

DISPENSER KEEPS JABBING WITH DIPPER ...MAKES A HOLE WAY DOWN IN CENTER....USES HEAVY PRESSURE....DIGS THE CREAM OUT BY MAIN FORCE

DISPENSER SHOVES ICE CREAM DOWN TO FILL UP HOLE....PACKS ICE CREAM STILL MORE FURTHER REDUCES NUMBER OF 'DIPS' OBTAINABLE

Fig. 21.2. How to dip ice cream. (Courtesy of C.P. Gundlach & Co.)

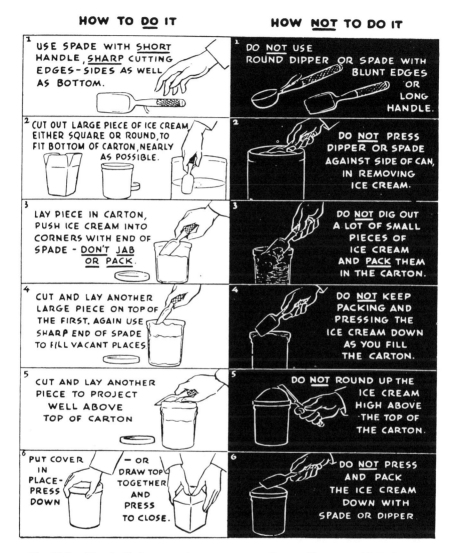

Fig. 21.3. How to dip ice cream into carry-out packages. (Courtesy of C.P. Gundlach & Co.)

The dipping temperature influences the number of servings that which can be dipped from a container of ice cream. Table 21.2 shows the effect of dipping temperatures on losses.

It appears from the above results that if dipping losses are to be kept at a minimum, ice cream of average composition (15% sugar) should be dipped at 8°F or lower. The dipping temperature should be varied inversely 1–1.5°F for each 1% difference in sugar content; to make dipping practical at 8°F or lower, the ice cream should contain approximately 90% overrun.

Table 21.1. How Overrun Affects Dipping Losses and Weight per Quart[a]

Average overrun (%)	Dealer dips from 20-qt containers (qt)	Average dipping loss (%)	Weight per quart (oz)	
			Before dipping	After dipping
60.3	16.96	15.18	22.95	27.05
80.6	15.37	23.14	20.37	26.52
100.8	14.07	29.66	18.30	26.25
118.6	13.45	32.76	16.81	25.14
Average:	14.96	25.18	19.61	26.24

[a]From Bierman (1926a).

Table 21.2. How Dipping Temperature Affects Dipping Losses and Weight per Quart[a,b]

Dipping temperature (°F)	Dealer dips from 20-qt containers (qt)	Average dipping loss (%)	Weight per quart after dipping (oz)
3–8	15.33	23.35	25.72
9–16	14.65	26.75	26.82
17–20	15.86	20.70	24.46

[a]Compiled from Bierman (1926).
[b]Average overrun, 90%; weight per quart before dipping, 19.34 oz.

The proper dipping temperature is determined by different factors. It must be low enough to keep dipping losses to a minimum and yet afford easy dipping. This is affected by the overrun and composition, especially the sugar content of the product.

Composition has only a slight effect on dipping losses when compared to the effect of overrun and dipping temperature. The dipping losses in high-fat ice cream are slightly less than in average- or low-fat ice cream. The loss encountered in high-MSNF ice cream is greater than in a low-MSNF product when dipped at the same temperature. This is caused by the increased sugar (lactose) content introduced in the mix when the MSNF content is increased. Ice cream with a high sugar content has a greater dipping loss than ice cream containing a lower percentage of sugar unless the dipping temperature is varied to give equal hardness to the ice cream; then the dipping loss will be approximately the same regardless of the sugar content.

Dipping studies indicate that two factors influence the weight of ice cream dipped: (1) the resistance offered by the ice cream, which prevents the expulsion of the air; (2) the amount of force applied to push the dipper into the ice cream.

The advantages of hand packing ice cream are completely outweighed by the disadvantages:

1. The greater chance for unintentional contamination by the retailer.
2. The wide variation in the amount of ice cream placed in containers of equal size. The main factors influencing this variation are (a) tempera-

tures of ice cream (3–8°F is generally recommended to make dipping easy but varies with freezing point, etc., of the ice cream); (b) individuality: variation from person to person doing the dipping is great; (c) the composition and air content of the ice cream.

3. The inevitable delay in serving customers.
4. The necessarily higher temperature of the ice cream when it leaves the retail store. It has to be softer for dipping and therefore does not reach the home in as good a condition.
5. The damaged quality, especially in body and texture, of the ice cream.
6. The inability of the retailer to control operating costs. Since it is impossible for the retailer completely to fill equal-sized containers with equal weights of dipped ice cream, it is impossible to operate on a narrow margin or to estimate profits.

The number of dipper portions per 72-oz gallon are given in Table 21.3.

BASIC SODA FOUNTAIN PREPARATIONS

Ice cream can be served in countless ways in tempting flavors with a combination of different toppings, syrups, whipped cream, or nuts. It has become the favorite fun food and few if any foods enjoy greater popularity with consumers of all ages.

Because of these attributes, ice cream provides such great potentials for merchandising at the fountain. Basic ice cream items of fountain service are the cone, the dish of ice cream with or without fruit, the sundae, the soda, the milkshake, the banana split, the parfait, and novelty items. The art of preparing and serving these items constitutes an important phase of ice cream merchandising.

Dish of Ice Cream with Fruit
1. Place two dippers in dish (glass or paper).
2. Surround with 1 oz fresh sliced fruit of preference.

Sundae
1. Place 1/2 oz crushed, sliced, or whole fruit into a dish.
2. Add two dippers of ice cream.
3. Surround ice cream with crushed, sliced, or whole fruit.

Table 21.3. Average Number of Dips per Gallon

Dipper size (no.)	Number of dips	Size of dip (oz)
10	19	3-3/4
12	23	3-1/8
16	29	2-1/2
20	38	1-7/8
24	44	1-5/8
30	60	1-3/16

4. Add nuts.
5. Top with whipped cream and a single item of fruit.

Soda
1. Place 1-1/2 oz syrup into 14-oz glass.
2. Stir spoon of ice cream or 1-1/2 oz coffee cream into syrup.
3. Fill glass three-quarters full with carbonated water.
4. Float two dippers of ice cream into mix.
5. Mix gently.
6. Top with whipped cream.

Milk Shake
1. Place two dippers of ice cream into chilled cup.
2. Add 1-1/2 oz syrup.
3. Add 6 oz milk.
4. Mix thoroughly and rapidly.
5. Pour into serving glass.

Banana Split
1. Split banana in half, lengthwise, with peel on. Place one half on each side of dish, flat side down, then remove peel.
2. Place three dippers of ice cream on banana halves. Vanilla in center and other flavors on each side.
3. Cover each dipper of ice cream with different topping.
4. Garnish the top and between dippers with whipped cream.
5. Add single piece of fruit.
6. Place slices of banana or fruit around center of item.

Parfait
1. Place 1 tbs of crushed fruit in parfait glass.
2. Add one dipper of ice cream.
3. Cover with 1 tbs crushed fruit.
4. Add one dipper ice cream.
5. Cover with 2 tbs crushed fruit.
6. Add one dipper ice cream.
7. Cover with 1 tbs. crushed fruit.
8. Top with whipped cream.
9. Decorate with single piece of fruit or nut.

SPECIALS FOR SEASONS AND SPECIAL OCCASIONS

One of the best ways to promote sales is by featuring specials and by having a "season-minded" approach. Many special days in every season will suggest to the imaginative soda fountain dispenser new ideas for taste-tempting formulas and decorative schemes. The intelligent manager must, of course, not only make these specials but see to it that they are well advertised so the public will know about them well in advance of the special day that is featured.

22
Formulas and Industry Standards

Basic mix formulas may have variations and modifications as demanded by the ingredients available, consumer buying habits, competition, costs, and finished product quality expected.

The recipes given are for 10 gal (approximately 92 lb) of flavored mix unless otherwise specified. Natural pure flavors are recocommended. The numbers in all of the formulas indicate percentages unless otherwise specified. The percentage of stabilizer–emulsifier may vary with manufacturer's recommendations.

PLAIN ICE CREAM

Formula

Fat	10.0	12.0	14.0	16.00	18.0
MSNF	11.5	11.0	10.0	8.50	7.0
Sugar	15.0	15.0	15.0	17.00	18.0
Stabilizer–emulsifier	0.3	0.3	0.3	0.25	0.2
TS	36.8	38.3	39.2	41.75	43.2

Variations

Vanilla. To 10 gal plain mix add 6–12 oz flavor and 8 ml yellow color. The amount of flavor needed varies with strength of vanilla, composition of the mix, and personal preference.

Coffee. To 10 gal plain mix add 1 qt coffee extract (a strong coffee cooked from 1 lb of ground coffee may be used in place of the coffee extract); 5–7 oz of 50% burnt sugar color may be added.

Maple. To 10 gal plain mix add 3 oz pure maple extract and 2 oz burnt sugar coloring. If maple sugar is used, a special mix is prepared with 10–12% sucrose and 3–6% maple sugar.

Caramel.   To 10 gal plain mix add enough caramel flavor to impart a satisfactory caramel taste and color. If a caramel syrup is used, 3 qt per 9-1/4 gal of plain mix (approximately 4 oz per gallon of ice cream) will impart caramel flavor. A caramel syrum may be made by using 5 parts sugar and 3 parts 20% cream and boiling until it becomes light brown.

Mint.   To 10 gal plain mix add 4–8 oz pure mint extract, or enough to flavor to desired intensity, and color to light green.

Butterscotch.   To 10 gal plain mix add 1 gal butterscotch syrup and color yellow.

Bisque ice cream.   To 9–9-1/2 gal plain mix add 4–8 lb macaroons, sponge cake, ladyfingers, grapenuts, or similar products broken into small pieces, added to the ice cream in the freezer or with a fruit feeder. The ice cream carries the name of the product used (such as grapenut, sponge cake, or macaroon).

Tortoni, biscuit.   To 10 gal 14–16% fat ice cream mix add 1 pt dark rum or rum flavoring. Freeze at overrun of 50% or lower. Place in small fluted cups, and spinkle with macaroon crumbs.

Candy or Confection Ice Cream

Numerous candy and confection combinations for various flavors occur on the market under various names. These contain 5–8% candy or confection.

Peppermint stick.   To 9-1/2 gal plain mix add 4–5 lb crushed peppermint candy to partially frozen ice cream in the freezer or with fruit feeder.

Butter crunch.   To 9-1/2 gal plain mix add 6 lb ground butter crunch candy.

Chocolate chip.   To 9-1/2 gal plain mix add 2 qt milk chocolate syrup.

Peanut brittle.   To 9-1/2 gal plain mix add 4–6 lb crushed peanut brittle.

Marshmallow.   To 9-1/2 gal plain mix add 4–6 lb marshmallows.

Chopped chocolate.   To 9-1/2 gal plain mix add 4–5 lb chopped milk chocolate.

Licorice.   To 10 gal plain mix add 4 oz licorice paste and 1-1/3 oz oil of anise. Color black.

Molasses taffy.   To 9-1/2 gal plain mix add 4–6 lb molasses taffy.

Toffee.   To 9-1/2 gal plain mix add 4–6 lb of broken toffee candy.

Mint chip.   To 9-1/2 gal plain mix add 4–6 lb green or red or mixture of mint chips.

English toffee.   To 9-1/2 gal plain mix add 4–6 lb crushed English toffee (consisting of 2 lb butter, 5 lbs sugar, 1-1/2 lb nutmeats and 1/2 tsp soda). Heat butter and sugar to 320°F. Remove from heat and add soda, stirring thoroughly. Mix in nutmeats and spread to cool.

Ginger.   To 9-1/2 gal plain mix add 8 lb preserved chopped ginger root, or add a no. 10 can of ginger root flavoring.

CHOCOLATE ICE CREAM

Formula

Fat	8.0	10.0	12.00	14.00	16.0
MSNF	12.5	12.0	11.00	10.00	8.0
Sugar	16.0	16.0	16.00	17.00	19.0
Cocoa	2.7	3.0	3.00	3.00	3.5
Stabilizer–emulsifier	0.3	0.3	0.25	0.25	0.2
TS	39.5	41.3	42.25	44.25	46.7

The quantity of cocoa needed to flavor chocolate ice cream ranges from 2.7 to 3 lb; cocoa–liquor blend, 3.5–4.5 lb; and chocolate liquor, 4.5–5.5 lb per 10 gal of mix.

Variations

Chocolate. To 9 gal plain mix add chocolate syrup made from 3 lb cocoa (or 4 lb chocolate liquor), 3 lb sugar, and 4–6 qt water. Mix the cocoa and sugar together and add enough water to make a paste. Heat in a steam-jacketed kettle. As the syrup thickens, add the water gradually, constantly stirring. Heat to 175°F, draw off the syrup, cool, and use. Just enough water to prevent an excessively thick syrup is needed. The syrup can be made up in quantities and stored for a few days in a cold storage room at 35–40°F.

Chocolate mint flake. To 9-1/2 gal chocolate mix add 4–6 mint flakes.

Chocolate malt. To 9 gal plain mix add half the chocolate syrup used for chocolate ice cream and 1 qt of malt syrup. If malt syrup is not available, use 1–2 lb of malted milk.

Chocolate almond. To 9-1/2 gal chocolate mix add 4–6 lb broken almonds.

Chocolate marshmallow. To 9-1/2 gal chocolate mix add 4–6 lb marshmallow.

Mocha. To 7-1/2 gal plain mix add 2-1/2 gal chocolate mix and 8–12 oz coffee syrup or enough coffee extract to give a mild coffee flavor.

German chocolate, Swiss chocolate, or other variations. These may be prepared by using chocolate flavoring or other flavorings typical of the product desired.

FRUIT ICE CREAM

The basic mixes containing 10, 12, 14, 16, or 18% fat may be flavored with fruit preparations, which are added at the rate of 10–15% or more depending on the kind of fruit and flavor intensity expected. Fruit:sugar ratios of 3:1 or 4:1 are best for frozen fruit. The ratio, however, varies with the type of fruit.

Variations

Strawberry.   To 8 gal plain mix add 2 gal berries, fresh or fresh frozen. Fruit: sugar ratios of 3:1 are preferred for frozen berries. Color to strawberry pink using approximately 16 ml red color.

Peach.   To 8 gal plain mix add 2 gal peaches. A portion of the peach is often added as a puree to gain flavor and intensity. Color light egg yellow.

Cherry.   To 8-1/2 to 9 gal plain mix add 4–6 qt cherries (usually maraschino cherries are used). If maraschino cherries are not used, it is necessary to select sour cherries and use cherry concentrate to strengthen the flavor. Color light red.

Apricot.   To 8 gal plain mix add 2 gal apricots. Color light egg yellow.

Pineapple.   To 9 gal plain mix add 1 gal crushed pineapple.

Apple.   To 8 gal plain mix add 2 gal sliced frozen apples, 7:1 fruit sugar ratio. Fortify apple flavor with 320 g apple essence per 10 gal mix.

Banana.   To 9 gal plain mix add 1 gal crushed banana. Color light yellow. Often a small amount of citric acid or lemon juice is added to prevent discoloration of the fruit and to enhance the flavor. A high fruit to sugar ratio gives best results.

Orange.   To 9 gal plain mix add 4 qt orange juice (fresh or canned or equivalent of orange concentrate frozen), plus 2 pt lemon juice. Add 3 lb sugar to the juice. Color light orange.

Orange–pineapple.   To 9 gal plain mix add 2 qt prepared flavor which consists of crushed pineapple mixed with orange concentrate or orange oil. Color light orange.

Lemon.   To 9 gal plain mix add 4 qt fresh lemon juice or the equivalent of lemon concentrate plus 2 pt orange juice, add 3 lb sugar to the juice. Color lemon yellow.

Raspberry.   To 9 gal plain mix add 1 gal red raspberry or black raspberry puree. Addition of true fruit raspberry extract to strengthen the flavor is often practical. Raspberry puree with 1:1 fruit:sugar ratio is preferred.

Fig.   To 9 gal plain mix add 4–6 qt canned figs. Color light tan. A good fig–nut ice cream can be made by using 4 qt canned figs and 2 lb chopped nutmeats.

Grape.   To 8 gal plain mix add 1 gal concentrated grape juice.

Blueberry.   To 8 gal plain mix add 1 gal concentrated grape juice.

Blueberry.   To 8 gal plain mix add 2 gal blueberry puree.

Cherry–vanilla.   To 8 gal plain mix add 2 gal nonbleeding cherries injected with fruit feeder.

Burgundy cherry.   To 8 gal plain mix add 2 gal Burgundy cherries injected with fruit feeder.

Date.   To 8 gal plain mix add 2 gal crushed dates.

NUT ICE CREAM

A basic mix of composition 10, 12, or 14% fat may be satisfactorily flavored with 3–6% nut preparations.

Variations

Burnt almond. To 9-1/2 gal plain mix add 4–5 lb burnt or roasted almonds. Almond flavor may also be added, as well as some burnt sugar or caramel color.

Pistachio. To 9-1/2 gal plain mix add 4 lb chopped pistachio nutmeats, pistachio extract to taste, and color light green. Frequently English walnuts or pecan nutmeats are used instead of pistachio nuts, in which case the pistachio flavor is secured from the extract.

Butter pecan. To 9-1/2 gal plain mix add 3 lb butter crunch candy plus 2 lb chopped pecans. Butter pecan ice cream may also be made by using 9 gal plain mix, adding 10 lb butter pecans, half chopped and half whole, or all ground to a coarse size.

Maple walnut. To 9-1/2 gal plain mix add 2–4 lb chopped nutmeats. Add 3 oz pure maple extract.

Maple pecan. To 9-1/2 gal plain mix add 2–4 lb chopped pecans. Add 3 oz pure maple extract.

Black walnut. To 9-1/2 gal plain mix add 4–5 lb broken black walnut meats.

Caramel nut. To 9-1/2 gal plain mix add 3 lb crushed nuts, 2 oz burnt sugar coloring, and caramel flavoring.

Pineapple nut. To 9 gal plain mix add 1 gal pineapple and 3 lb nuts.

Pecan crunch. To 9-1/2 gal plain mix add 6 lb ground pecan crunch candy.

Banana nut. To 9-1/4 gal plain mix add 3/4 gal crushed bananas and 2 lb chopped nuts.

Chocolate almond. To 9-1/2 gal chocolate mix add 4 lb whole and broken almonds.

Almond toffee. To 9-1/2 gal plain mix add 4 lb broken toffee candy and 2 lb broken almonds.

Coconut pineapple. To 9 gal plain mix add 3 qt crushed pineapple and 4 lb ground coconut.

Peanut. To 9-1/2 gal plain mix add 4–6 lb peanuts, crushed or peanut butter.

PUDDINGS

Variations

Nesselrode pudding. To 8–8-1/2 gal 14–16% fat mix, add 6–8 qt special commercial fruit mixture suitable for nesselrode pudding. This should be added after the mix is partly frozen by use of a fruit feeder. A nesselrode mixture may be prepared from the following chopped fruits: 1 qt crushed pineapple, 1 qt candied cherries, 1 qt maraschino cherries, 1 qt raisins, 12 oz candied orange peel, 2 lb each walnuts, almonds, and pecans, chopped or coarsely ground. Color light orange. Standard plain mix is often used instead of the richer mix in making puddings.

Tutti-frutti. To 9 gal plain mix add 4–8 qt of a mixture of several fruits of a suitable mixture for tutti-frutti. Color to a light pink. Usually a prepared mixture consists of the following fruits, chopped into small pieces: 2 qt red cherries, 2 qt green pineapple, 2 lb raisins, 2 qt crushed pineapple, 2 lb nuts. Add red coloring.

Frozen pudding.   Usually a prepared mixture is used. However, if nut-meats and rum, or rum flavor, are added to tutti-frutti ice cream, a frozen pudding flavor is the result.

English plum pudding.   To 8 gal parfait mix (16% fat) add 3 lb chocolate syrup, and the following fruits and nuts after the mix is partially frozen: 2 lb figs, 2 lb dates, 8 lb mixed candied fruits, 2 lb walnuts, 8 oz vanilla extract, 2 lb pecans, 6 tsp cinnamon, 1 tsp each ginger, allspice, and cloves. Fruits and nuts should be chopped and may be mixed with the spices before they are added to the partly frozen mix, or the spices may be added to the mix before freezing begins.

Plum pudding.   To 8 gal plain mix add 8 lb egg yolks, 6 lb sugar, 4 qt orange juice, 4 lb pecans, 4 lb walnuts, and 8 oz vanilla.

Date pudding.   To 9 gal plain mix add 6 lb dates, pitted and ground, 2 lb chopped walnuts.

CUSTARD

Custards may be of the same formula as ice cream, except 1.4% minimum egg yolk solids for plain flavors and 1.12% for bulky flavors are added.

Formula

Fat	10.0	12.0
MSNF	11.5	11.0
Sugar	15.0	15.0
Stabilizer–emulsifier	0.3	0.3
Dried egg yolks	1.5	1.5
TS	37.3	39.8

PARFAIT

To 9 gal high fat (16%) mix add 8 lb fresh whole eggs or 2-1/2 lb dried egg yolk. Mix egg yolk with 2 gal of the mix, which is then cooked to a custard (about 106° for 30 min), and cool to about 100°F. This custard is then added to the remaining part of the 9 gal of high-fat mix. The resulting 10 gal of parfait mix can be used like an ordinary ice cream mix to make any flavor desired.

MOUSSE

For a small quantity, whip 1 gal 40% cream to a stiff consistency. Gently stir in 2 lb sugar, 1–2 drops desired color, and 1/2–1 oz vanilla. Dates, nuts, and fruits, free from excessive juice and chopped into rather small pieces, can also be gently stirred in. The mixture is then placed in molds of the desired shape and is frozen in the hardening room without further agitation. This will yield about 2–2-1/2 gal finished mousse. For a larger quantity, use 6 lb 40% cream, 18 lb whole milk, 14 lb sugar, 6 oz stabilizer, and 6 oz vanilla. Chill mousse mix in the freezer to about 32°F and keep cool until whipped. Care should be taken to avoid cooling at too low temperature or whipping excessively in the freezer. Draw at low percentage overrun and harden.

VARIEGATED ICE CREAM

The base syrup used in making the fruit syrup and the base fruit syrup used in the variegated ice cream are as follows:

Base syrup	(lb)	Base fruit syrup	(%)
Sugar	55.0	Base syrup	66.7
Water	42.5	Citric acid	0.3
Pectin	2.5	Fruit puree	33.0
Total	100.0	Total	100.0

The base fruit syrup is injected into the ice cream at the rate of 20% of the volume of mix for most fruit flavors. The 20% level is approximately 9-1/2 lb fruit in 4 gal mix, and the 10% level is about 4-3/4 lb fruit in 4-1/4 gal mix. A chocolate base may be prepared by using 10% cocoa, 54% sugar, 35.25% water, and 0.75% pectin stabilizer. The stabilizer is mixed with a portion of the sugar and stirred into the water. The cocoa is mixed with the remaining sugar and added to the stabilizer–water mixture. The mixture is then heated to 190°F for about 20 min and cooled to 40°F.

As the plain vanilla ice cream is drawn from the freezer into the package, specially prepared syrups (such as chocolate and butterscotch) are added by means of a special nozzle so as to produce a marbled effect. Thus a stream of soft ice cream and a stream of the specially prepared syrup enter the package in the desired ratio and are slightly stirred to give a marbled effect. The syrups usually contain about 0.5% stablizer.

RAINBOW ICE CREAM

Carefully mix six or more differently colored ice creams while they are soft (as drawn from the freezer) to give a marbled or rainbow effect. Then set in the hardening room to harden.

GELATIN CUBE ICE CREAM

To 6-1/2 gal plain ice cream mix add 3/4 gal red gelatin cubes and 3/4 gal green gelatin cubes (gelatin cubes of other colors may also be used if desired).

ICE MILK

Formula

Fat	4.0
MSNF	12.0
Cane sugar	15.0
Stabilizer–emulsifier	0.4
TS	31.4

The ice milk mix may be made from 30% condensed skim milk, 40% cream, cane sugar, stabilizer–emulsifier product, and water. The mixes may be pasteurized at 160°F for 30 min or 175°F for 25 sec, or at a time and temperature equivalent to these. Homogenization should be at pasteurization temperatures at 2000 and 700 lb/in.^{2} on the first and second stages, respectively. The mix should be cooled to 40°F and aged and frozen at an overrun of 90%.

ICE

Formula

Cane sugar	16.0
Corn syrup solids	10.0
Stabilizer (pectin)	0.4
Fruit	20.0
Water, acid, and color	As required
Total	100.0

The ice mix may be pasteurized at 160°F for 30 min or at 175°F for 25 sec, or the equivalent of these times and temperatures, cooled to 40°F, and stored at this temperature until used. The addition of the fruits to the mix and the acid adjustment may be made just prior to freezing time. The ice should be drawn at approximately 25% overrun.

FRAPPÉS

Frappés are made in much the same manner as sherbets except that frappés are served in a soft condition. The juice of 3 doz lemons and 1 doz oranges, 2 qt grape juice, 2 lb sugar may be used for 5 gal base mix. The frappé is made in the same manner as an ice except that it is not hardened. Since frappés are served in a soft condition they are preferably frozen just prior to serving. Many other fruit mixtures, pleasing to the taste, may be easily developed. If a frappé is to be stored, it should be held at 20°F.

PUNCH

Punch is an ice in which fruit juices have been reinforced with an alcoholic beverage. Often rum flavoring (nonalcoholic) is used instead of liquor. The following formula is used extensively: To about 7 gal water add 20 lb sugar, 1 qt lemon juice, 1 qt grape juice, and rum flavoring as desired. If it is to be served in a frozen form, 5 oz stablizer should be added.

GRANITE

This is made from the same ingredients as an ice, but it is frozen much harder and with little whipping or stirring during the freezing process. The result is a coarser-textured product than an ice.

SHERBET

Formula

Cane sugar	16.0
Corn syrup solids	10.0
Stabilizer (pectin)	0.4
Ice cream mix (12% fat, 11% MSNF, 15% sugar[1])	17.4
Fruit	20.0
Water, acid, and color	As required
Total	100.0

The mix may be pasteurized at 160°F for 30 min or 175°F for 25 sec, cooled to 40°F, and stored at this temperature until used. The sherbet should be frozen at approximately 35% overrun.

Base mix	(lb)
Cane or beet sugar	21–25
Corn sugar	7–9
Stabilizer	0.4–0.6
Milk or other dairy product in amount to supply 2–5% milk solids	35–40
Enough water to make 80 lb base mix	

To 8 gal base mix, add 2 gal fruits, water, acid, and color.

For a small batch of sherbet dissolve 11 lb sugar and 4 oz stabilizer in 2.75 gal water. When cooled below 50°F, add 3.25 qt ice cream mix and 1 gal corn syrup. At the freezer, add 1 gal pureed fruit or fruit juices together with the desired amount of color and citric acid solution. When frozen, this mixture will yield about 9 gal finished sherbet.

---

[1]Sugar supplied by the ice cream mix is included as part of 16% cane sugar.

SOUFFLÉ

This product is made from sherbet mixes, except that whole eggs are added and the freezing is done with sufficiently high overrun to give a fluffy product. The following formula is often used for small batches: 42 eggs, 12 lb sugar, 1 gal strawberries (frozen pack), 3 gal skim milk or 3 gal water. By substituting only the fruit used as flavoring many other soufflées can be made. If larger batches are desired use 7-1/2 gal base sherbet mix, 8 lb whole eggs and 2 gal pureed fruit.

LACTO

This product is a milk sherbet made from cultured sour milk, buttermilk, or fermented milk. For grape lacto, use 3 gal cultured sour milk, 9 lb sugar, 12 eggs, 1.5 pt lemon juice, 1 qt grape juice. Dissolve the sugar in the milk, and add fruit juices and beaten egg yolk. Whip egg whites and add at the freezer. Other popular flavors can be made by substituting raspberry, cherry, or orange juice for the grape juice.

FRUIT SALAD

As generally made, this usually consists of fairly large pieces of mixed fruits in combination with whipped cream or ice cream. Pineapple (sliced or cubed), red cherries, apricots, peaches, pears, or prunes (properly pitted and sliced) are generally folded into the stiffly whipped cream, which has been flavored to taste with a good brand of mayonnaise. This mixture is set to stiffen somewhat before it is placed in molds to harden. A good formula is about 1 gal fruit mixture to 2/3 gal whipped cream (mayonnaise flavored). For variation, 2/3 gal soft vanilla ice cream may be substituted for the whipped cream. The mayonnaise may be prepared as follows; 1/2 lb dried egg yolk, 2 lb sugar, 6 tsp salt, 3 tsp mustard, 1/2 lb butter, 2/3 pt vinegar, 1/2 pt water. Mix ingredients and heat to about 185°F. If practical, prepare in large quantities and homogenize. Add enough cold mayonnaise to the whipped cream to give it the desired flavor. The above quantity should be used with about 2/3 gal ice cream. A small quantity of gelatin will improve the body. About 4 qt of fruit should be used with the above amount of mayonnaise.

FANCY MOLDED ICE CREAM

Aufait

This is a molded ice cream and fruit combination consisting of two or more layers of ice cream with pectinized fruit spread between the layers. For strawberry aufait fill strawberry mold half full with vanilla ice cream, harden, spread over this a layer of pectinized strawberries (not too thick since it is difficult to cut through the fruit layer when it hardens), and finish filling the mold with vanilla or strawberry ice cream. Many variations both as to number of layers and combinations of fruits are possible. Aufaits are also made in bulk by gently stirring the pectinized fruit into the ice cream as it comes from the freezer. The fruit should be heavy enough and cold enough so that it will make a more or less continuous line in the ice cream giving a marbled effect.

Spumoni

A special spumoni cup should be used. Press spumoni cup one-quarter full of vanilla ice cream around the edges and bottom to line the cup, add chocolate ice cream to half fill the cup. Finish filling with a mixture of fruit and whipped cream and then place in the hardening room. The fruit–whipped cream mixture is prepared by whipping 1 lb confectioners sugar with 1 gal heavy cream and gently stirring in the fruit, from which excessive juice has been drained.

QUIESCENTLY FROZEN DAIRY CONFECTIONS

These include products made from water, milk products, and sugar, with added flavoring, with or without added stabilizer–emulsifier or coloring, and freezing is accomplished without stirring or agitation. This confection is manufactured in the form of servings individually packaged for the consumer. The product should contain not less than 13% by weight of total milk solids and 33% by weight of total food solids, and not more than 0.5% by weight of stabilizer and 0.2% by weight of emulsifier. The freezing process should be such as not to develop physical expansion in excess of 10%. Quiescently frozen confections contain not less than 17% by weight of total food solids and not more than 0.5% by weight of stabilizer–emulsifier.

Formulas

Frozen dairy confection	(lb)	Frozen confection	(lb)
Water	36.00	Water	83.00
MSNF	4.00	Sugar	17.00
Sugar	10.00	Stabilizer	0.31
Ice cream mix, 10%	50.00		
Stabilizer	0.31		

SOFT-SERVE ICE CREAM AND ICE MILK

The distinguishing features of soft-serve products are (1) different procedures and equipment are used in their preparation; (2) the temperature at which they are served (18–20°F); (3) the overrun (30–50%); and (4) they are usually frozen on the premises of the retailer. The mix for soft-serve products is usually prepared by commercial plants and sold to the retailers for freezing in special soft-serve freezers. The soft-serve product may be of the same composition as ice cream or ice milk. Soft-serve products may also be of vegetable fat composition (formulas for such are shown under mellorine-type products).

Formula

	Ice cream	Ice milk
Fat	10.0	4.0
MSNF	13.0	13.0
Sucrose	13.0	12.0
Corn syrup solids	—	4.5
Stabilizer	0.5	0.4
Emulsifier	—	0.1
TS	36.5	34.0

FROSTED MALTED

To 3.5 gal ice milk mix add 1 qt syrup (or 1–2 lb malted milk powder) and chocolate syrup made of 1/2 lb cocoa (or 1 lb chocolate liquor), 3/4 lb sugar, and 1–1-1/2 qt water. Make syrup as directed for chocolate ice cream. Freeze and serve from freezer.

IMITATION ICE CREAM

This product is any frozen substance mixture or compound, regardless of the name under which it is represented, that is made in imitation or semblance of ice cream or is prepared or frozen as ice cream is prepared or frozen but is not ice cream.

Artificially Sweetened Frozen Dairy Foods

An artificial sweetener is a pure edible product made synthetically and with no calorie value. Artificially sweetened ice cream or ice milk means the pure, clean, frozen products for use by persons who must restrict their intake of ordinary sweets made from a combination of milk products, sorbitol, calcium and nonnutritive artificial sweeteners, with or without harmless coloring, and with or without added stabilizer or emulsifier composed of wholesome edible material. The composition, weight per gallon, of food solids, and weight per gallon of artificially sweetened products are the same as for the regular products.

Label declaration must include the words "artificially sweetened" immediately preceding the product and "intended for diabetics, under medical advice." The label must also contain a statement in terms of percentage by weight of protein, fat, and carbohydrates, the total number of calories per ounce, the number of calories contributed by carbohydrates other than lactose, and the name of each ingredient entering into the composition other than flavors.

Formula

Butterfat	10.2	6.0
MSNF	10.5	10.5
Diabetic base solids	14.0	14.0
TS	34.7	30.5

Regulations regarding composition and labeling of artificially sweetened ice cream or ice milk vary in different states. Label declaration may include the following: (1) Intended for use by diabetics. (2) List of ingredients: cream, milk, MSNF, sorbitol, stabilizer, name of flavoring, and name and amount of nonnutritive artificial sweetener, which should be used only by persons who must restrict their intake of ordinary sweets. (3) Contains no sugar.

Examples of the analysis that should appear on the label for the formulas given above are as follows:

Protein	4.0	4.20
Total carbohydrates	18.0	17.36
Milkfat	10.2	6.00
Total calories per avoirdupois ounce	52.5	42.40
Total calories from carbohydrates	19.8	19.73
Total calories from non-lactose carbohydrates	15.3	13.40

LOW SODIUM OR LOW PHENYLALANINE

Buchanan (1964) reports that commercial ice cream in Australia contains about 0.21% (60 mg/oz) of phenylalanine and 0.11% (31 mg/oz) of sodium chloride. He states these levels are too high to allow ice cream to be included in diets for phenylketonurics or for patients requiring very low salt intake. The following formula was therefore devised to provide an ice cream that was low in the two constituents, attractive in flavor and texture, and readily prepared for home or hospital use: 1/2 pt cream, 1/2 pt water, 3 oz sugar, 3/4 oz corn flour (1 oz wheat starch), and vanilla to taste. (For phenylketonurics 1 tsp salt may be added.) If a 42% cream is used the ice cream contains 0.033% (9 mg/oz) phenylalanine, and 0.013% (4 mg/oz) sodium chloride.

MELLORINE-TYPE PRODUCTS

Vegetable fat products are typical of imitation ice cream.[2] There is no federal standard but some states have composition regulations for imitation ice cream. The milkfat is replaced with hydrogenated vegetable oil.

---

[2]The vegetable fats used for imitation ice cream are special processed and refined hydrogenated coconut, soybean, corn oil, cottonseed oil, or blends of these. Vitamin A and D fortification is remommended.

Formulas

	Imitation ice cream	4.0% Imitation ice milk
Vegetable fat	10.0	4.0
MSNF	12.0	13.0
Sucrose	12.0	12.0
Corn syrup solids	5.0	5.0
Stabilizer	0.3	0.3
Emulsifier	0.1	0.2
Vitamins A and D	Optional	Optional
TS	39.4	34.5

SUPERPREMIUM ICE CREAM

Characteristics

The aspects of superpremium ice cream in the United States include the following: (a) it frequently has a prestigious, European-sounding name; (b) it has a high composition of good-quality ingredients; (c) it has low overrun (20%); (d) it is fast-hardened (2 hr); (e) it is packaged in small, attractive units; (f) it carries a high price.

Formula

Fat	18
MSNF	7
Sugar (all cane)	18
Egg yolk	2
TS	45

The proof sheet for a superpremium ice cream is given in Table 22.1.

SORBETS

Sorbets are usually manufactured on a small scale by specialized retail stores. A sorbet is similar in composition to an ice. It has a relatively high sugar (30%)

Table 22.1. Proof Sheet for Superpremium Ice Cream

Ingredients	Quantity	Fat	MSNF	Sugar	Egg yolk solids	TS
Cream (40%)	45.0	18.0	2.4	—	—	20.4
Skim milk	31.9	—	1.7	—	—	1.7
Nonfat dry milk	3.0	—	2.9	—	—	2.9
Sugar	17.0	—	—	17.0	—	17.0
Dry egg yolk	3.0	—	—	—	3.0	3.0
Total (16)	99.9	18.0	7.0	17.0	3.0	45.0
Check with desired weight	100.0	18.0	7.0	17.0	3.0	45.0

and fruit (30–50%) or flavor content, generally contains egg whites, and has a low overrun (20% or less). Sorbet products are often of exotic flavor.

Formula

	(lb)
Cane sugar	30.0
Stabilizer (pectin or gum)	0.4
Egg white solids	2.6
Fruit puree, juice, citric acid and water	67.0
TS	100.0

ALL-VEGETABLE FROZEN DESSERTS

The introduction and successful utilization of 100% corn-sweetened ice cream has led to the introduction of an all-vegetable frozen dessert.

Formulas

	10% Fat	4% Fat	2% Fat
Vegetable fat	10.0	4.00	2.0
Soy protein	3.0	4.00	2.0
Corn sweetener (36DE)	10.0	13.00	14.0
Fructose (5/S)	10.0	12.00	14.0
Stabilizer–emulsifier	0.3	0.45	0.5
TS	33.3	32.75	32.5

SPECIALS

Egg nog.   To 9 gal plain mix add 1 gal egg nog base (can be a commercial preparation). An egg nog base may be prepared by using 15 lb whole fresh eggs, 7-1/2 lb fresh egg yolks, 4 lb dry eggs, 8 lb sugar, and 45 lb 20% cream. This mixture is heated to 160°F for 20–30 min and homogenized at about 2000 lb/in.^{2} Egg nog ice cream may also be prepared by using 10 gal plain mix, 1-1/2 lb dry egg yolks, 3 oz vanilla extract, 2 oz lemon extract, 1 pt rum, 3 oz egg color, and spices if desired.

Rum raisin.   To 9 gal plain mix add 25 lb soft seedless raisins and 4–6 oz roman punch or rum flavor and yellow color. The raisins should be soft when added to the ice cream. If the preserved raisins are not in this condition, they should be soaked in water for a time and drained before adding to the ice cream.

Date walnut.   To 9 gal mix add 15 lb soft pitted dates, 3–4 lb English walnuts, and color as desired. The soft pitted dates and English walnut pieces may be blended with a small amount of sugar and added to the mix at the above rate. The rate may be decreased as desired.

Sweet potato.   To 7 gal plain mix add 28 lb sweet potato puree (7:1 sugar pack), 2 pt lemon chip, 2 oz vanilla extract, and 4 oz Prussian orange color.

Avocado.   Grind finely and add 1 lb sugar to 4 lb fruit. Mix well and add 16 lb of mixture to 90 lb of mix.

Honey.   Approximately half the sugar on a cane sugar basis can be replaced by honey to obtain a honey flavor:

Fat	10
MSNF	11
Sugar	8
Honey	9–7.4% honey solids
Stabilizer	0.3
TS	36.7

This formula would provide 8% cane sugar solids and 7.4% honey solids. If more honey is used, freezing and hardening difficulties may be experienced. There is the possibility of using honey in combination with a medium-DE corn syrup solids. Since a low- or medium-DE corn syrup solids does not depress the freezing point as much as other sweeteners, this combination would allow the use of a greater percentage of honey without freezing difficulties. Under these conditions, the following formula should give a good product:

Fat	10
MSNF	11
Corn syrup solid (low or medium DE)	8
Honey	12–9.8% honey solids
Stabilizer	0.25
TS	39.05

The milder flavored and lighter colored honeys are preferred for ice cream. Sweet clover, alfalfa, or clover honey are desirable.

Persimmon.   To 8 gal plain mix add 2 gal persimmon pulp (4:1 sugar pack), 1 pt grated orange rind, and 2 oz vanilla. The persimmon should be prepared by separating the peel and seed from the pulp. Pulp should be medium coarse. The fruit gives a golden yellow product that is smooth in texture and rich in flavor.

Watermelon.   To 10 gal plain mix add 10–12 oz watermelon flavor. Color pink.

Rhubarb.   To 8-1/2 gal plain mix, add 1-1/2 gal cooked, crushed rhubarb (3:1 sugar pack), 2 lb broken pecans, 2 pt orange chips (or 1 pt preserved orange peel, or orange rind), 2 oz vanilla, and 1/2 oz mace. Color pink.

Pumpkin.   To 8 gal plain mix add 2 gal cooked pumpkin puree, 2 pt orange chips (or 1 pt preserved orange peel or orange rind), 2 oz vanilla, 1/2 oz cinnamon, and 1/4 oz nutmeg.

HOME MADE ICE CREAM

Each of the following basic formulas will produce about 1 gal of ice cream when frozen in a salt and ice freezer and when an extract flavor is used. (The gelatin must be dissolved in 1/2 cup cold water).

Basic Formulas

(a)	Quantity	(b)	Quantity
Light cream	1-3/4 qt	Cream (30–40%)	1-1–3 qt
Evaporated milk	1/2 pt	Milk	1-1/2 pt
Gelatin	1 tsp	Sugar	2 cups
Salt	Pinch	Gelatin	1 tsp
Vanilla	1 tbl		

(c)	Quantity	(d)	Quantity
Cream (30–40%)	1-1/2 qt	Cream (30–40%)	1-1/2 qt
Milk	1-1/2 pt	Evaporated milk	15 oz
Sweetened condensed milk	15 oz	Sugar	2 cups
Sugar	1 cup	Gelatin	1 tsp
Gelatin	1 tsp		

(e) Cooked base	Quantity	(f) Diabetic formula	Quantity
Cream (30–40%)	1-1/2 qt	Cream (30–40%)	1 qt
Milk	1 pt	Milk	1 qt
Sugar	2 cups	Saccharin	4 grains
Eggs or yolks of 8 eggs)	6	Gelatin	1 tsp

Other flavors as desired may be developed by using these formulas and recipes as a guide. In using the above formulas, it should be kept in mind that package labeling statements must be in compliance with the laws.

FROZEN YOGURT

Frozen yogurt is a food that is prepared by freezing while stirring a pasteurized mix, containing one or more of the following ingredients: whole milk, partially defatted milk, skim milk, other milk products, and with or without fruits, nuts, flavoring materials, sweeteners, stabilizers, emulsifiers, and any other safe or suitable ingredient approved by the regulatory official, which is cultured after pasteurization by one or more strains of *Lactobacillus bulgaricus* and *Strepto-coccus thermophilus*, provided, however, fruits, nuts, and other flavoring materials are added before or after the mix is pasteurized and cultured. The provisions regarding pasteurization, cooling, and standard plate count apply only to the mix prior to culturing. The finished frozen yogurt must weigh not less than 5 lb/gal. The label on a package of frozen yogurt, in addition to other required information, must include a complete listing of all ingredients in descending order of predominance. The strains of bacteria may be collectively referred to as yogurt culture (see appendix for specifications).

This frozen dairy dessert has all the refreshing qualities of a sherbet combined with the unusual tanginess and depth of flavor character contrib-uted by the presence of the cultured yogurt. It will handle and freeze much the same as sherbet, and at a profit margin equal to or better than that of a comparable frozen sherbet.

Formula (10 gal)

	(lb)
Yogurt or whole milk	55.0
Sugar	17.0
Stabilizer	0.2
Fruit	17.8
Total	90.0

Place whole pasteurized, homogenized milk in vat and innoculate with 1% yogurt culture; hold at 90°F until set; or place milk, sugar, and stabilizer in vat, pasteurize and homogenize, and then innoculate and hold. Mix stabilizer with 5 times its weight of sugar and disperse carefully with good agitation. Add remainder of sweeteners and fruit and allow to mix well. Pump to freezer flavor tank. In continuous freezers use a temperature of 21°F. Freeze to 50% overrun or 13 oz/pt. Harden at −20°F in the usual manner.

Parevine

Parevine is a nondairy frozen dessert for those who want to avoid mixing meat and dairy products because of religious or other reasons.

It is a pure, clean, frozen product made from a combination of food fats; water; one or more protein or carbohydrate food ingredients from other than milk, milk products, meat or their derivatives; optional sweeting ingredients other than lactose as approved by the State Department of Health; with or without eggs or egg products; harmless flavoring; with or without harmless coloring; and with or without added vegetable stabilizer or vegetable emulsifier. It must contain not more than 0.5% by weight of stabilizer, not more than 0.2% by weight of emulsifier, and not less than 10% food fat except when fruit, nuts, cocoa, chocolate, maple syrup, cakes, or confections are used for the purpose of flavoring—then such reduction in food fat as is due to the addition of such flavors shall be permitted, but in no such case shall it contain less than 8% by weight of food fat. In no case may any Parevine weigh less than 4-1/2 lb/gal and contain less than 1.3 lb of total food solids per gallon. Parevine sold, held, or offered for sale by any manufacturer, wholesaler, retailer or any other seller only in properly labeled, factory-filled containers not larger than 1 gal. Parevine may be served for consumption on the premises, provided the individual service is taken from a properly labeled factory-filled container no larger than 1 gal. When Parevine is served on the premises a sign must be displayed that reads "Parevine served here" in letters that can be read by consumers' under normal conditions of use. It must include a list of all ingredients in a manner prescribed by the State Department of Health, provided, however, that the type of food fat used must be specified in letters that can be read by consumers and, provided further, that the type of food fat intgredient or ingredients shall be identified as to specific source. Optionally, all information required to be printed on the sign may be printed on a menu when a menu is provided each consumer. The label on packages of parevine shall, in addition to other required information, include the name "Parevine" in a conspicuous manner and shall include a complete list of all ingredients in a manner prescribed by the regulatory official, provided, however, that the type of food fat used must be specified.

The following mixes involve the ingredients permitted for use in parevine mix (Arbuckle 1969) for 100 lb of mix.

Formulas

Economy mix no. 1	(lb)
Vegetable fat (pure)	10.00
Sugar	15.00
Low-DE corn syrup solid or hydrolized cereal solids	3.00
Microcrystalline cellulose	1.50
Vegetable protein	2.00
Stabilizer	0.35
Salt	0.15
TS	32.00

Medium mix no. 2	(lb)
Vegetable fat (pure)	10.00
Sugar	16.00
Whole egg solids or dry whole eggs (or 18 fresh whole eggs)	4.50
Low-DE corn syrup solid or hydrolized cereal solids	2.00
Stabilizer	0.35
Salt	0.15
TS	33.50

Deluxe mix no. 3	(lb)
Vegetable fat (pure)	10.00
Sugar	16.00
Whole egg solids or dry whole eggs (or 26 fresh whole eggs)	9.00
Stabilizer	9.00
Salt	0.35
TS	0.15
	35.50

1. All equipment and utensils generally used in the manufacture and processing of dairy products require proper steaming prior to their use in the manufacture of parevine. Steaming is essential and may be required under religious supervision so as to insure the necessary license, which indicates that the product is kosher-parevine.

2. Dry blend the nonfat dry ingredients and add them to water in the pasteurizing vat.

3. Heat to 120°F and add the fat.

4. Pasteurize at 160°F for 30 min.

5. Homogenize at 2700 lb pressure; 1800 lb on the first stage and 900 lb on the second stage.

6. Cool to at least 40°F.

7. Hold for 4 hr.
8. Flavor and freeze to 90% overrun.

Reduced- or Low-Lactose Ice Cream

Lactose-reduced ice cream is now being marketed. The lactose enzymes are the result of recent technology, but the first commercial application was in hydrolyzing the lactose in whole milk. The commercial lactose enzymes have potential for use in other products, including ice cream. Benefits claimed for lactose reduction in ice cream include the following: (a) reduced lactose content for lactose-intolerant consumers, (b) smoother texture, (c) flavor quality enhancement, (d) potential for calorie reduction and position of sugar in the label (reduced amount of sucrose).

The methods of treatment for lactose hydrolysis may be (1) low-temperature–long-time—40–50°F for 12 hr or longer, or (2) high-temperature–short-time—100–115°F for 2–4 hr. The lactose-containing ingredients in the ice cream mix are milk, NFDM, whey, cream, and condensed skim milk.

The extent of hydrolysis of the lactose may be 35, 50 or 75%, with reduction in pounds sucrose per 100 lb mix of 1.05, 1.50, and 2.25, respectively. The theoretical reduction of added sucrose per 100 lb mix may be as shown in Table 22.2.

The low-temperature–long-time hydrolysis method is best suited for ice cream mix. The use rate of the enzyme is based on the assumption that dairy products contain 5% lactose and the amount of enzyme varies with temperature, time, percentage hydrolysis, and percentage lactose in the product to be treated. The amount of lactose may vary from 7 to 46 ml per 100 lb of mix, with approximately 11 ml for 35% hydrolysis to 46 ml for 75% hydrolysis (see Pfizer 1985, Bannar 1984).

PRODUCT IDENTITY AND LABEL STATEMENTS

Examples of product identity and label statements for artificially sweetened ice cream and ice milk and a number of other products are as follows.

Butterfat Mix Products

Butterfat mix products have been defined in the literature as a blend of milkfat with either sucrose alone or a blend of sucrose and MSNF. The interest in these butterfat mix products has been due to the price structure that has existed at certain times (Arbuckle 1967).

The following formulas for 100 lb of mix are examples of the use of these products:

Fresh cream and butter-powder mix	(lb)
Cream	15.0
Butter-powder mix	
(44% fat, 46% MSNF, 10% water)	13.7
Nonfat dry milk	5.0
Sugar	15.0
Stabilizer–emulsifier	0.3
Water	51.0
Total	100.0

Table 22.2. Reduction of Added Sucrose per 100 lb of Mix at Different Levels of Hydrolysis

Sugar	Relative sweetness	Unhydrolyzed		Hydrolized 35%		Hydrolized 50%		Hydrolized 75%	
		lb	Sweetness	lb	Sweetness	lb	Sweetness	lb	Sweetness
Sucrose	1.0	16.0	16.00	14.95	14.95	14.5	14.50	13.75	13.75
Lactose	0.2	5.0	1.00	3.25	0.65	0.5	1.25	1.25	0.25
Glucose and galactose	0.8	0.0	0.00	1.75	0.40	2.50	2.00	3.75	3.00
Total			17.00		17.00		17.00		17.00

Fresh cream and butter-powder–sucrose mix	(lb)
Cream	15.0
Butter-powder–sucrose mix	
(44% fat, 26% MSNF, 20% sugar, 10%	13.7
water)	7.3
Nonfat dry milk	12.3
Sugar	0.3
Stabilizer–emulsifier	51.4
Water	100.0
Total	

Usage rates at levels providing all the fat in the ice cream from butterfat mix products are feasible only when the very best quality products are available.

The use of cream to provide 50% of the fat in combination with the butterfat mix may be expected to produce more desirable results.

Mellorine

Mellorine conforms to the definition and standard of identity, and is subject to the requirements for optional ingredients, prescribed for ice cream, except that in place of optional dairy ingredients containing butterfat as permitted, edible fats or oils other than milkfat are used, and provided further that the weight of edible fats or oils other than milkfat, is not less than 10% of the weight of the finished Mellorine and the weight of the MSNF is not less than 10% of the weight of the finished Mellorine, except that when one or more of the bulky optional ingredients as specified are used, the weight of the edible fats or oils other than milkfat and the combined weight of edible fats or oils other than milkfat and MSNF (exclusive of any fat and MSNF in any malted milk used) are not less than 10 and 20%, respectively, of the remainder obtained by subtracting the weight of such optional ingredients as provided for, from the weight of the finished Mellorine, but in no case is the weight of edible fats or oils other than milkfat, or the combined weight of edible fats and oils other than milkfat and MSNF to be less than 8 and 16%, respectively, of the weight of the finished Mellorine, and that wherever provisions appear referring to milkfat, it shall be understood to be edible fats or oils other than milkfat in case of Mellorine.

When any artificial color is used in Mellorine, directly or as a component of any other ingredient, the label must bear the statement "artificially colored," "artifical coloring added," "with added artificial color," or "_____, an artificial color added," the blank to be filled in with the common or usual name of the artificial color, or in lieu thereof, in case the artifical color is a component of another ingredient, "_____, artificially colored."

If both artificial color and artificial flavoring are used, the label statements may be combined.

Mellorine can be sold, held, offered for sale by any manufacturer, wholesaler, retailer, or any other seller only in factory-filled containers not larger than 1/2 gal.

The label on a package of Mellorine must include the name "Mellorine" in a conspicuous manner and include a complete list of all ingredients in descending order or predominance, provided, however, that the specific vegetable fat used is specified. Mellorine may not be designated by the use of the word "cream" or its phonetic equivalent.

Lo-Mel

Lo-Mel means a pure, clean, wholesome, semiviscous drink prepared by stirring while freezing in a dispensing freezer a mixture of vegetable fat, MSNF, water, optional sweetening ingredients as approved with or without egg or egg products, with harmless flavoring, with or without harmless coloring, and with or without stabilizer or emulsifier as approved. It must contain 6% vegetable fat, not less than 10% MSNF, not more than 0.5% by weight of stabilizer, and not more than 0.2% of emulsifier. Lo-Mel may only be served or sold from a dispensing freezer and may not be sold hard frozen. When Lo-Mel is sold from a dispensing freezer a sign must be displayed that can be read by consumers under normal conditions of purchase and must read "Lo-Mel served here," in letters at least 3 in. in height, and also must include a list of all ingredients in descending order of predominance, provided, however, that the specific vegetable fat used must be specified in letters that can be read by consumers under normal conditions of purchase. No such list of ingredients need be included on the sign if the list of ingredients is printed on the side of the container in which the product is served to the customer.

Freezer-Made Milk Shakes

Freezer-made milk shake means a pure, clean, wholesome, semiviscous drink prepared by stirring while freezing in a dispensing freezer a pasteurized mix obtained from an approved source consisting of milkfat, MSNF, water, optional sweetening ingredients, with or without egg or egg products, with harmless flavoring, with or without harmless coloring, and with or without approved stabilizer or emulsifier. It must contain not less than 2% milkfat, not less than 10% MSNF, not more than 0.5% by weight of stabilizer, and not more than 0.2% of emulsifier. Freezer-made milk shakes may only be sold or served from a dispensing freezer and may not be sold hard frozen.

Quiescently Frozen Confection

Quiescently frozen confection means the frozen, sweetened, flavored product in the manufacture of whch freezing has not been accompanied by stirring or agitation (generally known as quiescent freezing). This confection may be acidulated with harmless organic acid, may contain milk solids, may be made with or without added harmless natural or artificial flavoring, with or without added harmless coloring. The finished product may contain not more than 0.5% by weight of stabilizing agents, and not less than 17% by weight of total food solids. This confection must be manufactured in the form of servings, individually packaged, bagged or otherwise wrapped, properly labeled, and purveyed to the consumer in its original factory-filled package. In the production of this quiescently frozen confection, no processing or mixing prior to quiescent freezing may be used that develops in the finished confection mix any physical expansion in excess of 10%.

Quiescently Frozen Dairy Confection

Quiescently frozen dairy confection means the frozen product made from water, milk products, and sweetening agents, with added harmless natural or artificial flavoring, with or without added harmless coloring, with or without stabilizing and emulsifying ingredients, and in the manufacture of which freezing has not been accompanied by stirring or agitation (generally known as quiescent freezing). It contains not less than 13% by weight of total milk solids, not less than 33% by weight of total food solids, not more than 0.5% by weight of stabilizing agents, not more than 0.2% by weight of monoglycerides or diglycerides or a combination of both, not more than 0.1% by weight of polyoxyethylene (20) sorbitan tristearate or polysorbate 80 [polyoxyethylene (20) sorbitan monooleate], or a combination of both. This confection must be manufactured in the form of servings, individually packaged, bagged, or otherwise wrapped, properly labeled, and purveyed to the consumer in its original factory-filled package. In the production of this quiescently frozen dairy confection no processing or mixing prior to quiescent freezing may be used that develops in the finished confection mix any physical expansion in excess of 10%.

Artificially Sweetened Ice Cream

Artificially sweetened ice cream or "frozen dietary dairy desert" means ice cream manufactured, prepared, or processed for consumption by persons who wish to restrict their intake of ordinary sweetening ingredients. It must conform to the definition and standard of identity prescribed for ice cream except that it must be sweetened with an artificial sweetening agent and contain edible carbohydrates other than sugar. The artificial sweetening agent and the edible carbohydrates must be approved ingredients and no sugars other than those naturally present in the milk solids or flavoring agent can be added to it.

The manufacturer must place the product in packages or containers that are conspicuously labeled either "artificially sweetened" immediately preceding the words "ice cream" in similar type at least half the size of the type used for the words "ice cream" and on the same contrasting background, or "frozen dietary dairy dessert."

The label shall also contain a statement in terms of percentage by weight of protein, fat, and carbohydrates, the total number of calories per ounce, the number of calories contributed by carbohydrates and any carbohydrates other than lactose, and the name of each ingredient entering into the composition other than flavors.

For the artificial sweetener saccharin, the following declaration must appear conspicuously on the product: "Use of this product may be hazardous to your health. This product contains saccharin which has been determined to cause cancer in laboratory animals."

The product may not be sold in any manner other than in sealed or unbroken packages or containers from one or more separate compartments of a refrigerated container or cabinet.

Artificially Sweetened Ice Milk

Artificially sweetened ice milk means ice milk manufactured, prepared, or processed for consumption by persons who wish to restrict their intake of ordinary sweetening ingredients and conforms to the definition and standard of identity prescribed for ice milk except that is sweetened with an artificial sweetening agent and contains edible carbohydrates other than sugar. The artificial sweetening agent and the edible carbohydrates must be approved ingredients and no sugars other than those naturally present in the milk solids or flavoring agent shall be added thereto.

The manufacturer must place the product in packages or containers conspicuously labeled "artificially sweetened" immediately preceding the words "ice milk" in similar type at least half the size of the type used for the words "ice milk" and on the same contrasting background.

The label also must contain a statement in terms of percentage by weight of protein, fat, and carbohydrates, the total number of calories per ounce, the number of calories contributed by carbohydrates and any carbohydrates other than lactose, and the name of each ingredient entering into the composition other than flavors. The same statement must also be made for ice milk as for ice cream, regarding the artificial sweetener saccharin.

The product must not be sold in any manner other than in sealed or unbroken packages or containers from one or more separate compartments of a refrigerated container or cabinet.

Manufactured Dessert Mixes

Manufactured dessert mix, whipped cream confection, and bisque tortoni indicate a frozen dessert made with milk products, sweetening agents, flavoring agents, stabilizing agents, emulsifying agents, with or without harmless coloring. It contains not less than 18% by weight of milkfat, not more than 0.5% by weight of stabilizing agents, not more than 0.2% by weight of monoglycerides or diglycerides of fat forming fatty acids or a combination of both, not more than 0.1% by weight of polyoxyethylene (20) sorbitan tristearate or polysorbate 80 [polyoxyethylene (20) sorbitan monooleate] or a combination of both, not more than 12% MSNF, and may be packaged with harmless gas causing it to fluff upon ejection from the package or container.

The standards of identity set forth in this chapter are for products not identified in the Federal Standards.

Bibliography

Alberts, R.A. 1905. Gelatin: Its manufacture and use in ice cream. Ice Cream Trade J. *1*, 15–16.

Alexander, J., and Rothwell, J. 1970. The effect of *E. Coli* and *B. Cereus* on methylene blue reduction times in ice cream. Proc. 18th Int. Dairy Congr. *1E*, 401. Australian Natl. Dairy Comm., Sydney.

American Dry Milk Institute. 1965. Standards for grades of dry milk including methods of analysis. Rev. Am. Milk Inst. Bull. *916*.

American Public Health Association 1967. Standard Methods for the Examination of Dairy Products, 12th edition. Am. Public Health Assoc., New York.

Anon. 1959. What whey is all about. Ice Cream Field *73*(4), 61–64, 66, 68, 70, 73.

Anon. 1964. Instant ice cream via freeze drying. Ice Cream Field *84*(5), 20–21, 24, 58.

Arbuckle, W.S. 1940. A microscopical and statistical analysis of texture and structure of ice cream as affected by composition, physical properties, and processing methods. Missouri AES Res. Bull. *320*.

Arbuckle, W.S. 1948a. Milk solids not fat in ice cream. Southern Dairy Prod. J. *43*(4), 32, 78–79.

Arbuckle, W.S. 1948b. Will egg improve ice cream? Ice Cream Field *52*(6), 24–25.

Arbuckle, W.S. 1950. Emulsifiers in ice cream. Ice Cream Trade J. *46*(10), 106, 114.

Arbuckle, W.S. 1952. Stabilized fruits for ice cream. Ice Cream Trade J. *48*(5), 34, 36, 86.

Arbuckle, W.S. 1955. High temperature processing and its effect on product properties— the Roswell heater. Proc. 51st Annu. Conv. Rept. IAICM Prod. Lab. Council.

Arbuckle, W.S. 1960. The microscopical examination of the texture and structure of ice cream. Ice Cream Trade J. *56*(10), 62–63, 66, 68, 168–172.

Arbuckle, W.S. 1964. The effects of low temperature freezing upon the texture of ice cream. Ice Cream World *71*(7), 26–28.

Arbuckle, W.S. 1967. Value of butterfat–sugar mix is shown by results of recent tests. Am. Dairy Rev. *29*(5), 61–64.

Arbuckle, W.S. 1968. Ice cream and other frozen dairy foods. *In* The Freezing Preservation of Foods, 4th edition, Vol. 4, D.K. Tressler *et al.* (Editors). AVI Publ. Co., Westport, CT.

Arbuckle, W.S. 1969a. Nonfat dry milk solids in ice cream. Dairy Ice Cream Field *152*(3), 48–50.

Arbuckle, W.S. 1969b. Parevine—a frozen non-dairy dessert. Am. Dairy Rev. *31*(8), 19, 22, 74.

Arbuckle, W.S. 1970. Advances in ingredients and technology in ice cream manufacture. Proc. 18th Int. Dairy Congr. *1E* 396. Australian Natl. Dairy Comm., Sydney.

Arbuckle, W.S. 1977. Ice Cream Services Handbook. AVI Publ. Co., Westport, CT.

Arbuckle, W.S., and Bell, R.W. 1963. Comparison of concentrated sweetened cream and conventional sources of milk fat on the properties of ice cream. Ice Cream Field *82*(5), 40.

Arbuckle, W.S., and Cremers, L.F.M. 1954. Chemistry and Testing of Dairy Products, 4th edition. AVI Publ. Co., Westport, CT.

Arbuckle, W.S., and Nisonger, J.W. 1951. The effect on mix of high temperature pasteurization. Ice Cream Field 58(6), 60–61, 68.

Arbuckle, W.S., Shepardson, C.H., and Walling, H.M. 1944. The utilization of skim milk in ice cream. Texas AES Bull. 656.

Arbuckle, W.S., Venter, W., Jr., Mattick, J.F., and Aceto, N.C. 1961. The technology of utilizing concentrated fruit juices and essences in ice cream and related products. Maryland AES Bull. A118.

Arbuckle, W.S., Blanton, L.F., Walter, H.E., and Sadler, A.M. 1967. Using heat-treated milk in frozen dairy foods. Ice Cream Field Trade J. 149(10), 38, 40.

Association of Official Agricultural Chemists. 1971. Methods of Analysis of the Association of Official Agricultural Chemists. Assoc. Official Agric. Chemists, Washington, DC.

Atherton, H.V., and Newlander, J.A. 1977. Chemistry and Testing of Dairy Products, 4th edition. AVI Publ. Co., Westport, CT.

Bannar, R. 1984. Lactose revisited. Dairy Record, August, 77–84.

Bassett, J.J. 1969. Use of proper emulsifiers and stabilizers. Am. Dairy Rev. 31(2), 44, 47, 79, 83.

Baumer, E.F., and Jacobson, R.E. 1969. Economic and marketing report on frozen desserts. IAICM, Washington, DC.

Bayer, A.H. 1963. Modern ice cream plant management. Reuben H. Donnelly Corp., New York, NY.

Bayer, A.H. 1965. Evaluating ice cream mix stabilizers. Ice Cream Trade J. 61(4), 34–35, 39.

Bell, R.W. 1959. Concentrated sweet cream—a simple and economical method of preserving milk fat. Proc. 15th Int. Dairy. Congr. 2, 979.

Bell, S.L. 1983. Use of Computers in Least-Cost Formulation of Ice Cream Mixes. Computer Concepts Corp., Knoxville, Tennessee.

Berger, K.G. 1973. Good Emulsion—Ice Cream, Chapter 4, 145, 146, 147, 152.

Berger, K.G., Bullimore, B.K., White, G.W., and Wright, R.C. 1972. A most comprehensive study of the structure of ice cream by use of the electron microscope. Dairy Ind. 37, 419–425.

Beuchat, L.R. 1978. Food and Beverage Mycology. AVI Publ. Co., Westport, CT.

Bierman, H.R. 1926a. How the composition of ice cream affects dipping. Ice Cream Trade J. 23(2), 45.

Bierman, H.R. 1926b. Effect of temperature on dipping. Ice Cream Rev. 10(8), 126.

Bierman, H.R. 1927. The effect of overrun, temperature and composition on dipping losses. Maryland AES Bull. 293.

Bird, E.W., Sadler, H.W., and Iverson, C.A. 1935. The preparation of a non-desiccated sodium caseinate sol and its use in ice cream. Iowa AES Bull. 187.

Blakely, L.E., and Stein, C.M. 1964. Foam spray-dried cottage cheese whey as a source of solids in sherbet. Missouri AES Quart. Bull. 47.

Bradley, R.L. Jr. 1984. Plotting freezing curves for frozen desserts. Dairy Record, July, 86–87.

Bruhn, J.C., Pecore, S., and Granke, A.A. 1980. Measuring proteins in frozen desserts by dye binding. Food Protection 43(10), 753–755.

Buchanan, R.A. 1964. An ice cream low in phenylalanine and in salt. J. Dietetic Assoc. Dairy Res. Pub. 209(2), 4, 14.

Bucheim, W. 1970. The submicroscopic structure of ice cream. Proc. 18th Int. Dairy Congr. 1E, 398. Australian Natl. Dairy Comm., Sydney.

Buzzell, F.M. 1909. Origin and development of the ice cream industry. Ice Cream Trade J. 5(3), 22.

Byars, L.L. 1969. Computerized linear programming for minimum cost ice cream blending. Proc. 65th Annu. Conv. IAICM, New Orleans.

Chou, T.C., and Tharp, B.W. 1963. A paper chromatographic method for determination of vanillin and ethyl vanilla flavoring. J. Dairy Sci. 46, 237–238.

Chou, T.C., and Tobias, J. 1960. Quantitative determination of carbohydrates in ice cream by paper chromatography. J. Dairy Sci. *43*, 1031–1041.

Clarke, F.J., and Goldsmith, T.L. 1965. Production of ice cream or the like. Dairy Sci. Abstr. *27*(8), 388.

Corbett, W.J., and Tracy, P.A. 1939. Dextrose in commercial ice cream. Univ. of Illinois AES Bull. *452.*

Corn Industry Research Foundation. 1958a. Corn Sweeteners in Ice Cream. Corn Ind. Res. Found., Washington, D.C.

Corn Industry Research Foundation. 1958b. Corn Syrups and Sugars. Corn Ind. Res. Found., Washington, D.C.

Cosgrove, C.J. 1967. Butterfat-sugar blends and their use in frozen desserts. Am. Dairy Rev. *29*(2), 44.

Coutler, S.T., and Thomas, E.L. 1943. Preparation of invert syrup. Ice Cream Rev. *26*(10), 67.

Cremers, L.F.M. 1954. The distribution and arrangement of fat globules in the internal structure of ice cream and the effect of fat–air orientation upon the smoothness of ice cream. M.S. Thesis, Univ. of Maryland, College Park.

Cremers, L.F.M., and Arbuckle, W.S. 1954. The identification of fat globules in the internal structure of ice cream. J. Dairy Sci. *37*(6), 642.

Crest Food Co. (no date). Dietetic and diabetic ice cream and ice milk. Crest Food Co., Tech. Bull. *B33*, Ashton, IL.

Dahlberg, A.C. 1926. A study of the manufacture of water ices and sherbets. New York State AES Bull. *536.*

Dahlberg, A.C., and Hening, J.C. 1928. Chocolate ice cream. Ice Cream Trade J. *24*(5), 42.

Dahlberg, A.C., and Penczek, E.S. 1941. The relative sweetness of sugars as affected by concentration. New York State AES Bull. *258.*

Dahle, C.D. 1927. The manufacure of chocolate ice cream. Ice Cream Rev. *11*, August, p. 90.

Dahle, C.D. 1930. The effect of aging the mix on the freezing time, overrun, and quality of ice cream. Pennsylvania AES Bull. *247.*

Dahle, C.D. 1941a. Frozen cream—a review. J. Dairy Sci. *24*(3), 245–264.

Dahle, C.D. 1941b. Variegated ice cream. Ice Cream World *37*(4), 14, 86.

Dahle, C.D. 1945a. How to make ice cream without fluid cream. Ice Cream Field *46*(6), 18.

Dahle, C.D. 1945b. Commercial ice cream manufacture. Pennsylvania State College AES Circ. *27.*

Dahle, C.D. 1946. Analysis of stabilizers. Ice Cream Field *48*(4), 62.

Dahle, C.D., Walts, C.C., and Keith, J.I. 1931. Dry skim milk in ice cream. Pennsylvania AES Bull. *271.*

Dairy Ice Cream Field. 1970. Dairy Industries Catalog, 43rd Annu. Edition.

Day, E.A., Arbuckle, W.S., and Seely, D.J. 1959. Quality sherbets. Ice Cream Field *73*(2), 28, 30, 78–79.

Deb, Jay. 1983. Rheological and high technology studies of the properties of ice cream (personal communications). Baskin-Robbins Ice Cream Co. Burbank, CA.

Decker, C.W. 1950. Chocolate ice cream. Ice Cream Rev. *34*(9), 46, 66, 68–69.

Der Hovanesian, J. 1960. Quick hardening of ice cream by liquid immersion. Ice Cream Rev. *43*(9), 98.

Desrosier, N.W. 1977. Elements of Food Technology. AVI Publ. Co., Westport, CT.

Desrosier, N.W., and Tressler, D.K. 1977. Fundamentals of Food Freezing. AVI Publ. Co., Westport, CT.

Dethmers, A.E. *et al.* 1981. Sensory evaluation guide for testing food and beverage products. Food Technol. *35* (11), 50–57.

Doan, F.J. 1958. Problems of lactose crystallization in concentrated milk products. J. Dairy Sci. *41*(2), 325–331.

Doan, F.J., and Keeney, P.G. 1965. Frozen dairy products. *In* Fundamentals of Dairy Chemistry, B.H. Webb and A.H. Johnson (Editors). AVI Publ. Co., Westport, CT.

Douglas, F.W., Jr., and Tobias, J. 1982. Casein and whey protein determination. Dairy Field *165*(6), 45, 46.

Drawbridge, R.F. 1951. The effect of developed and adjusted acidity on the various properties of ice cream mix and the finished ice cream. M.S. Thesis, Univ. of Maryland, College Park.

Drusendahl, L.G. 1963a. Corn syrup as a source of economical ice cream solids. Ice Cream Rev. 46(6), 25.

Drusendahl, L.G. 1963b. Trends in corn syrup usage. Ice Cream Field 81(1), 96.

Elliker, P.R. 1964. Effective use of modern bactericides. Klenzade's 25th Educational Seminar.

England, C.W. 1947. Some practical aids in maintaining quality in ice cream. Ice Cream Rev. 31(5), 52, 82–83.

England, C.W. 1953. Practical application of the vacreator in continuous pasteurization of ice cream mix. Proc. 13th Int. Dairy Congr., The Hague 3, 465.

England, C.W. 1968. The control of overrun in ice cream. Ice Cream—Short Course. Univ. of Maryland, College Park (mimeo).

England, C.W. 1968. Calculating the percent overrun in ice cream. Ice Cream Short Course, Univ. of Maryland, College Park (mimeo).

Erb, J.H. 1942. Stretching your supply of chocolate. Ice Cream Trade J. 38(10), 26.

Ess-Dee Craft Industries. 1968. Sanitary bakelite stencils for ice cream. Ess-Dee Craft Ind., Philadelphia, PA.

Fabricius, N.E. 1930. Improving chocolate ice cream. Ice Cream Rev. 14, August, p. 72.

Fabricius, N.E. 1931. Strawberries for ice cream manufacture. Iowa AES Circ. 132.

Farrall, A.W. 1963. Engineering for Dairy and Food Products. Wiley, NY.

FDA. 1961. Food and Drug Administration additives. Fed. Reg. 24, 9368–9370.

FDA. 1976. Frozen Desserts—Definitions and Standards of Identity. U.S. Food and Drug Administration, Washington, DC.

FDA. 1979. Fed. Reg. 44 (53), March.

FDA. 1981. Code of Federal Regulations, Title 21. U.S. Food and Drug Administration, Washington, D.C.

Foster, E.M., et al. 1957. Dairy Microbiology. Prentice Hall, Englewood Cliffs, NJ.

Frandsen, J.H. 1958. Dairy Handbook and Dictionary. Published by the author, Amherst, MA.

Frandsen, J.H., and Markham, E.A. 1915. The Manufacture of Ice Cream and Ices. Orange Judd Publ. Co., New York.

Frazeur, D.R. 1959. Some factors affecting churning of butterfat in soft-serve ice cream. Part I. Effect of certain salts. Ice Cream Field 73(3), 18.

Frieschknect, C. 1945. Use of dried eggs in ice cream. Ice Cream Rev. 28(10), 41.

Garard, I.D. 1976. Introductory Food Chemistry. AVI Publ. Co., Westport, CT.

Gavin, R.R. 1969. Studies of emulsifier action in ice cream utilizing the HLB concept. Dairy Sci. Abstr. 32(3), 156–157.

Glazier, L.R., and Mack, M.J. 1941. Corn syrup solids improve dairy products. Food Ind. 13(6), 68.

Glickman, M. 1969. Gum technology in the food industry. Adv. Food. Res., 417–423.

Graham, H.S. 1977. Food Colloids. AVI Publ. Co., Westport, CT.

Guadagni, D.G. 1956. Some quality factors in strawberries for ice cream. Quick Frozen Foods 18(7), 211–212.

Gunderson, F.L., Gunderson, H.W., and Ferguson, E.R., Jr. 1963. Food Standards and Definitions in the United States—A Guide Book, Academic Press, Orlando, FL.

Hall, C.W., and Hedrick, T.I. 1971. Drying of Milk and Milk Products, 2nd edition. AVI Publ. Co., Westport, CT.

Hall, C.W., and Trout, G.M. 1968. Milk Pasteurization. AVI Publ. Co., Westport, CT.

Hall, R.L. 1971. GRAS review and food additive legislation. Food technol. 25(5), 12–16.

Hall, R.L., and Oser, B.L. 1970. Recent progress in the consideration of flavoring ingredients under the food additives amendment. 4. ARAS substances survey of flavoring ingredient usage level. Food Technol. 24(5), 25–28, 30–32, 34.

Haller, H.S., and Bell, R.W. 1950. Improving the keeping quality of frozen homogenized milk. Milk Dealer 40(1), 98.

Hammer, B.W., and Babel, F.J. 1957. Dairy Bacteriology, 4th edition. Wiley, New York.

Harper, W.J., and Hall, C.W. 1976. Dairy Technology and Engineering. AVI Publ. Co., Westport, CT.

Harris, R.S., and Karmas, E. 1975. Nutritional Evaluation of Food Processing, 2nd edition. AVI Publ. Co., Westport, CT.

Heath, H. 1977. Flavors: Profiles, Products, Applications. AVI Publ. Co., Westport, CT.

Hedrick, T.I., Armitage, A.V., and Stein, C.M. 1964. A comparison of high-heat and low-heat nonfat dry milk as the sole source of serum solids in ice cream and ice milk. Michigan AES Quart. Bull. 47(2), 153–158.

Heldman, D.R., and Hedrick, T.I. 1968. Refrigeration requirements for ice cream freezing. J. Dairy Sci. 51(6), 931.

Henderson, J.L. 1971. The Fluid-Milk Industry, 3rd edition. AVI Publ. Co., Westport, CT.

Hening, J.C. 1930. A comparison of aging periods for ice cream mixes. New York State AES Bull. 161.

Hening, J.C. 1935. Using frozen cherries in cherry ice cream. Ice Cream Trade J. 30(11), 16.

Hening, J.C. 1949. Apple ice and apple ice cream. Fruit Prod. J. 28, 365, 381.

Hening, J.C., and Dahlberg, A.C. 1933. Frozen fruits for ice cream. New York State AES Bull. 634.

Hilker, L.D., and Caldwell, W.R. 1961. A method for calculating the weight per gallon of fluid dairy products. J. Dairy Sci. 44(1) 183–188.

Hill, R.L., and Stone, W.K. 1964. Procedure for determination of protein in ice milk and ice cream by formol titration. J. Dairy Sci. 47, 1014–1015.

IAICM. 1951. The History of Ice Cream. Int. Assoc. Ice Cream Mfrs., Washington, DC.

IAICM. 1953. Flavor preference and other products sold analysis. Spec. Bull. 87. Int. Assoc. Ice Cream Mfrs., Washington, DC.

IAICM. 1961a. Chocolate ice cream calculations under the Federal Standards. Ice Cream News Letter 854. Int. Assoc. Ice Cream Mfrs., Washington, DC.

IAICM. 1961b. Fruit and nut ice cream calculations under the Federal Standards. Ice Cream News Letter 855. Int. Assoc. Ice Cream Mfrs., Washington, DC.

IAICM. 1965a. Ice Cream Labeling Guidelines. Int. Assoc. Ice Cream Mfrs., Washington, DC.

IAICM. 1965b. Production index of ice cream and related products, 1964. Spec. Bull 110. Int. Assoc. Ice Cream Mfrs., Washington, DC.

IAICM. 1968. Let's Sell Ice Cream. Dairy Training and Merchandising Cust., Int. Assoc. Ice Cream Mfrs., Washington, DC.

IAICM. 1984. The Latest Scoop, 1984 edition. Int. Assoc. Ice Cream Mfrs., Washington, DC.

Igol, R.S. 1982. Hydrocolloid interaction useful in food systems. Food Technol. 36(4), 72–74.

Jacobson, R.E., and Bartlett, R.W. 1963. The ice cream and frozen dessert industry— Changes and challenges. Univ. of Illinois AES Bull. 694.

Jenness, R., and Patton, S. 1959. Principles of Dairy Chemistry. Wiley, New York.

Jensen, R.G., Sampugna, J., and Gardner, G.W. 1961. Glyceride and fatty acid composition of some mono- and diglycerides in ice cream emulsifiers. J. Dairy Sci. 44(6), 1057.

Jones, R.E. 1948. Industry Builder. Pacific Books, Palo Alto, CA.

Josephson, D.V., and Dahle, C.D. 1949. A new cellulose gum stablizer for ice cream. Ice Cream Rev. 28, 11–32.

Josephson, D.V., Dahle, C.D., and Patton, S. 1943. A comparison of some ice cream stabilizers. Southern Dairy Prod. J. 33(4), 34.

Keeney, P.G. 1958. Fat stability problems. Ice Cream Field 72(1), 20, 60–65.

Keeney, P.G. 1962. Effect of some citrate and phosphate salts on stability of fat emulsion in ice cream. J. Dairy Sci. 45(3), 430.

Keeney, P.G., and Dahle, C.D. 1960. Commercial ice cream and other frozen desserts. Penn. State Univ. Circ. 495.

King, N. 1950. The physical structure of ice cream. Dairy Ind. 15(10), 1052–1055.

King, N. 1955. The milk fat membrane. Commonwealth Agric. Bur. Dairy Sci. Tech. Commun. 2. Farmham Royal, Bucks, England.

Klose, R.E., and Glickman M. 1968. Gums. (1), 20, 60–65.

Keeney, P.G. 1962. Effect of some citrate and phosphate salts on stability of fat emulsion in ice cream. J. Dairy Sci. 45(3), 430.

Keeney, P.G., and Dahle, C.D. 1960. Commercial ice cream and other frozen desserts. Penn. State Univ. Circ. *495*.

King, N. 1950. The physical structure of ice cream. Dairy Ind. *15*(10), 1052–1055.

King, N. 1955. The milk fat membrane. Comm20. 1963. Speaking of chocolate soft-serve ice cream. Ice Cream Rev. *46*(9), 28, 38, 40–42.

Knightly, W.H. 1959. The role of liquid emulsifier in relation to recent research on ice cream emulsification. Ice Cream Trade J. *55*(6), 24.

Knightly, W.H. 1962. Fluid emulsifier for ice cream. Dairy Sci. Abstr. *24*(7), 338.

Koerver, C. 1958. The role of neutralizers in soft-serve ice milk mixes. Ice Cream Trade J. *54*(6), 20.

Kracauer, P. 1969. Ice cream mix. Dairy Sci. Abstr. *32*(4), 218.

Kramer, A., and Arbuckle, W.S. 1965. Getting greater economy in your filling operation. Ice Cream World *72*(12), 10, 14–15.

Kreider, E.L., and Snyder, J.C. 1964. Computer control for ice cream production. Purdue Univ. AES Res. Prog. Rep. *94*.

Langley, P. 1967. The argument for whey solids. Univ. Maryland Ice Cream Conf., College Park.

Laskin, M. 1969. Freeze-drying ice milk confections. Dairy Sci. Abstr. *32*(5), 279.

Lazar, J.T., Jr. 1970. Flavoring ice cream with freezer-dried fruits. Production Tips, Natl. Ice Cream Retailers Assoc. Bull, July.

Lee, F.A. 1975. Basic Food Chemistry. AVI Publ. Co., Westport, CT.

Leighton, A. 1927. On the calculation of the freezing point of ice cream mixes and of quantities of ice separated during the freezing process. J. Dairy Sci. *10*(4), 300–308.

Leighton, A. 1941. Some newer ice cream stabilizers and their functions. Ice Cream Trade J. *37*(12), 12, 48.

Leighton, A. 1942. A method for saving sugar in the manufacture of ice cream. Ice Cream Trade J. *38*(9), 12, 32–34.

Leighton, A. 1944a. Use of whey solids in ice cream and sherbets. Ice Cream Rev. *27*(6), 18.

Leighton, A. 1944b. A method for calculating commercial ice cream mixes. USDA, BDIM Inform. *12*.

Leighton, A. 1945. Commercial ice cream formulas. USDA BDIM Inform. *11*. [Reissued in 1956 by Agr. Res. Service as Circ. CA-E-7.]

Leighton, A., and Leviton, A. 1939. Whipping capacity of ice cream mixes. Ind. Eng. Chem. *31*(6), 779–783.

Leighton, A., Leviton, A., and Williams, O.E. 1934. The apparent viscosity of ice cream. J. Dairy Sci. *17*(9), 639–650.

Leo, A.J. 1967. Frozen dessert stabilizers. Am. Dairy Rev. *29*(8), 42, 91–96.

Lindamood, J.B., and Gould, I.A. 1964a. Chocolate flavor materials and their use in ice cream. Ice Cream Trade J. *60*(7), 24, 26–27.

Lindamood, J.B., and Gould, I.A. 1964b. Chocolate flavoring materials for ice cream. IV. Basic and flavor bean products. J. Dairy Sci. *47*(12), 1432–1435.

Lombard, S.H. 1965. Soft-frozen dairy products. Dairy Ind. J. *5*(2), 72–76.

Lucas, P.S. 1929. Vanilla won't freeze out. Ice Cream Trade J. *25*(8), 48.

Lucas, P.S. 1941. Monoglyceride—Gelatin as an ice cream stabilizer. J. Dairy Sci. *24*, 536.

Ludwig, K.G., and Gakenheimer, W.C. 1967. Modern emulsifiers—the basis of improving dryness in ice cream. Dairy Sci. Abstr. *30*(3), 141.

Mack, M.J. 1927. Defects of high solids mixes and their cure. Ice Cream Field *27*, 44–45.

Mack, M.J. 1930. Frozen cream as an ingredient for ice cream. Massachusetts AES Bull. *368*.

Mack, M.J. 1936. Sodium alginate as a stabilizer for ice cream. Ice Cream Rev. *20*(4), 60.

Mack, M.J., and Fellers, C.R. 1932. Frozen fruits and their utilization in frozen dairy products. Massachusetts AES Bull. *287*.

MacKinney, G., and Little, A. 1962. Color of Foods. AVI Publ. Co., Westport, CT.

Macy, I.G., Kelly, H.J., and Sloan, R.E. 1953. The composition of milks. Nat. Acad. Sci. Bull. *254*.

Maeno, M., Ogasa, K., and Okonogi, T. 1968. Equipment and method for making ice cream. Dairy Sci. Abstr. *30*(7), 370.

Mahdi, S.R., and Bradley, R.L., Jr. 1968. Fat destabilization in ice cream and ice milk containing low D.E. corn sweeteners. J. Dairy Sci. *51*, 931.

Martin, W.H. 1931. The selection and use of flavoring in making chocolate ice cream. Ice Cream Trade J. *27*(4), 39.

Masurovsky, B.I. 1945. Egg solids improve ice cream quality. Ice Cream Trade J. *41*(9), 56.

Masurovsky, B.I. 1946. Butter oil as a fat for ice cream. Ice Cream Trade J. *42*(6), 68.

Mattick, J.F. 1965. Steps in calculation of mix using serum-point method. Ice Cream—Short Course, Univ. of Maryland, College Park (mimeo).

Merory, J. 1968. Food Flavorings: Composition, Manufacture, and Use, 2nd edition. AVI Publ. Co., Westport, CT.

Milk Industry Foundation 1974. Laboratory Manual Methods of Analysis of Milk and Its Products, 4th edition. Milk Ind. Found., Washington, DC.

Milk Industry Foundation. 1981. Milk Facts, 1981 edition. Milk Ind. Found. Washington, D.C.

Minifie, B.W. 1970. Chocolate, Cocoa, and Confectionary. AVI Publ. Co., Westport, CT.

Mitten, H.L., Jr. 1958. Ultra-high temperature pasteurization of the ice cream mix. Ice Cream Trade J. *54*(7), 18, 20, 83–85.

Moresl, C. 1969. The aging of ice cream mixes. Dairy Sci. Abstr. *32*(5), 278.

Morrison, W.L. 1960. Method of preparing and handling ice cream, sherbet, ices, and the like. Dairy Sci. Abstr. *22*(9), 445.

Mortensen, M. 1911. Classification of ice cream and related frozen products. Iowa AES Bull. *123*.

Moss, J.R. 1955. Stabilizers and ice cream quality. Ice Cream Trade J. *51*(1), 22, 24.

Mueller, W.S., and Frandsen, J.H. 1933. Higher aging temperatures in the manufacture of ice cream. Massachusetts, AES Bull. *302*.

Mull, L.E., and Krienke, W.A. 1968. Tropical fruits in frozen desserts. Am. Dairy. Rev. *30*(3), 23.

National Dairy Council. 1946. Ice Cream through the Years. National Dairy Council, Chicago, IL.

National Dairy Council. 1952. Ice Cream for a Nation. National Dairy Council, Chicago, IL.

Nelson, J.A., and Trout, G.M. 1964. Judging Dairy Products, 4th edition. AVI Publ. Co., Westport, CT.

Nickerson, T.A. 1956. Lactose crystallization in ice cream. J. Dairy Sci. *39*(10), 1342–1350.

Nickerson, T.A. 1962. Lactose crystallization in ice cream. IV. Factors responsible for reduced incidence of sandiness. J. Dairy Sci. *45*(3), 354–359.

Nickerson, T.A., and Pangborn, R.M. 1961. Influence of sugar in ice cream. III. Effect on physical properties. Food Technol. *15*(3), 105.

Nickerson, T.A., and Tarassuk, N.P. 1955. How to control shrinkage in ice cream. J. Dairy Sci. *38*(11), 1305–1306.

Nielsen, A.J. 1963. Dry whey an optional ingredient. Ice Cream Field 81(4), 34.

Nieman, C. 1960. Sweeteners of glucose, dextrose, and sucrose. Manuf. Confect. *50*(8), 2–11.

Noonan, J. 1968. Color additives in food. *In* Handbook of Food Additives. Chem. Rubber Co., Cleveland.

Pangborn, R.M., Simone, M., and Nickerson, T.A. 1957. Influence of sugar in ice cream. I. Consumer preference for vanilla ice cream. Food Technol. *11*, 679–682.

Pearson, A.M. 1963. Liquid nitrogen immersion for ice cream hardening. Ice Cream World *69*(10), 20, 34.

Pfizer, Inc. 1985. Lactose treatment of dairy products. Pfizer, Inc., Milwaukee, Wisconsin (company brochure).

Pierce, H.B., Combs, W.B., and Borst, W.F. 1924. The use of true and imitation vanilla extracts in ice cream. J. Dairy Sci. *7*(6), 585.

Potter, F.E. 1966a. Effect of temperature on dipping. Ice Cream Rev. *10*(8), 126.

Potter, F.E. 1966b. Purchasing dairy products for food service establishments. Food Mgmt. Program Leaflet *15*. Univ. of Mass, Amherst.

Potter, F.E., and Williams, D.H. 1949a. Dried ice cream mixes. USDA BDIM Inform. 74, 3.

Potter, F.E., and Williams, D.H. 1949b. Use of whey in sherbets. Ice Cream Rev. 32(12), 102–104.

Potter, F.E., and Williams, D.H. 1949c. Use of whey in sherbets. Ice Cream Trade J. 45(9), 54–55, 86–88.

Potter, F.E., and Williams, D.H. 1950. Stabilizers and emulsifiers in ice cream. Milk Plant Monthly 39(4), 76.

Price, W.V. 1926. An algebraic method of proportioning ice cream mixes. J. Dairy Sci. 9(2), 243–250.

Price, W.V., and Whittier, R. 1931. Dry skim milk in ice cream. Cornell Univ. AES Bull. 516.

Prittle, T.R. 1926. History of Dairying. Mojonnier Bros., Chicago, IL.

Ramachandran, K.S., and Gould, I.A. 1961. Organic evaluation of chocolate. J. Dairy Sci. 44(6), 1172.

Ramachandran, K.S., Gould, I.A., and Lindamood, J.B. 1961. A review—Cocoa and chocolate, with particular reference to flavor in ice cream. Ice Cream Field 78(5), 18, 20, 22, 24. 57–60.

Redfern, R.B., and Arbuckle, W.S. 1949. Stabilizers and emulsifiers—their use in the production of ice cream. Southern Dairy Prod. J. 46(3), 32–34, 36–39.

Reid, W.H.E., and Arbuckle, W.S. 1938. The effects of serving temperature upon consumer acceptance of ice cream and sherbets. Missouri AES Res. Bull 272.

Reid, W.H.E., and Garrison, E.R. 1929. The effect of processing ice cream mixtures at different pressures when the milk solids-not fat content is varied. Missouri AES Bull. 128.

Reid, W.H.E., and Minert. K.R. 1942. Effect of dextrose and sucrose sugars upon the properties of ice cream. Missouri AES Bull. 339.

Reid, W.H.E., and Mosely, W.K. 1926. The effect of processing on the dispersion of fat in an ice cream mixture. Missouri AES Bull. 91.

Reid, W.H.E., and Painter, W.E. 1931. Freezing properties, stability, and physical qualities of chocolate ice cream. Ice Cream Rev. 15(12), 40.

Reid, W.H.E., and Russell, L.B. 1930. The effect of different homogenization processes on the physical properties of an ice cream mixture and the resulting ice cream when the percentage of fat is varied and the solids not fat remain constant. Missouri AES Bull. 134.

Reid, W.H.E., and Skinner, G.R. 1929. The effect of homogenization at different pressures on the physical properties of ice cream mixture and resulting ice cream. Missouri AES Bull. 127.

Reid, W.H.E., and Smith, L.E. 1942. The effect of cultures and the relation of acid standardization to several of the physical and chemical properties. Missouri AES Bull. 340.

Reid, W.H.E., Decker, C.W., and Arbuckle, W.S. 1940. The relation of acidity solids per gallon and different sources of serum solids on the physical and chemical properties of high serum solids ice cream. Missouri AES Bull. 322.

Rochow, T.G., and Mason, C.W. 1936. Breaking emulsions by freezing. Ind. Eng. Chem. 28, 1926.

Ross, O.E. 1963. Sherbets for tomorrow's market. Ice Cream Field 81(4), 48, 72, 74, 76, 78.

Rothwell, J., and Palmer, M.M. 1965. Modern trends in ice cream stabilizers. Dairy Ind. 30(2), 107–108, 118.

Sacharow, S. 1976. Handbook of Package Materials. AVI Publ. Co., Westport, CT.

Sacharow, S., and Griffin, R.C., Jr. 1970. Food Packaging. AVI Publ. Co., Westport, CT.

Sanders, F. 1932. How the soda fountain developed. Ice Cream Rev. 15(8), 50–51.

Sherfy, C.B., and Smallwood, N.W. 1928. Bibliography on ice cream up to and including the year 1926. US Dep. Agr. Bibliogr. Contrib. 17.

Sherman, P. 1961. Rheological methods for studying the physical properties of emulsifier films at the oil–water interface in ice cream. Food Technol. 15, 394–399.

Shipe, W.F., Roberts, W.M., and Blanton, L.F. 1963. Effect of ice cream stabilizers on the freezing characteristics of various aqueous systems. J. Dairy Sci. *46*(3), 169–175.

Simpfendorfer, S., and Martin, W.H. 1964. Effect of corn-syrup solids on quality and properties of ice milk. Food Technol. *18*. 12.

Snyder, W.E. 1949. Emulsifiers are useful. Milk Plant Monthly *38*(6), 30–33, 43–44.

Sommer, H.H. 1951. Theory and Practice of Ice Cream Making, 6th edition. Olson Publ. Co., Milwaukee, WI.

Speck, M.L., Grosche, C.A., Lucas, H.L., and Hankin, L. 1954. Bacteriological studies on high-temperature short-time pasteurizer. J. Dairy Sci. *37*(1), 37–44.

Sperry, G.D. 1955. Stabilizers and H.T.S.T. Ice Cream Field *65*(5), 10.

Spooner, D.R. 1980. Federal and state standards for the composition of milk products. US Dep. Agric., Agric. Handb. *51*, 12–15, 22–25.

Stebnitz, V.C., and Sommer, H.H. 1938. Stabilization of ice cream with sodium alginate. Ice Cream Rev. *21*(7), 36–37, 64.

Stein, C.M., Barnes, J., and Hedrick, T.I. 1963. Contact hardening of ice cream between vertical refrigerated plates. Food Technol. *17*(8), 105–107.

Steinetz, W.S. 1958. Stabilizer for frozen sweet aqueous base comestibles and product and method of utilizing same. Dairy Sci. Abstr. *20*(10), 826.

Steinetz, W.S. 1965. Guide to labeling of frozen desserts under new standards of identity. Am. Food Lab., Brooklyn, NY.

Stistrup, K., and Julin, B. 1970. The influence of some emulsifiers on the physical properties of ice cream. Proc. 18th Int. Dairy Congr. *1E*, 397. Australian Natl. Dairy Comm., Sydney.

Struble, E.B. 1951. How the ice cream industry uses frozen fruits. Quick Frozen Foods *13*(9), 72–73.

Struble, E.B. 1952. Improving the quality of fruits for ice cream use. Quick Frozen Foods *14*(8), 121–122, 316, 318.

Tallman, K.L. 1958. Stabilizers for continuous systems. Ice Cream Trade J. *54*(12), 16–18, 27.

Tamsma, A., and Bell, R.W. 1957. Concentrated sweetened cream—a new dairy product for ice cream. Rept. Proc. 53rd Annu. Conv. IAICM.

Taylor, J.C. 1961. Ice cream manufacturing plants in the midwest—methods, equipment, and layout. USDA, AMRS Rept. *477*.

Tharp, B.W. 1961. The use of low-conversion corn sweeteners in ice cream. Ice Cream World *65*(2), 25, 27.

Tharp, B.W. 1982. Use of freezing point calculations in evaluating dry mix compositions. J. Dairy Sci. *65, Suppl. 1*, 19.

Tharp, B.W., and Gould, I.A. 1962. A survey of vanilla-type flavoring materials for ice cream. Ice Cream Trade J. *58*(8), 46, 48, 50, 91–92.

Thorner, M.E., and Herzberg, R.J. 1970. Food Beverage Service Handbook. AVI Publ. Co., Westport, CT.

Tobias, J., Kaufman, O.W., and Tracy, P.H. 1955. Pasteurization equivalents of high-temperature short-time heating with ice cream mix. J. Dairy Sci. *38*(9), 959–968.

Tracy, P.H. 1945. Powdered whole milk and mix. Ice Cream Trade J. *41*(4), 22.

Tracy, P.H. 1966. Layouts and operating criteria for automation of dairy plants manufacturing ice cream and ice cream novelties. US Dep. Agric. Mark. Res. Rep. *750*.

Tracy, P.H., and Corbett, W.J. 1939. Preparation and use of low lactose skim milk. Food Res. *5*, 493–498.

Tracy, P.H., and Edman, G. 1940. Tests of enzyme converted corn syrup reveal desirable properties. Food Ind. *12*, 43.

Tracy, P.H., and Hahn A.J. 1938. A comparison of concentrated and superheated skim milk in the manufacture of ice cream. Dairy Mfg. Conf. Manual, Univ. of Illinois, Chicago.

Tracy, P.H., and McCown, C.Y. 1934. A study of factors related to the hardening of ice cream. J. Dairy Sci. *17*(1), 47–60.

Tracy, P.H., and McGarrahan, E.T. 1957. How to Plan and Operate a Soft-Frozen Dairy Products Store. Garrard Press, Champaign, IL.

Tracy, P.H., Ruehe, H.A., and Shanmann, F.P. 1930. Use of honey in ice cream. Univ. of Illinois AES Bull. *345*.

Traugott, H.N. 1965. A study of consumer use of frozen desserts. Ice Cream World Spec. Suppl.

Trempel. L.G. 1964. New developments in the processing of corn sweeteners for use in ice cream. Ice Cream Trade J. *60*(4), 42, 44, 49, 86, 88.,

Tressler, D.K. 1946. Frozen fruit purees in ice cream. Ice Cream Field *47*(1), 32, 60–61.

Tressler, D.K., Van Arsedl, W.B., and Copley, M.J. (Editors). 1968. The Freezing Preservation of Foods, 4th edition, Vol. 3. AVI Publ. Co., Westport, CT.

Tuckey, S.L., Tracy, P.H., and Ruehe, R.A. 1932. Studies in the manufacture of chocolate ice cream. Ice Cream J. *28*(8), 39.

Turnbow, G.D., and Nielson, K.W. 1928. Viscosity and ice cream. J. Ind. Eng. Chem. *20*, 376.

Turnbow, G.D., Tracy, P.H., and Raffetto, L.A. 1946. The Ice Cream Industry, 2nd edition, Wiley, NY.

Union Starch and Refining Co., Ice cream and frozen desserts, Union Starch and Refining Co., Tech., Serv. Dept., E. St. Louis, IL.

USDA. 1980. Agric. Handb. *51*.

USDA. 1966. US Dep. Agric. Mark. Res. Rep.

USDA. 1970. Nutritive value of foods. US Dep. Agric. Home Gard. Bull. *72*.

U.S. Government, 1973. Food nutrition labeling, Fed. Reg. *38*(9).

U.S. Public Health Service. 1965. Grade "A" pasteurized milk ordinance. U.S. Public Health Serv. Bull. *229*.

Valaer, E.P., and Arbuckle, W.S. 1961. The state of dispersion of butterfat in ice cream. Ice Cream Field *77*(1), 10, 30–32, 36–38.

Washburn, R.M. 1910. Principles and practices of ice cream making. Vermont AES Bull. *155*.

Watt, B.K., and Merrill, A.L. 1963. Composition of Foods—Raw, Processed, and Prepared. US Dep. Agric., Agric. USDA Handb. *8*.

Webb, B.H., Johnson, A.H., and Alford, J.A. 1974. Fundamentals of Dairy Chemistry, 2nd edition, AVI Publ. Co., Westport, CT.

Webb, B.H., and Whittier, E.O. 1971. By-products from Milk, 2nd edition. AVI Publ. Co., Westport CT.

Webb, B.H., and Williams, O.E. 1934. The manufacture of low-lactose skim milk for use in ice cream. J. Dairy Sci. *17*, 103–114.

Weidner, H.E. 1967a. Using buttermix products in ice cream. Part I. Ice Cream World *77*(3), 26.

Weidner, H.E. 1967b. Using buttermix products in ice cream. Part II. *77*(4), 14.

Weidner, H.E. 1967c. Using buttermix products in ice cream. Part III. *77*(5), 26.

Weinstein, B.R. 1963. Understanding the difference between diabetic and dietetic. Ice Cream Field *82*(1), 17, 52, 54.

Whitaker, R. 1930. The influence of using butter on the freezing properties of ice cream mix. J. Dairy Sci. *13*(1), 1–7.

Whitaker, R., and Hilker, L.D. 1938. The viscosity of ice cream mix made with plain and superheated skim milk. J. Dairy Sci. *21*, 569–573.

Williams, O.E., and Hall, S.A. 1931. Effect of heat treatment upon the quality of dry skim milk for ice cream. US Dep. Agric. Circ. *179*.

Willingham, J.J. 1963. Imitation frozen desserts. Ice Cream Field *82*(1), 12, 56, 58.

Wolff, I.A. 1982. Handbook of Processing and Utilization in Agriculture, Vol. 1, pp. 323–325. CRC Press, Boca Raton, FL.

Wolfmeyer, H.J. 1963. Wide screen analysis of corn sweeteners in frozen desserts. Ice Cream Field *81*(6), 17, 19, 46, 49–50, 52.

Woodruff, J.G. 1967. Tree Nuts—Production, Processing, and Products, Vols. 1 and 2. AVI Publ. Co., Westport, CT.

Woolrich, W.R. 1965. Handbook of Refrigerating Engineering, 4th edition, Vols. 1 and 2. AVI Publ. Co., Westport, CT.

Woolrich, W.R., and Hallowell, E.R. 1970. Cold and Freezer Storage Manual. AVI Publ. Co., Westport, CT

Wright, K.E. 1930. The effect of initial cooling temperature on gelatin in the aging of ice cream mix. J. Dairy Sci. *13*(9), 406–415.

Ziemer, K.A., Amundsen, C.H., Winder, W.C., and Swanson, A.M. 1962. Dried butter-
    milk and its properties in ice cream. J. Dairy Sci. *45*, 659.
Zuczkowa, J. 1970. An investigation into the effect of some technological factors on
    lactose crystalization in ice cream. Proc. 18th Intern, Dairy Congr. *1E*, 399. Au-
    stralian Natl. Dairy Comm., Sydney.

Appendix A
Historical Chronology of Ice Cream Industry

The development of the ice cream industry can be most quickly told by listing the approximate dates of some important methods of processing and merchandising.

1700   Ice cream probably came to America with the English colonists. A letter written in 1744 by a guest of Governor Bladen of Maryland described having been served ice cream.

1774   First public recorded mention of ice cream in America was made by Philip Lenzi, a caterer, announcing in a New York newspaper that he was prepared to supply various confections including ice cream.

1777–1800   Early advertisement of ice cream by Philip Lenzi, *New York Gazette Mercury*, May 19, 1777, and November 24, 1777; by J. Corree in 1779 and 1781 in the *Gazette*; by Joseph Crowe in the *New York Post Bay*, June 8, 1786; by A. Pryor on May 18, 1789. Mr. Hall was selling ice cream in New York in 1785 and Mr. Bosio, in Germantown, Pennsylvania, established a retail business in 1800.

1789   Mrs. Alexander Hamilton, wife of the Secretary of the Treasury, served ice cream at a dinner attended by George Washington.

1811   Ice cream was served in the White House by Mrs. Dolly Madison, wife of the fourth President.

1848   Patents were granted on a revolving household type of hand freezer with dasher.

1851   The father of the wholesale ice cream industry of America, Jacob Fussell, a Baltimore milk dealer, began to manufacture ice cream in Baltimore. He established plants in Washington, D.C., in 1856; and in New York in 1864.

1856   Patent granted Gail Borden in August 1856 for the process of condensing milk. The first condensed milk factory was established in Wolcottville, Connecticut.

1858   Ice cream plant opened in St. Louis by Perry Brazelton, who learned the business from Jacob Fussell.

1864   The Horton Ice Cream Company was started in New York.

1879   Ice cream soda was introduced at Centennial Exposition, Philadelphia.

1892 The Pennsylvania State College established the first course in ice cream making.

1895 Pasteurizing machines were introduced.

1892–1906 Investigation and development of the dry milk industry in America. One of the first dry milk plants was established by Merrell Soule Company at Arcade, New York, in May 1906. The first spray process plant was built in Ferndale, California, in 1911.

1899 The homogenizer was invented in France and was in use within two years. The US patent was dated April 11, 1904.

1900 The Association of Ice Cream Manufacturers was formed; later the name was changed to International Association of Ice Cream Manufacturers (IAICM).

1902 The horizontal circulating brine freezer was invented.

1904 The ice cream cone appeared at the World's Fair, St. Louis.

1904 The *Ice Cream Trade Journal* was made the official organ of IAICM.

1910 First State Agricultural Experiment Station Bulletins concerning ice cream were published, including R. W. Washburn, 1910: "Principles and Practices of Ice Cream Making," Vermont State Bull. *155*, M. Mortensen, 1911: "Classification of Ice Cream and Related Frozen Products—Score Cards for Judging Ice Cream," Iowa State Bull. *123*: B. W. Hammer, 1912: "Bacteria in Ice Cream," Iowa State Bull. *134*.

1911 The homogenizing process was applied to condensed or evaporated milk.

1913 The direct expansion freezer was introduced. The continuous freezing process was patented.

1915 Textbooks on ice cream were published in the United States: J. H. Frandsen and E. A. Markham, 1915: "The Manufacture of Ice Creams and Ices," W. W. Fisk and H. B. Ellenberger, 1917: "The Ice Cream Laboratory Guide," W. W. Fisk, 1919: "The Book of Ice Cream."

1920 Ice cream was generally recognized as a protective and essential food.

1921 The Eskimo Pie was patented by C. Nelson, Waukon, Iowa. This was the first of the coated ice cream and novelty sticks.

1922 Development of direct expansion refrigeration adapted to freezers.

1925 Dry ice (solid CO_2) was used to facilitate delivery of ice cream.

1926 The counter freezer for soft ice cream appeared.

1928 The Vogt continuous freezer was developed by Henry Vogt of Louisville, Kentucky.

1929–1935 Development and acceptance of continuous freezers. The Vogt instant freezer was first introduced by Cherry Burrell and installed commercially in 1929. The Creamery Package continuous freezer was introduced in 1935.

1940–1945 Development of low-temperature storage units for the home.

1946 Carry-home packages marketed through chain grocery stores gained popularity. Soft ice cream and drive-in stores appeared.

1950 Appearance of vegetable fat products in the ice cream industry.

1942–1953 FDA hearings on federal standards for ice cream.

1951 Ice cream centennial held in Baltimore, June 15.

1953 High-temperature–short-time pasteurization of ice cream mix (175°F, 25 sec) approved by U.S. Public Health Service, February 13.

1960 Definitions and Standards for Frozen Desserts approved by FDA of the U.S. Dept. of Health, Education, and Welfare.

1965–1970 Introduction and development of highly automated, high volume processing equipment.

1974–1981 Revision of definitions and standards of idenity for frozen desserts.

1983 Ice cream standards and regulations revised.

1983 Ice Cream for America Day.

1984 July, National Ice Cream Month.

Appendix B
Federal Standards for Frozen Desserts

Federal standards for frozen desserts were first issued in 1960 by the U.S. Department of Health, Education and Welfare, Food and Drug Administration under the Federal Food, Drug, and Cosmetic Act, Part 20, Title 21, Code of Federal Regulations. The purpose of the act was to promulgate reasonable definitions and standards for food to promote honesty and fair dealing in the interest of consumers. In 1974, the identity standards were rewritten to reflect changes in the industry, and the new standards were issued as part 135. As published in the 1982 Code of Federal Regulations, 1982, the new standards are as follows:

PART 135—FROZEN DESSERTS

Subpart A—General Provisions

Sec.
135.3 Definitions.

Subpart B—Requirements for Specific Standardized Frozen Desserts

135.110 Ice cream and frozen custard.
135.120 Ice milk.
135.130 Mellorine.
135.140 Sherbet.
135.160 Water ices.

AUTHORITY: Secs. 401, 701(e), 52 Stat. 1046 as amended, 70 Stat. 919, 1055-1056 as amended (21 U.S.C. 341, 371).

Subpart A—General Provisions

§ 135.3 Definitions.

For the purposes of this part, a pasteurized mix is one in which every particle of the mix has been heated in properly operated equipment to one of the temperatures specified in the table in this section and held continuously at or above that temperature for the specified time (or other time/temperature relationship which has been demonstrated to be equivalent thereto in microbial destruction):

Temperature	Time
155° F	30 min.
175° F	25 sec.

[42 FR 19132, Apr. 12, 1977]

Subpart B—Requirements for Specific Standardized Frozen Desserts

§ 135.110 Ice cream and frozen custard.

(a) *Description.* (1) Ice cream is a food produced by freezing, while stirring, a pasteurized mix consisting of one or more of the optional dairy ingredients specified in paragraph (b) of this section, and may contain one or more of the optional caseinates specified in paragraph (c) of this section subject to the conditions hereinafter set forth, and other safe and suitable

420

nonmilk-derived ingredients; and excluding other food fats, except such as are natural components of flavoring ingredients used or are added in incidental amounts to accomplish specific functions. Ice cream is sweetened with nutritive carbohydrate sweeteners and may or may not be characterized by the addition of flavoring ingredients.

(2) Ice cream contains not less than 1.6 pounds of total solids to the gallon, and weighs not less than 4.5 pounds to the gallon. Ice cream contains not less than 10 percent milkfat, nor less than 10 percent nonfat milk solids, except that when it contains milkfat at 1 percent increments above the 10 percent minimum, it may contain the following milkfat-to-nonfat milk solids levels:

Percent milkfat	Minimum percent nonfat milk solids
10	10
11	9
12	8
13	7
14	6

Except that when one or more bulky flavors are used, the weights of milkfat and total milk solids are not less than 10 percent and 20 percent, respectively, of the remainder obtained by subtracting the weight of the bulky flavors from the weight of the finished food; but in no case is the weight of milkfat or total milk solids less than 8 percent and 16 percent, respectively, of the weight of the finished food. Except in the case of frozen custard, ice cream contains less than 1.4 percent egg yolk solids by weight of the food, exclusive of the weight of any bulky flavoring ingredients used. Frozen custard shall contain 1.4 percent egg yolk solids by weight of the finished food: *Provided, however,* That when bulky flavors are added the egg yolk solids content of frozen custard may be reduced in proportion to the amount by weight of the bulky flavors added, but in no case is the content of

egg yolk solids in the finished food less than 1.12 percent. A product containing egg yolk solids in excess of 1.4 percent, the maximum set forth in this paragraph for ice cream, may be marketed if labeled as specified by paragraph (e)(1) of this section.

(3) When calculating the minimum amount of milkfat and nonfat milk solids required in the finished food, the solids of chocolate or cocoa used shall be considered a bulky flavoring ingredient. In order to make allowance for additional sweetening ingredients needed when certain bulky ingredients are used, the weight of chocolate or cocoa solids used may be multiplied by 2.5; the weight of fruit or nuts used may be multiplied by 1.4; and the weight of partially or wholly dried fruits or fruit juices may be multiplied by appropriate factors to obtain the original weights before drying and this weight may be multiplied by 1.4.

(b) *Optional dairy ingredients.* The optional dairy ingredients referred to in paragraph (a) of this section are: Cream, dried cream, plastic cream (sometimes known as concentrated milkfat), butter, butter oil, milk, concentrated milk, evaporated milk, sweetened condensed milk, superheated condensed milk, dried milk, skim milk, concentrated skim milk, evaporated skim milk, condensed skim milk, superheated condensed skim milk, sweetened condensed skim milk, sweetened condensed part-skim milk, nonfat dry milk, sweet cream buttermilk, condensed sweet cream buttermilk, dried sweet cream buttermilk, skim milk that has been concentrated and from which part of the lactose has been removed by crystallization, skim milk in concentrated or dried form that has been modified by treating the concentrated skim milk with calcium hydroxide and disodium phosphate, and whey and those modified whey products (e.g., reduced lactose whey, reduced minerals whey, and whey protein concentrate) that have been determined by FDA to be generally recognized as safe (GRAS) for use in this type of food. Water may be added, or water may be evaporated from the mix. The sweet cream buttermilk and the concentrated sweet cream buttermilk or dried sweet cream buttermilk, when adjusted with water to a total solids content of 8.5 percent, has a titratable acidity of not more than 0.17 percent, calculated as lactic acid. The term "milk" as used in this section means cow's milk. Any whey and modified whey products used contribute, singly or in combination, not more than 25 percent by weight of the total nonfat milk solids content of the finished food. The modified skim milk, when adjusted with water to a total solids content of 9 percent, is substantially free of lactic acid as determined by titration with $0.1N$ NaOH, and it has a pH value in the range of 8.0 to 8.3.

(c) *Optional caseinates.* The optional caseinates referred to in paragraph (a) of this section that may be added to ice cream mix containing not less than 20 percent total milk solids are:

Casein prepared by precipitation with gums, ammonium caseinate, calcium caseinate, potassium caseinate, and sodium caseinate. Caseinate may be added in liquid or dry form, but must be free of excess alkali.

(d) *Methods of analysis.* The fat content shall be determined by the method prescribed in "Official Methods of Analysis of the Association of Official Analytical Chemists," 12th Ed. (1975), section 16.228, under "Fat: Roese-Gottlieb Method—Official Final Action," which is incorporated by reference. Copies are available from the Division of Food Technology, Bureau of Foods (HFF-210), Food and Drug Administration, 200 C St. SW., Washington, DC 20204, or available for inspection at the Office of the Federal Register, 1100 L St. NW., Washington, DC 20408.

(1) Fat content shall be determined by the method: "Fat; Roese-Gottlieb Method—Official Final Action," section 16.255.

(e) *Nomenclature.* (1) The name of the food is "ice cream"; except that when the egg yolk solids content of the food is in excess of that specified for ice cream by paragraph (a) of this section, the name of the food is "frozen custard" or "french ice cream" or "french custard ice cream".

(2) (i) If the food contains no artificial flavor, the name on the principal display panel or panels of the label shall be accompanied by the common or usual name of the characterizing flavor, e.g., "vanilla", in letters not less than one-half the height of the letters used in the words "ice cream".

(ii) If the food contains both a natural characterizing flavor and an artificial flavor simulating it, and if the natural flavor predominates, the name on the principal display panel or panels of the label shall be accompanied by the common name of the characterizing flavor, in letters not less than one-half the height of the letters used in the words "ice cream", followed by the word "flavored", in letters not less than one-half the height of the letters in the name of the characterizing flavor, e.g., "Vanilla flavored", or "Peach flavored", or "Vanilla flavored and Strawberry flavored".

(iii) If the food contains both a natural characterizing flavor and an artificial flavor simulating it, and if the artificial flavor predominates, or if artificial flavor is used alone the name on the principal display panel or panels of the label shall be accompanied by the common name of the characterizing flavor in letters not less than one-half the height of the letters used in the words "ice cream", preceded by "artificial" or "artificially flavored", in letters not less than one-half the height of the letters in the name of the characterizing flavor, e.g., "artificial Vanilla", or "artifically flavored Strawberry" or "artificially flavored Vanilla and artificially flavored Strawberry".

(3)(i) If the food is subject to the requirements of paragraph (e)(2)(ii) of this section or if it contains any artificial flavor not simulating the characterizing flavor, the label shall also bear the words "artificial flavor added" or "artificial ———— flavor added", the blank being filled with the common name of the flavor simulated by the artificial flavor in letters of the same size and prominence as the words that precede and follow it.

(ii) Wherever the name of the characterizing flavor appears on the label so conspicuously as to be easily seen under customary conditions of purchase, the words prescribed by this paragraph shall immediately and conspicuously precede or follow such name, in a size reasonably related to the prominence of the name of the characterizing flavor and in any event the size of the type is not less than 6-point on packages containing less than 1 pint, not less than 8-point on packages containing at least 1 pint but less than one-half gallon, not less than 10-point on packages containing at least one-half gallon but less than 1 gallon, and not less than 12-point on packages containing 1 gallon or over: *Provided, however,* That where the characterizing flavor and a trademark or brand are presented together, other written, printed, or graphic matter that is a part of or is associated with the trademark or brand, may intervene if the required words are in such relationship with the trademark or brand as to be clearly related to the characterizing flavor: *And provided further,* That if the finished product contains more than one flavor of ice cream subject to the requirements of this paragraph, the statements required by this paragraph need appear only once in each statement of characterizing flavors present in such ice cream, e.g., "Vanilla flavored, Chocolate, and Strawberry flavored, artificial flavors added".

(4) If the food contains both a natural characterizing flavor and an artificial flavor simulating the characterizing flavor, any reference to the natural characterizing flavor shall, except as otherwise authorized by this paragraph, be accompanied by a reference to the artificial flavor, displayed with substantially equal prominence, e.g., "strawberry and artificial strawberry flavor".

(5) An artificial flavor simulating the characterizing flavor shall be deemed to predominate:

(i) In the case of vanilla beans or vanilla extract used in combination with vanillin if the amount of vanillin used is greater than 1 ounce per unit of vanilla constituent, as that term is defined in § 169.3(c) of this chapter.

(ii) In the case of fruit or fruit juice used in combination with artificial fruit flavor, if the quantity of the fruit or fruit juice used is such that, in relation to the weight of the finished ice cream, the weight of the fruit or fruit juice, as the case may be (including water necessary to reconstitute partially or wholly dried fruits or fruit juices to their original moisture content) is less than 2 percent in the case of citrus ice cream, 6 percent in the case of berry or cherry ice cream, and 10 percent in the case of ice cream prepared with other fruits.

(iii) In the case of nut meats used in combination with artificial nut flavor, if the quantity of nut meats used is such that, in relation to the finished ice cream the weight of the nut meats is less than 2 percent.

(iv) In the case of two or more fruits or fruit juices, or nut meats, or both, used in combination with artificial flavors simulating the natural flavors and dispersed throughout the food, if the quantity of any fruit or fruit juice or nut meat is less than one-half the applicable percentage specified in paragraph (e)(5) (ii) or (iii) of this section. For example, if a combination ice cream contains less than 5 percent of bananas and less than 1 percent of almonds it would be "artificially flavored banana-almond ice cream". However, if it contains more than 5 percent of bananas and more than 1 percent of almonds it would be "banana-almond flavored ice cream".

(6) If two or more flavors of ice cream are distinctively combined in one package, e.g., "Neapolitan" ice cream, the applicable provisions of this paragraph shall govern each flavor of ice cream comprising the combination.

(f) *Label declaration.* Each of the optional ingredients used shall be declared on the label as required by the applicable sections of Part 101 of this chapter, except that sources of milkfat or milk solids not fat may be declared in descending order of predominance either by the use of all the terms "milkfat and nonfat milk" when one or any combination of two or more of the ingredients listed in § 101.4(b) (3), (4), (8), and (9) of this chapter are used or alternatively as permitted in § 101.4 of this chapter. Under section 403(k) of the Federal Food, Drug, and Cosmetic Act, artificial color need not be declared in ice cream, except as required by § 101.22(c) of this chapter. Voluntary declaration of all colors used in ice cream and frozen custard is recommended.

[43 FR 4598, Feb. 3, 1978, as amended at 45 FR 63838, Sept. 26, 1980; 46 FR 44433, Sept. 4, 1981; 47 FR 11826, Mar. 19, 1982]

EFFECTIVE DATE NOTE:

1. Paragraph (b) of § 135.110 was revised at 46 FR 44432, Sept. 4, 1981, effective date for compliance July 1, 1981. The confirmation of the effective date for compliance appears at 47 FR 1287, Jan. 12, 1982. Paragraph (b) published at 43 FR 4598, Feb. 3, 1978, and set forth below is currently effective.

§ 135.110   Ice cream and frozen custard.

*   *   *   *   *

(b) *Optional dairy ingredients.* The optional dairy ingredients referred to in paragraph (a) of this section are: Cream, dried cream, plastic cream (sometimes known as concentrated milk fat), butter, butter oil, milk, concentrated milk, evaporated milk, sweetened condensed milk, superheated condensed milk, dried milk, skim milk, concentrated skim milk, evaporated skim milk, condensed skim milk, superheated condensed skim milk, sweetened condensed skim milk, sweetened condensed part-skim milk, nonfat dry milk, sweet cream buttermilk, condensed sweet cream buttermilk, dried sweet cream buttermilk, skim milk that has been concentrated and from which part of the lactose has been removed by crystallization, skim milk in concentrated or dried form which has been modifed by treating the concentrated skim milk with calcium hydrox-

ide and disodium phosphate, concentrated cheese whey, and dried cheese whey. Water may be added, or water may be evaporated from the mix. The sweet cream buttermilk and the concentrated sweet cream buttermilk or dried sweet cream buttermilk, when adjusted with water to a total solids content of 8.5 percent, has a titratable acidity of not more than 0.17 percent, calculated as lactic acid. The term "milk" as used in this section means cow's milk. Any concentrated cheese whey and dried cheese whey used contribute not more than 25 percent by weight of the total nonfat milk solids content of the finished food. Dried cheese whey is uniformly light in color, free from brown and black scorched particles, and has an alkalinity of ash, not more than 225 milliliters 0.1N HCl per 100 grams, a bacterial count of not more than 50,000 per gram, and, as adjusted with water to a total solids content of 6.5 percent, a titratable acidity of not more than 0.16 percent, calculated as lactic acid. Concentrated cheese whey has an alkalinity of ash, not more than 115 milliliters 0.1N HCl per 100 grams, a bacterial count of not more than 50,000 per gram, and, as adjusted with water to a total solids content of 6.5 percent, a titratable acidity of not more than 0.18 percent, calculated as lactic acid. The modified skim milk, when adjusted with water to a total solids content of 9 percent is substantially free of lactic acid as determined by titration with

0.1N NaOH, and it has a pH value in the range of 8.0 to 8.3.

2. Paragraph (f) of § 135.110 was revised at 45 FR 63838, Sept. 26, 1980, effective date for compliance July 1, 1981. The compliance date was extended to July 1, 1982, at 46 FR 31004, June 12, 1981. Paragraph (f) published at 43 FR 4598, Feb. 3, 1978, and set forth below is currently effective.

§ 135.110   Ice cream and frozen custard.

*   *   *   *   *

(f) *Label declaration.* Each of the optional ingredients used shall be declared on the label as required by the applicable sections of Part 101 of this chapter, except that sources of milkfat or milk solids not fat may be declared in descending order of predominance either by the use of all the terms "milkfat and nonfat milk" when one or any combination of two or more of the ingredients listed in § 101.4(b) (3), (4), (8), and (9) of this chapter are used or alternatively as permitted in § 101.4 of this chapter. Pursuant to section 402(k) of the Federal Food, Drug, and Cosmetic Act artificial color need not be declared in ice cream. Voluntary declaration of such color in ice cream is recommended.

*   *   *   *   *

§ 135.120   Ice milk.

(a) *Description.* Ice milk is the food prepared from the same ingredients and in the same manner prescribed in § 135.110 for ice cream and complies with all the provisions of § 135.110 (including the requirements for label statement of optional ingredients), except that:

(1) Its content of milkfat is more than 2 percent but not more than 7 percent.

(2) Its content of total milk solids is not less than 11 percent.

(3) Caseinates may be added when the content of total milk solids is not less than 11 percent.

(4) The provision for reduction in milkfat and nonfat milk solids content from the addition of bulky flavors in § 135.110(a) applies, except that in no case will the milkfat content be less than 2 percent, nor the nonfat milk solids content be less than 4 percent. When the milkfat content increases in increments of 1 percent above the 2 percent minimum, it may contain the following milkfat-to-nonfat milk solids levels:

Percent milkfat	Minimum percent nonfat milk solids
2	9
3	8
4	7
5	6
6	5
7	4

(5) The quantity of food solids per gallon is not less than 1.3 pounds.

(6) When any artificial coloring is used in ice milk, directly or as a component of any other ingredient, the label shall bear the statement "artificially colored", "artificial coloring added", "with added artificial color", or "————, an artificial color added", the blank being filled in with the common or usual name of the artificial color; or in lieu thereof, in case the artificial color is a component of another ingredient, "—————— artificially colored".

(7) If both artificial color and artificial flavoring are used, the label statements may be combined.

(b) *Nomenclature.* The name of the food is "ice milk".

[43 FR 4599, Feb. 3, 1978]

§ 135.130   Mellorine.

(a) *Description.* (1) Mellorine is a food produced by freezing, while stirring, a pasteurized mix consisting of safe and suitable ingredients including, but not limited to, milk-derived nonfat solids and animal or vegetable fat, or both, only part of which may be milkfat. Mellorine is sweetened with nutritive carbohydrate sweetener and is characterized by the addition of flavoring ingredients.

(2) Mellorine contains not less than 1.6 pounds of total solids to the gallon, and weighs not less than 4.5 pounds to the gallon. Mellorine contains not less than 6 percent fat and 2.7 percent protein having a protein efficiency ratio (PER) not less than that of whole milk protein (108 percent of casein) by weight of the food, exclusive of the weight of any bulky flavoring ingredients used. In no case shall the fat content of the finished food be less than 4.8 percent or the protein content be less than 2.2 percent. The protein to meet the minimum protein requirements shall be provided by milk solids, not fat and/or other milk-derived ingredients.

(3) When calculating the minimum amount of milkfat and protein required in the finished food, the solids

of chocolate or cocoa used shall be considered a bulky flavoring ingredient. In order to make allowance for additional sweetening ingredients needed when certain bulky ingredients are used, the weight of chocolate or cocoa solids used may be multiplied by 2.5; the weight of fruit or nuts used may be multiplied by 1.4; and the weight of partially or wholly dried fruits or fruit juices may be multiplied by appropriate factors to obtain the original weights before drying and this weight may be multiplied by 1.4.

(b) *Fortification.* Vitamin A is present in a quantity which will ensure that 40 international units (IU) are available for each gram of fat in mellorine, within limits of good manufacturing practice.

(c) *Methods of analysis.* Fat and protein content, and the PER shall be determined by following the methods contained in "Official Methods of Analysis of the Association of Official Analytical Chemists," 12th Ed. (1975), which is incorporated by reference. Copies are available from the Division of Food Technology, Bureau of Foods (HFF-210), Food and Drug Administration, 200 C St. SW., Washington, DC 20204, or available for inspection at the Office of the Federal Register, 1100 L St. NW., Washington, DC 20408.

(1) Fat content shall be determined by the method: "Fat, Roese-Gottlieb Method—Official Final Action," section 16.255.

(2) Protein content shall be determined by one of the following methods: "Nitrogen—Official Final Action," Kjeldahl Method, section 16.253, or Dye Binding Method, section 16.254.

(3) PER shall be determined by the method: "Biological Evaluation of Protein Quality—Official Final Action" sections 43.183–43.187.

(d) *Nomenclature.* The name of the food is "mellorine". The name of the food on the label shall be accompanied by a declaration indicating the presence of characterizing flavoring in the same manner as is specified in § 135.110(c).

(e) *Label declaration.* The common or usual name of each of the ingredients used shall be declared on the label as required by the applicable sections of Part 101 of this chapter, except that sources of milkfat or milk solids not fat may be declared, in descending order of predominance, either by the use of the terms "milkfat, and nonfat milk" when one or any combination of two or more ingredients listed in § 101.4(b) (3), (4), (8), and (9) of this chapter are used, or alternatively as permitted in § 101.4 of this chapter.

[42 FR 19137, Apr. 12, 1977, as amended at 47 FR 11826, Mar. 19, 1982]

§ 135.140 Sherbet.

(a) *Description.* (1) Sherbet is a food produced by freezing, while stirring, a pasteurized mix consisting of one or more of the optional dairy ingredients specified in paragraph (b) of this section, and may contain one or more of the optional caseinates specified in paragraph (c) of this section subject to the conditions hereinafter set forth, and other safe and suitable nonmilk-derived ingredients; and excluding other food fats, except such as are added in small amounts to accomplish specific functions or are natural components of flavoring ingredients used. Sherbet is sweetened with nutritive carbohydrate sweeteners and is characterized by the addition of one or more of the characterizing fruit ingredients specified in paragraph (d) of this section or one or more of the non-fruit-characterizing ingredients specified in paragraph (e) of this section.

(2) Sherbet weighs not less than 6 pounds to the gallon. The milkfat content is not less than 1 percent nor more than 2 percent, the nonfat milk-derived solids content not less than 1 percent, and the total milk or milk-derived solids content is not less than 2 percent nor more than 5 percent by weight of the finished food. Sherbet that is characterized by a fruit ingredient shall have a titratable acidity, calculated as lactic acid, of not less than 0.35 percent.

(b) *Optional dairy ingredients.* The

optional dairy ingredients referred to in paragraph (a) of this section are: Cream, dried cream, plastic cream (sometimes known as concentrated milkfat), butter, butter oil, milk, concentrated milk, evaporated milk, superheated condensed milk, sweetened condensed milk, dried milk, skim milk, concentrated skim milk, evaporated skim milk, condensed skim milk, sweetened condensed skim milk, sweetened condensed part-skim milk, nonfat dry milk, sweet cream buttermilk, condensed sweet cream buttermilk, dried sweet cream buttermilk, skim milk that has been concentrated and from which part of the lactose has been removed by crystallization, and whey and those modified whey products (e.g., reduced lactose whey, reduced minerals whey, and whey protein concentrate) that have been determined by FDA to be generally recognized as safe (GRAS) for use in this type of food. Water may be added, or water may be evaporated from the mix. The sweet cream buttermilk and the concentrated sweet cream buttermilk or dried sweet cream buttermilk, when adjusted with water to a total solids content of 8.5 percent, has a titratable acidity of not more than 0.17 percent calculated as lactic acid. The term "milk" as used in this section means cow's milk.

(c) *Optional caseinates.* The optional caseinates referred to in paragraph (a) of this section which may be added to sherbet mix are: Casein prepared by precipitation with gums, ammonium caseinate, calcium caseinate, potassium caseinate, and sodium caseinate. Caseinates may be added in liquid or dry form, but must be free of excess alkali, such caseinates are not considered to be milk solids.

(d) *Optional fruit-characterizing ingredients.* The optional fruit-characterizing ingredients referred to in paragraph (a) of this section are any mature fruit or the juice of any mature fruit. The fruit or fruit juice used may be fresh, frozen, canned, concentrated, or partially or wholly dried. The fruit may be thickened with pectin or other optional ingredi-

ents. The fruit is prepared by the removal of pits, seeds, skins, and cores, where such removal is usual in preparing that kind of fruit for consumption as fresh fruit. The fruit may be screened, crushed, or otherwise comminuted. It may be acidulated. In the case of concentrated fruit or fruit juices, from which part of the water is removed, substances contributing flavor volatilized during water removal may be condensed and reincorporated in the concentrated fruit or fruit juice. In the case of citrus fruits, the whole fruit, including the peel but excluding the seeds, may be used, and in the case of citrus juice or concentrated citrus juices, cold-pressed citrus oil may be added thereto in an amount not exceeding that which would have been obtained if the whole fruit had been used. The quantity of fruit ingredients used is such that, in relation to the weight of the finished sherbet, the weight of fruit or fruit juice, as the case may be (including water necessary to reconstitute partially or wholly dried fruits or fruit juices to their original moisture content), is not less than 2 percent in the case of citrus sherbets, 6 percent in the case of berry sherbets, and 10 percent in the case of sherbets prepared with other fruits. For the purpose of this section, tomatoes and rhubarb are considered as kinds of fruit.

(e) *Optional nonfruit characterizing ingredients.* The optimal nonfruit characterizing ingredients referred to in paragraph (a) of this section include but are not limited to the following:

(1) Ground spice or infusion of coffee or tea.

(2) Chocolate or cocoa, including sirup.

(3) Confectionery.

(4) Distilled alcoholic beverage, including liqueurs or wine, in an amount not to exceed that required for flavoring the sherbet.

(5) Any natural or artificial food flavoring (except any having a characteristic fruit or fruit-like flavor).

(f) *Nomenclature.* (1) The name of each sherbet is as follows:

(i) The name of each fruit sherbet is "——— sherbet", the blank being filled in with the common name of the fruit or fruits from which the fruit ingredients used are obtained. When the names of two or more fruits are included, such names shall be arranged in order of predominance, if any, by weight of the respective fruit ingredients used.

(ii) The name of each nonfruit sherbet is "——— sherbet", the blank being filled in with the common or usual name or names of the characterizing flavor or flavors; for example, "peppermint", except that if the characterizing flavor used is vanilla, the name of the food is "——— sherbet", the blank being filled in as specified by § 135.110(e)(2) and (5)(i).

(2) When the optional ingredients, artificial flavoring, or artificial coloring are used in sherbet, they shall be named on the label as follows:

(i) If the flavoring ingredient or ingredients consists exclusively of artificial flavoring, the label designation shall be "artificially flavored".

(ii) If the flavoring ingredients are a combination of natural and artificial flavors, the label designation shall be "artificial and natural flavoring added".

(iii) The label shall designate artificial coloring by the statement "artificially colored", "artificial coloring added", "with added artificial coloring", or "———, an artificial color added", the blank being filled in with the name of the artificial coloring used.

(g) *Characterizing flavor(s).* Wherever there appears on the label any representation as to the characterizing flavor or flavors of the food and such flavor or flavors consist in whole or in part of artificial flavoring, the statement required by paragraph (f)(2) (i) and (ii) of this section, as apprpriate, shall immediately and conspicuously precede or follow such representation, without intervening written, printed, or graphic matter (except that the word "sherbet" may intervene) in a size reasonably related to the prominence of the name of the characterizing flavor and in any event the size of the type is not less than 6-point on packages containing less than 1 pint, not less than 8-point on packages containing at least 1 pint but less than one-half gallon, not less than 10-point on packages containing at least one-half gallon but less than 1 gallon, and not less than 12-point on packages containing 1 gallon or over.

(h) *Display of statements required by paragraph (f)(2).* Except as specified in paragraph (g) of this section, the statements required by paragraph (f)(2) of this section shall be set forth on the principal display panel or panels of the label with such prominence and conspicuousness as to render them likely to be read and understood by the ordinary individual under customary conditions of purchase and use.

(i) *Label declaration.* Each of the optional ingredients used shall be declared on the label as required by the applicable sections of Part 101 of this chapter.

[43 FR 4599, Feb. 3, 1978, as amended at 46 FR 44434, Sept. 4, 1981]

EFFECTIVE DATE NOTE: Paragraph (b) of § 135.140(b) was revised at 46 FR 44434, Sept. 4, 1981, effective date for compliance July 1, 1983. The confirmation of the effective date for compliance appears at 47 FR 1287, Jan. 12, 1982. Paragraph (b) published at 43 FR 4599, Feb. 3, 1978, and set forth below is currently effective.

§ 135.140 Sherbet.

*   *   *   *   *

(b) *Optional dairy ingredients.* The optional dairy ingredients referred to in paragraph (a) of this section are: Cream, dried cream, plastic cream (sometimes known as concentrated milk fat), butter, butter oil, milk, concentrated milk, evaporated milk, superheated condensed milk, sweetened condensed milk, dried milk, skim milk, concentrated skim milk, evaporated skim milk, condensed skim milk, sweetened condensed skim milk, sweetened condensed part-skim milk, nonfat dry milk, sweet cream buttermilk, condensed sweet cream buttermilk, dried sweet cream buttermilk, skim milk that has been concentrated and from which part of the lactose has been removed by crystallization, concentrated cheese whey, and dried cheese whey. Water may be added, or water may be evaporated from the mix. The sweet cream buttermilk and the concentrated sweet cream buttermilk or dried sweet cream buttermilk, when adjusted with water to a total solids content of 8.5 percent, has a titratable acidity of not more than 0.17 percent, calculated as lactic acid. The term "milk" as used in this section means cow's milk. Dried cheese whey is uniformly light in color, free from brown and black scorched particles, and has an alkalinity of ash, not more than 225 milliliters 0.1N HCl per 100 grams, a bacterial count of not more than 50,000 per gram, and, as adjusted with water to a total solids content of 6.5 percent, a titratable acidity of not more than 0.16 percent calculated as lactic acid. Concentrated cheese whey has an alkalinity of ash, not more than 115 milliliters 0.1N HCl per 100 grams, a bacterial count of not more than 50,000 per gram, and, as adjusted with water to a total solids content of 6.5 percent, a titratable acidity of not more than 0.18 percent, calculated as lactic acid.

* * * * *

§ 135.160 Water ices.

(a) *Description.* Water ices are the foods each of which is prepared from the same ingredients and in the same manner prescribed in § 135.140 for sherbets, except that the mix need not be pasteurized, and complies with all the provisions of § 135.140 (including the requirements for label statement of optional ingredients) except that no milk or milk-derived ingredient and no egg ingredient, other than egg white, is used.

(b) *Nomenclature.* The name of the food is "——— ice", the blank being filled in, in the same manner as specified in § 135.140(f)(1) (i) and (ii), as appropriate.

[42 FR 19132, Apr. 12, 1977]

§135.115 Goat's milk ice cream.

(a) *Description.* Goat's milk ice cream is the food prepared in the same manner prescribed in § 135.110 for ice cream, and complies with all the provisions of § 135.110, except that the only optional dairy ingredients that may be used are those in paragraph (b) of this section; caseinates may not be used; and paragraphs (e)(1) and (f) of § 135.110 shall not apply.

(b) *Optional dairy ingredients.* The optional dairy ingredients referred to in paragraph (a) of this section are goat's skim milk, goat's milk, and goat's cream. These optional dairy ingredients may be used in liquid, concentrated, and/or dry form.

(c) *Nomenclature.* The name of the food is "goat's milk ice cream" or, alternatively, "ice cream made with goat's milk", except that when the egg yolk solids content of the food is in excess of that specified for ice cream in paragraph (a) of § 135.110, the name of the food is "goat's milk frozen custard" or, alternatively, "frozen custard made with goat's milk", or "goat's milk french ice cream", or, alternatively, "french ice cream made with goat's milk", or "goat's milk french custard ice cream", or, alternatively, "french custard ice cream made with goat's milk".

(d) *Label declaration.* Each of the optional ingredients used shall be declared on the label as required by the applicable sections of Part 101 of this chapter.

§ 135.125 Goat's milk ice milk.

(a) *Description.* Goat's milk ice milk is the food prepared in the same manner prescribed in § 135.115 for goat's milk ice cream, except that paragraph (c) shall not apply, and which complies with all the requirements of §135.120(a) (1), (2), (4), (5), (6), and (7) for ice milk.

(b) *Nomenclature.* The name of the food is "goat's milk ice milk" or, alternatively, "ice milk made with goat's milk".

Any person who will be adversely affected by the foregoing regulation may at any time on or before October 21, 1982 submit to the Dockets Management Branch (address above), written objections thereto and may make a written request for a public hearing on the stated objections. Each objection shall be separately numbered and each numbered objection shall specify with particularity the provision of the regulation to which objection is made. Each numbered objection on which a hearing is requested shall specifically so state; failure to request a hearing for any particular objection shall constitute a waiver of the right to a hearing on that objection. Each numbered objection for which a hearing is requested shall include a detailed description and analysis of the specific factual information intended to be presented in support of the objection in the event that a hearing is held; failure to include such a description and analysis for any particular objection shall constitute a waiver of the right to a hearing on the objection. Three copies of all documents shall be submitted and shall be identified with the docket number found in brackets in the hearing of this regulation. Received objections may be seen in the office above between 9 a.m. and 4 p.m., Monday through Friday.

Effective date: Except as to any provisions that may be stayed by the filing of proper objections, compliance with the final regulation, including any required labeling changes, may begin November 22, 1982, and all affected products initially introduced or initially delivered for introduction into interstate commerce on or after July 1, 1985, shall fully comply. Notice of the filing of objections or lack thereof will be published in the Federal Register.

(Secs. 401, 701(e), 52 Stat. 1046, 70 Stat. 919 amended (21 U.S.C. 341, 371(e)))

Dated: September 13, 1982.

William F. Randolph,
Acting   Associate   Commissioner   for Regulatory Affairs.

Appendix C
Nutrition Labeling Requirements

The labeling of frozen dessert products generally conforms to the regulations set forth in the Code of Federal Regulations, Section 101.9. The relevant portions are reproduced below:

§101.9 Nutrition labeling of food

(a) Nutrition information relating to food may be included on the label and in the labeling of a product: *Provided*, That it conforms to the requirements of this section. *Except as provided in paragraph (h) of this section*, inclusion of any added vitamin, mineral, or protein in a product or of any nutrition claim or information, other than sodium content, on a label or in advertising for a food subjects the label to the requirements of this section, and in labeling for a food subjects the label and that labeling to the requirements of this section.

(b) All nutrient quantities (including vitamins, minerals, calories, protein, carbohydrate, and fat) shall be declared in relation to the average or usual serving or, where the food is customarily not consumed directly, in relation to the average or usual portion. Another column of figures may be used to declare the nutrient quantities in relation to the average or usual amount consumed on a daily basis, in the same format required in paragraph (c) of this section for the serving (portion), where reliable data have established that the food is customarily consumed more than once during the day and the average or usual amount so consumed.

(c) The declaration of nutrition information on the label and in labeling shall contain the following information in the following order, using the headings specified, under the overall heading of "Nutrition Information Per Serving (Portion)." The terms "Per Serving (Portion)" are optional and may follow or be placed directly below the terms "Nutrition Information."

(h) The following foods are exempt from this section or are subject to special labeling requirements:

(8) Food products shipped in bulk form for use solely in the manufacture of other foods and not for distribution to consumers in such bulk form or container.

(9) Food products containing an added vitamin, mineral, or protein, or for which a nutritional claim is made on the label or in labeling or in advertising, which are supplied for institutional food service use only: *Provided*, That the manufacturer or distributor provides the nutrition information required by this section directly to those institutions on a current basis.

Appendix D
Whey and Whey Products —General Specifications and Definitions

The U.S. standards for whey and whey products were first published in the Federal Register, April 1980, and went into effect on June 22, 1980. The relevant portions (Part 2858, Subpart O) follow:

Subpart O—United States Standards for Dry Whey

Definitions

§2858.2601   Whey.
"Whey" is the fluid obtained by separating the coagulum from milk, cream, and/or skim milk in cheesemaking. The acidity of the whey may be adjusted by the addition of safe and suitable pH adjusting ingredients. Salt drippings (moisture removed from cheese curd as a result of salting) shall not be collected for further processing as whey.

§2858.2602   Dry Whey.
"Dry Whey" is the product resulting from drying fresh whey which has been pasteurized and to which nothing has been added as a preservative. It contains all constituents, except moisture, in the same relative proportions as in the whey.

U.S. Grade

§2858.2603   Nomenciature   of   U.S. grade.
The nomenclature of the U.S. grade is U.S. Extra.

§2858.2604   Basis for determination of U.S. grade.
The U.S. grade of dry whey is determined on the basis of flavor, physical appearance, bacterial estimate, coliform, milkfat content, and moisture.

§2858.2605   Requirements   for   U.S. grade.
(a) *U.S. Extra.* U.S. Extra Grade dry whey conforms to the following requirements:
(1) *Flavor* (applies to the reliquefied form). Shall have a normal whey flavor free from undesirable flavors, but may possess the following flavors, to a slight degree: bitter, fermented, storage, and utensil: and the following to a definite degree: feed and weedy.
(2) *Physical appearance.* Has a uniform color, and is free flowing, free from lumps that do not break up under slight pressure, and is practically free from visible dark particles.
(3) *Bacterial estimate.* Not more than 50,000 per gram standard plate count.
(4) *Coliform.* Not more than 10 per gram.
(5) *Milkfat content.* Not more than 1.50 percent.
(6) *Moisture content.* Not more than 5.0 percent.

§2858.2606   Basis for acidity classification.
Acidity classification is not a U.S. grade requirement. Acidity classification will be made available only upon a U.S. graded product and the results will be shown on the grading certificate. The dry whey will be classified for acidity as follows:
(a) *Dry sweet-type whey.* Dry whey

not over 0.16 percent titratable acidity on a reconstituted basis.

(b) *Dry whey—% titratable acidity.* Dry whey over 0.16 percent, but below 0.35 percent titratable acidity on a reconstituted basis. The blank being filled with the actual acidity.

(c) *Dry acid-type whey.* Dry whey with 0.35 percent or higher titratable acidity on a reconstituted basis.

§2858.2607 [Reserved].

§2858.2608 Optional tests.

There are certain optional requirements in addition to those specified in section 2858.2605. Tests for these requirements may be run occasionally at the option of the Department and will be run whenever they are requested by an interested party. These optional requirements are as follows:

(a) *Protein content (N×6.38).* Not less than 11 percent.

(b) *Alkalinity of ash (sweet-type whey only).* Not more than 225 ml. of 0.1 N HC1 per 100 grams.

(c) *Scorched particle content.* Not more than 15.0 mg.

§2858.2609 U.S. grade not assignable.

(a) Dry whey which fails to meet the requirements of U.S. Extra Grade shall not be assigned a U.S. grade.

(b) Dry whey which fails to meet the requirements of any optional test, when tests have been made, shall not be assigned a U.S. grade.

(c) Dry whey produced in a plant found on inspection to be using unsatisfactory manufacturing practices, equipment, or facilities, or to be operating under unsanitary plant conditions shall not be assigned a U.S. grade.

§2858.2610 Test methods.

All required tests, and optional tests when specified, shall be performed in accordance with the following methods:

(a) "Methods of Laboratory Analysis," DA Instruction series 918-103-2, 918-103-5, 918-109-2, and 918-109-3, Dairy Grading Branch, Poultry and Dairy Quality Division, Food Safety and Quality Service, U.S. Department of Agriculture, Washington, DC 20250, or the latest revision thereof. Explanation of Terms

§2858.2611 Explanation of terms.

(a) *With respect to flavor.*

(1) *Slight.* An attribute barely identifiable and present only to a small degree.

(2) *Definite.* An attribute readily identifiable and present to a substantial degree.

(3) *Undesirable.* Identifiable flavors in excess of the intensity permitted, or those flavors not otherwise listed.

(4) *Bitter.* Distasteful, similar to taste of quinine.

(5) *Feed.* Feed flavors such as alfalfa, sweet clover, silage, or similar feed.

6) *Fermented.* Flavors, such as fruity or yeasty, produced through unwanted chemical changes brought about by microorganisms or their enzyme systems.

(7) *Storage.* Lacking in freshness and imparting a "rough" or "harsh" aftertaste.

(8) *Utensil.* A flavor that is suggestive of improper or inadequate washing and sterilization of utensils or factory equipment.

(9) *Weedy.* Aromatic flavor characteristic of the weeds eaten by cows carried through into the dry whey.

(b) *With respect to physical appearance.*

(1) *Slight pressure.* Only sufficient pressure to readily disintegrate the lumps.

(2) *Practically free.* Present only upon very critical examination.

(3) *Free flowing.* Capable of being poured continuously without interruption.

(4) *Lumps.* Loss of powdery consistency but not caked into hard chunks.

(5) *Uniform color.* Free from variation in shades or intensity of color.

(6) *Visible dark particles.* The presence of scorched or discolored specks capable of being seen by the eye.

Appendix E
Other Related Frozen Desserts
—Definitions and Labeling

The following definitions and labeling requirements, while not official, represent generally accepted industry standards.

Frozen Yogurt

Description. Frozen yogurt is the food prepared by freezing while stirring a pasteurized mix consisting of the same ingredients permitted for ice cream in the CFR, Title 21, Part 135.110 (Appendix B). These ingredients are cultured after pasteurization by one or more strains of *Lactobacillus bulgarius* and *Streptococcus thermophilus*, provided, however, fruits, nuts, or other flavoring materials may be added before or after the mix is pasteurized and cultured. Bacteria and coliform requirements for frozen yogurt shall apply to the mix before culturing. Coliform requirements for frozen yogurt also shall apply to the mix after culturing. Frozen yogurt shall contain not less than 3.25% milkfat and not less than 8.25% MSNF and has a titratable acidity of not less than 0.5%, expressed as lactic acid. This characteristic acidity, developed as the result of bacterial activity, shall be applied to the product after culturing. No heat or bacteriostatic treatment (other than refrigeration), which results in the total destruction of the microorganisms, may be applied to the product after culturing. The finished yogurt shall weigh not less than 5 lb/gal.

Labeling. In addition to all other required information, the label shall comply with the applicable provisions prescribed in the CFR, Title 21.

Lowfat Frozen Yogurt

Description. Lowfat frozen yogurt is the food prepared from the same ingredients and in the same manner prescribed in the CFR for frozen yogurt. Lowfat frozen yogurt, exclusive of any flavorings, shall not contain less than 0.5 or more than 2% milkfat.

Labeling. In addition to all other required information, the label shall comply with the applicable provisions prescribed in the CFR, Title 21.

Nonfat Frozen Yogurt

Description. Nonfat frozen yogurt is the food prepared from the same ingredients and in the same manner prescribed in the Regulation for frozen yogurt. Nonfat frozen yogurt, exclusive of any flavorings, shall contain less than 0.5% milkfat.

Labeling. In addition to all other required information, the label shall comply with the applicable provisions prescribed in the CFR, Title 21.

Quiescently Frozen Confection

Description. Quiescently frozen confection means the frozen product made from sweetening agents, harmless natural or artificial flavoring, and water; and it may contain milk solids, harmless coloring, organic acids, and any safe and suitable functional ingredient approved. The finished product shall contain not less than 17% by weight of total food solids. In the manufacture of this product, freezing has not been accompanied by stirring or agitation (generally known as quiescent freezing). In the production of this quiescently frozen confection, no processing or mixing before quiescent freezing may be used that develops in the finished confection mix any physical expansion in excess of 10%. This confection shall be manufactured in the form of servings, individually packaged, bagged or otherwise wrapped, properly labeled, and purveyed to the consumer in its original factory-filled package.

Labeling. In addition to all other required information, the label shall comply with the applicable provisions prescribed in the CFR, Title 21.

Quiescently Frozen Dairy Confection

Description. Quiescently frozen dairy confection means the frozen produce made from milk products, sweetening agents, harmless natural or artificial flavoring, and water; and it may contain harmless coloring, and any safe and suitable functional ingredient. The finished product contains not less than 33% by weight of total foods solids. In the manufacture of this product, freezing has not been accompanied by stirring or agitation (generally known as quiescent freezing). In the production of this quiescently frozen dairy confection, no processing or mixing before quiescent freezing may be used that develops in the finished confection mix any physical expansion in excess of 10%. This confection shall be manufactured in the form of servings, individually packaged, bagged, or otherwise wrapped, properly labeled, and purveyed to the consumer in its original factory-filled package. The individually wrapped confection need not be labeled if it is contained in a multiple package that is properly labeled and purveyed unopened to the consumer.

Labeling. In addition to all other required information, the label shall comply with the applicable provisions prescribed in the CFR, Title 21.

Lowfat Frozen Dairy Dessert

Description. (1) Lowfat frozen dairy dessert is the food prepared by freezing while stirring, a pasteurized mix consisting of the ingredients permitted for ice cream. The finished product contains less than 2% by weight of fat: its content of total milk solids is not less than 7% by weight. The product weighs no less than 4.5 lb/gal and the quantity of food solids is not less than 1.1 or more than 1.55 lb/gal, exclusive of any microcrystalline cellulose used as an ingredient.

(2) One or more vitamins or minerals, or both, prescribed in the CFR, Title 21, Part 101.9, may be added to the product. If vitamins or minerals, or both, are added, each 4-oz serving of finished product shall provide not less than 8 or more than 20% of the U.S. Recommended Daily Allowance of these vitamins or minerals or both.

(3) Lowfat frozen dairy dessert may be sold in properly labeled factory-filled containers, except it may be sold directly from a dispensing freezer at the time of a direct request from a customer. When sold directly from a dispensing freezer, each container shall be labeled with the name of the product and with nutritional and ingredient information as prescribed in the CFR, Title 21.

Nomenclature. The name of the food is "nonfruit dessert."

Labeling. (1) If vitamins or minerals, or both, are added, the name of the food on the principal display panel and each alternate principal display panel shall be immediately preceded or follwed by the word "fortified" in the same style and at least one-half the size of the type used for the name "dietary frozen dessert" and on the same contrasting background.

(2) In addition to all other required information, the label shall comply with the applicable provisions prescribed in the CFR, Title 21.

Parevine

Description. (1) Parevine is the food prepared by freezing while stirring a pasteurized mix composed of one or more edible vegetable oils or fats, protein and carbohydrate food ingredients from other than milk or meat sources, nutritive sweeteners other than lactose, characterizing ingredients except any containing meat or milk, and any other safe and suitable ingredient that is not milk or meat or a product or a derivative of milk or meat. This product may not contain any milk, milk product, meat, or meat products, or any of their derivatives of any kind.

(2) Its fat content shall be not less than 10%, except that when bulky optional characterizing ingredients are used, the fat content may be reduced, as a result of the addition of these ingredients, but may not be less than 8%.

(3) Its content of food solids shall be not less than 1.3 lb/gal of finished product.

(4) Parevine shall be sold, held, offered for sale by any manufacturer, wholesaler, retailer, or any other seller only in factory-filled containers. Parevine may be served for consumption on the premises provided that the individual service is taken from a properly labeled factory-filled container. When parevine is served for consumption on the premises, a sign shall be conspicuously displayed on the sale premises or vehicle where it can be clearly read by customers under normal conditions of purchase, stating "PAREVINE SOLD HERE." Letters on the sign shall be boldface capitals at least 3 in. high and in contrasting color to the background. The sign need not be displayed if each customer is provided with a menu wherein is stated "PAREVINE

SERVED HERE" in boldface capitals as large as those in listing most food items.

Labeling. In addition to all other required information, the label shall comply with the applicable provisions prescribed in the CFR, Title 21.

Manufactured Desserts Mix

Description. "Manufactured desserts mix," whipped cream confection, or bisque tortoni, means a frozen dessert made with milk products, sweetening agents, flavoring agents, with or without harmless coloring, or any other safe and suitable ingredients. It contains not less than 18% by weight of milkfat, and not more than 12% of MSNF, and may be packaged with harmless gas, causing it to fluff upon ejection from the package or container.

Labeling. In addition to all other required information, the label shall comply with the provisions prescribed in the CFR, Title 21.

Freezer-Made Shake: Freezer-Made Milk Shake

Description. "Freezer-made milk shake" means a pure, clean wholesome semiviscous drink prepared by stirring while freezing in a dispensing freezer a pasteurized mix consisting of the ingredients prescribed in the CFR, Title 21, Part 135.120, except that:

(1) It shall contain not less than 3-1/4 and not more than 6% milkfat.

(2) Its contents of milk solids not fat shall be not less 10%. Freezer-made milk shake may only be sold or served from a dispensing freezer and may not be sold hard-frozen.

Other freezer-made shakes, including jumbo shake, thick shake, TV shake, or any coined or trade name containing the word "shake," shall meet the requirements above, except that the minimum percentage of milk fat may be less than 3-1/4%. "Shakes" not meeting the requirements for "milk shakes" may not be advertised, sold, or served as milk shakes.

When any freezer-made milk shake or other freezer-made shake purports to be or is represented for any special dietary use by humans, it shall be sold only in a container labeled in accordance with all applicable provisions of the CFR, Title 21.

Lactose-Reduced Ice Cream

Description. Lactose-reduced ice cream is the product resulting from the treatment of ice cream, as defined in the CFR, Title 21, by the addition of safe and suitable enzyme(s) to convert sufficient amounts of lactose to glucose and galactose so that the remaining lactose is 30% or less of the lactose in ice cream.

Labeling. The label on lactose-reduced ice cream in addition to all other required information shall contain a complete list of ingredients in accordance with the provisions of CFR, Title 21, Section 101.4, and contain nutrition information as required by CFR, Title 21, Section 101.9.

Wherever the name appears on the container, the words "lactose-reduced" shall be in the same type style and size and in the same color and contrasting background as the words "ice cream."

Lactose-Reduced Ice Milk

Description. Lactose-reduced ice milk is the product resulting from the treatment of ice milk, as defined in the CFR, Title 21, by the addition of safe and suitable enzyme(s) to convert sufficient amounts of lactose to glucose and galactose so that the remaining lactose is 30% or less of the lactose in ice milk.

Labeling. The label on lactose-reduced ice milk in addition to all other required information shall contain a complete list of ingredients in accordance with the provisions of CFR, Title 21, Section 101.4, and contain nutrition information as required by CFR, Title 21, Section 101.9.

Wherever the name appears on the container, the words "lactose-reduced" shall be in the same type style and size and in the same color and contrasting background as the words "ice milk."

Appendix F
Dairy Associations and Trade Journals that Promote the Ice Cream Industry

Associations

American Dairy Association,
Alden R. Grimes, Executive
  Vice-President
6300 North River Road
Rosemont, Ill. 60018

American Dairy Science
  Association,
Executive Secretary
309 W. Clark St.
Champaign, Ill. 61820

Dairy & Food Industries Supply
  Association, Inc.,
Fred J. Greiner Jr., Executive
  Vice President
6245 Executive Boulevard
Rockville, MD 20852

International Association of Ice
  Cream Manufacturers,
John F. Speer Jr., President
888 16th Street N.W.
Washington, DC 20006

The National Association of Retail
  Ice Cream Manufacturers, Inc.,
Craig E. Peterson, Executive
  Director
1800 Pickwick Avenue
Glenview, Ill 60025

National Dairy Council,
M.F. Brink, President
6300 North River Road
Rosemont, Ill 60018

National Ice Cream Mix
  Association, Inc.,
Walter Holm, Executive Director
5610 Crofordsville Road
Indianapolis, Ind 46224

Publications

Canadian Dairy and Ice Cream
  Journal,
122 Richmont St. West,
Toronto, Canada

Dairy Field,
757 Third Avenue
New York, NY 10017

Dairy Record
O'Hare Plaza
5725 East River Road
Chicago, Ill 60631

Appendix G
Miscellaneous Tables

Example I. Required to make 50 gal of 30° Baumé sugar syrup.

Formula. Read directly from Table A.1 the Baumé degree and the amount of sugar and water needed to make 1 gal of that degree syrup. Note also the weight per gallon of syrup. Multiply each of these amounts by the number of gallons to be made:

$$5.80 \times 50 = 290 \text{ lb sugar}$$
$$4.70 \times 50 = 235 \text{ lb water}$$
$$10.50 \times 50 = 525 \text{ lb, 50 gal 30° Baumé syrup}$$

Example II. To find the amount of water required to dilute 1 gal of 34° Baumé syrup to 30° Baumé syrup.

Solution. Use the formula

$$\frac{(\text{lb water per gal dilute syrup}) \times (\text{lb sugar gal original syrup})}{\text{lb sugar per gal dilute syrup}}$$

$$- (\text{lb water per gal original syrup} = \text{lb water required}$$

From Table A.1 substitute into the formula:

$$\frac{4.70 \times 6.85}{5.80} - 4.03 = 1.52 \text{ lb water}$$

For any larger quantity multiply 1.52 by the number of gallons to be diluted.

Example III. To find the amount of sugar required to thicken 1 gal of 30° Baumé syrup to 34° Baumé.

Solution.   Use the formula.

$$\frac{\text{(lb sugar per gal thickened syrup)} \times \text{(lb water gal original syrup)}}{\text{lb water per gal thickened syrup}}$$

$$- \text{(lb sugar per gal original syrup} = \text{lb sugar required}$$

From Table A.1 substitute into the formula:

$$\frac{6.85 \times 4.70}{4.03} - 5.80 = 2.19 \text{ lb sugar}$$

For any larger quantity multiply 2.19 lb by the number of gallons to be thickened.

HOW TO USE TABLE A.2

Example IV.   Find Baumé of syrup wanted in leftmost column. Read across to column beneath Baumé of syrup to be diluted. The figure given is the amount of water, in fluid ounces, to be added to 1 gal of syrup.

WEIGHT, MEASURE AND FOOD SOLIDS
IN VARIOUS ICE CREAMS

All foods contain water, and everything not water is called a "solid."

In producing ice cream having certain characteristics (for example, weighing so much per gallon or quart, having certain volume per unit of weight, or certain food solids per gallon, and having at all times 12% fat), the relationships in Tables A.5 and A.6 will be helpful.

A mix of 31–48% TS, having the weights per gallon as shown, then made to take on 100% overrun, or to have 1.6 lb of food solids per gallon, or to weigh 4.5 lb per finished gallon, will give the figures shown in Table A.6.

TABLE A.13

Table A.13 gives the Federal and State Standards for the composition of milk products and various frozen desserts, according to USDA Handbook 51.

TABLE A.15—FROZEN DESSERTS PLANT
INSPECTION FORM

The FDA has recommended good manufacturing practices in manufacturing, processing, packaging and holding human food. It includes general provisions for definitions and personnel; building and facilities involving plants and grounds, sanitation facilities and controls, and sanitation operations; equipment and procedures; and production and process controls. Table A.14 shows a city, county, or district frozen dessert plant inspection form.

Table A.1. How to Make Sugar Solutions and Determine Their Concentration Using the Baumé and Brix Hydrometers[a]

Degrees Baumé at 68°F[b]	Degrees Brix at 68°F	Weight in air at 68°F (lb/gal)	Weight of sugar (lb/gal)	Weight of water (lb/gal)
30.0	55.2	10.50	5.80	4.70
30.5	56.2	10.54	5.92	4.62
31.0	57.1	10.59	6.05	4.54
31.5	58.1	10.64	6.18	4.46
32.0	59.1	10.68	6.31	4.37
32.5	60.0	10.73	6.44	4.29
33.0	61.0	10.78	6.58	4.20
33.5	62.0	10.83	6.71	4.12
34.0	63.0	10.88	6.85	4.03
34.5	63.9	10.92	6.98	3.94
35.0	64.9	10.97	7.12	3.85
35.5	65.9	11.02	7.26	3.76
36.0	66.9	11.07	7.41	3.66
36.5	67.9	11.13	7.56	3.57
37.0	68.9	11.18	7.70	3.48
37.5	69.9	11.23	7.85	3.38
38.0	70.9	11.28	8.00	3.28
38.5	71.9	11.33	8.15	3.18
39.0	72.9	11.39	8.30	3.09
39.5	73.9	11.44	8.45	2.99
40.0	74.9	11.49	8.61	2.88

[a]This table is based on information given in U.S. Bureau of Statistics Circular No. 375, Table I.
[b]The relationship of Baumé degrees (B) to specific gravity (sp.gr.) is given by $B = 145 - (145/\text{sp.gr.})$, and sp.gr. $= 145/(145 - B)$.

Table A.2. Fountain Syrup Dilution per Gallon of Syrup[a]

Syrup wanted (Baumé degrees)	Syrup to be diluted (Baumé degrees)			
	31	32	33	34
30	6	11.5	17.5	23.5
31	—	6	11.5	17.5
32	—	—	5.5	11.0
33	—	—	—	5.5

[a]Numbers indicate amount (fluid ounces) of water to be added.

Table A.3. Fountain Syrup Manufacture—Based on Size of Batch Wanted

Baumé (degrees)	10-gal batch	
	Sugar (lb)	Water (gal)
30	58	5⅝
31	60½	5⅜
32	63½	5¼
33	66	5
34	69	4¾

Table A.4. Fountain Syrup Manufacture—Based on 100 lb of Sugar at 77°F

Baumé wanted (degrees)	Amount of water to add (gal–oz)	Amount of syrup made (gal–oz)
34	6–119	14–61
33	7–68	15–8
32	8–23	15–84
31	8–111	16–47
30	9–74	17–10

Table A.5. Weight of Finished Ice Cream, with Various Weights of Mix and Various Overruns

Overrun (%)	Mix weight (lb/gal)				
	8.75	9.00	9.25	9.50	9.75
50	5.80	6.00	6.17	6.33	6.50
60	5.47	5.63	5.78	5.94	6.09
70	5.15	5.29	5.44	5.59	5.74
75	5.00	5.14	5.29	5.43	5.57
80	4.86	5.00	5.14	5.28	5.42
85	4.73	4.86	5.00	5.14	5.27
90	4.60	4.74	4.85	5.00	5.13
95	4.48	4.63	4.74	4.97	5.00
100	4.38	4.50	4.62	4.75	4.87
105	4.27	4.39	4.51	4.63	4.76
110	4.17	4.29	4.40	4.52	4.64
115	4.07	4.19	4.30	4.41	4.53
120	3.98	4.09	4.20	4.32	4.43
125	3.88	4.00	4.11	4.22	4.33
130	3.80	3.91	4.02	4.13	4.24
135	3.72	3.38	3.93	4.04	4.15
140	3.65	3.75	3.85	3.96	4.06

Table A.6. Relationships of Mix Factors

TS (%)	Mix		Yield 100%		Food solid weight 1.6 lb/gal		Weight 4.25 lb/gal	
	Weight (lb/gal)	TS weight (lb/gal)	Weight frozen (lb)	Weight of food solids (lb)	Yield (%)	Weight frozen (lb)	Yield (%)	Weight of food solids (lb/gal)
21	8.92	2.77	4.49	1.39	73.1	5.20	109.8	1.32
31	8.95	2.95	4.49	1.62	84.4	4.85	110.5	1.40
36	8.98	3.23	4.49	1.71	102.0	4.45	110.0	1.53
38	9.00	3.42	4.50	1.85	114.0	4.21	111.8	1.62
40	9.03	3.61	4.52	1.88	126.0	4.01	112.6	1.70
42	9.07	3.81	4.53	1.90	138.1	3.81	113.4	1.79
46	9.14	4.20	4.57	2.10	162.5	3.48	115.0	1.96
48	9.16	4.40	4.58	2.20	175.0	3.33	115.4	2.04

Table A.7. Composition, Relations, and Densities of Milks and Creams

Fat (%)	MSNF (%)	TS (%)	Ratio of fat to MSNF	Fat, percentage of solids	Specific gravity at 68°F	Weight lb/gal	lb/gal
Milk							
3.0	8.33	11.33	1:2.77	25.20	1.034	8.61	2.15
3.1	8.40	11.50	1:2.71	26.95			
3.2	8.46	11.66	1:2.64	27.47			
3.3	8.52	11.82	1:2.58	27.93			
3.4	8.55	11.95	1:2.52	28.41			
3.5	8.60	12.10	1:2.46	28.90	1.033	8.60	2.15
3.6	8.65	12.25	1:2.40	29.40			
3.7	8.69	12.39	1:2.35	29.85			
3.8	8.72	12.52	1:2.30	30.30			
3.9	8.76	12.66	1:2.25	30.77			
4.0	8.79	12.79	1:2.20	31.25	1.032	8.59	2.15
4.1	8.82	12.92	1:2.15	31.74			
4.2	8.86	13.06	1:2.11	32.15			
4.3	8.89	13.19	1:2.07	32.57			
4.4	8.92	13.32	1:2.03	33.00			
4.5	8.95	13.45	1:1.99	33.44	1.032	8.58	2.14
4.6	8.98	13.58	1:1.59	33.90			
4.7	9.01	13.71	1:1.92	34.25			
4.8	9.04	13.84	1:1.88	34.72			
4.9	9.07	13.97	1:1.85	35.09			
5.0	9.10	14.10	1:1.82	35.46	1.031	8.58	2.14
Cream							
18.0	7.31	25.31	1:0.41	71.11	1.015	8.48	2.12
20.0	7.13	27.13	1:0.36	73.71	1.013	8.43	2.11
22.0	6.95	28.95	1:0.31	75.30	1.011	8.42	2.11
25.0	6.68	31.68	1:0.27	78.91	1.008	8.37	2.10
30.0	6.24	36.24	1:0.21	82.78	1.004	8.36	2.09
35.0	5.79	40.79	1:0.16	85.81	1.000	8.32	2.08
40.0	5.35	45.35	1:0.13	88.20	0.995	8.28	2.07
45.0	4.90	49.90	1:0.09	90.11	0.985	8.22	2.05

Table A.8. Relationship of Baumé to TS in Sweetened Condensed Skim Milk[a]

Baumé at 120°F (degrees)	Sucrose (%)	MSNF (%)	TS (%)
37.4	45.63	27	72.63
37.6	45.00	28	73.00
37.8	44.38	29	73.38
38.0	43.75	30	73.75
38.2	43.13	31	74.13
38.4	42.50	32	74.50

[a]Assumes a sucrose:water ratio of approximately 62%. While the Baumé reading for TS is approximately right, too much value should not be given this test for there may be considerable variation due to varying proportions of serum solids and sucrose of different types, the amount of fat content, etc.

Table A.9. Sodium Chloride (Salt) Solution

Degrees Baumé at 60°F	Specific gravity at 39°F	Degrees Salometer at 60°F	Salt per gallon of solution (lb)	Salt per cubic foot (lb)	Salt by weight (%)	Freezing point (°F)	Specific heat[a]	Weight at 39°F (lb/gal)
1	1.007	4	0.084	0.628	1	31.8	0.992	8.40
2	1.015	8	0.169	1.264	2	29.3	0.984	8.46
3	1.023	12	0.256	1.914	3	27.8	0.976	8.53
4	1.030	16	0.344	3.573	4	26.6	0.968	8.59
5	1.037	20	0.433	3.238	5	25.2	0.960	8.65
6	1.045	24	0.523	3.912	6	23.9	0.946	8.72
7	1.053	28	0.617	4.615	7	22.5	0.932	8.78
8	1.061	32	0.708	5.295	8	21.2	0.919	8.85
9	1.068	36	0.802	5.998	9	19.9	0.905	8.91
10	1.076	40	0.897	6.709	10	18.7	0.892	8.97
12	1.091	48	1.092	8.168	12	16.0	0.874	9.10
15	1.115	60	1.389	10.389	15	12.2	0.855	9.26
20	1.155	80	1.928	14.421	20	6.1	0.829	9.64
24	1.187	96	2.376	17.772	24	1.2	0.795	9.90
25	1.196	100	2.488	18.610	25	0.5	0.783	9.97
26	1.204	104	2.610	19.522	26	1.1	0.771	10.04

[a]Specific heat is the ratio between the amount of heat required to raise a given weight of substance to a given temperature and the amount of heat required to raise the same amount of water to the same temperature.

Table A.10. The Freezing Point Relationships of Calcium Chloride Brine

Calcium chloride anhydrous (%)	Calcium chloride hydrous CaCl–6H₂O (%)	Specific gravity 18/4 C	Weight (lb/gal)	Degrees Baumé	Degrees Salometer	Freezing point (°F)
1	1.98	1.0070	8.41	1.0	4	31.6
2	3.96	1.0154	8.45	2.2	8	31.3
3	5.94	1.0239	8.54	3.4	12	30.6
4	7.92	1.0319	8.61	4.5	16	29.8
5	9.90	1.0409	8.67	5.7	22	28.9
6	11.88	1.0495	8.75	6.8	26	27.9
7	13.86	1.0582	8.82	8.0	32	26.8
8	15.84	1.0660	8.89	9.0	36	25.5
9	17.82	1.0757	8.96	10.2	40	24.3
10	19.80	1.0847	9.04	11.3	44	22.8
11	21.78	1.0937	9.12	12.4	48	21.6
12	23.76	1.1029	9.19	13.5	52	20.1
13	25.74	1.1121	9.28	14.6	58	18.3
14	27.72	1.1214	9.35	15.7	62	16.7
15	29.70	1.1307	9.42	16.8	68	14.7
16	31.68	1.1402	9.50	17.8	72	12.9
17	33.66	1.1497	9.58	18.9	76	10.8
18	35.64	1.1594	9.67	19.9	80	8.4
19	37.62	1.1692	9.75	21.0	84	5.5
20	39.60	1.1791	9.83	22.0	88	2.7
21	41.58	1.1890	9.91	23.1	92	−0.6
22	43.56	1.1990	10.00	24.1	96	−4.4
23	45.54	1.2090	10.08	25.1	100	−8.3
24	47.52	1.2192	10.16	26.0	104	−13.2
25	49.50	1.2294	10.24	27.1	108	−18.8
26	51.48	1.2398	10.34	28.1	112	−25.1
27	53.46	1.2503	10.42	29.0	116	−32.8
28	55.44	1.2610	10.51	30.0	120	−42.2
29	57.42	1.2718	10.60	31.0	124	−54.4
29.8	58.80	1.2804	10.67	31.8	128	−67.0

Table A.11. Cost of Bulk Ice Cream by Scoops (cents/serving)

Price ($/gal)	Size of scoop (average servings/gallon)						
	30 (59)	24 (51)	20 (41)	16 (34)	12 (26)	10 (25)	8 (23)
1.20	2.03	2.35	2.92	3.52	4.61	4.80	5.22
1.25	2.12	2.45	3.05	3.67	4.81	5.00	5.43
1.30	2.20	2.55	3.17	3.82	5.00	5.20	5.65
1.35	2.29	2.65	3.29	3.97	5.19	5.40	5.87
1.40	2.37	2.75	3.41	4.12	5.38	5.60	6.09
1.45	2.46	2.84	3.54	4.26	5.58	5.80	6.30
1.50	2.54	2.94	3.66	4.41	5.77	6.00	6.52
1.55	2.63	3.04	3.78	4.56	5.96	6.20	6.74
1.60	2.71	3.14	3.90	4.71	6.15	6.40	6.96
1.65	2.80	3.24	4.02	4.85	6.35	6.60	7.17
1.70	2.88	3.33	4.15	5.00	6.54	6.80	7.39
1.75	2.97	3.43	4.27	5.15	6.73	7.00	7.61
1.80	3.05	3.53	4.39	5.29	6.92	7.20	7.83
1.85	3.14	3.63	4.51	5.44	7.11	7.40	8.04
1.90	3.22	3.73	4.63	5.59	7.30	7.60	8.26
1.95	3.31	3.82	4.76	5.74	7.50	7.80	8.48
2.00	3.39	3.92	4.88	5.88	7.69	8.00	8.70
2.05	3.47	4.02	5.00	6.03	7.88	8.20	8.91
2.10	3.56	4.12	5.12	6.18	8.08	8.40	9.13
2.15	3.64	4.22	5.24	6.32	8.27	8.60	9.35
2.20	3.73	4.31	5.37	6.47	8.46	8.80	9.57
2.25	3.81	4.41	5.49	6.62	8.65	9.00	9.78
2.30	3.90	4.51	5.61	6.76	8.85	9.20	10.00
2.35	3.98	4.61	5.73	6.91	9.04	9.40	10.22
2.40	4.07	4.71	5.85	7.06	9.23	9.60	10.43
2.45	4.15	4.80	5.98	7.21	9.42	9.80	10.65
2.50	4.24	4.90	6.10	7.35	9.62	10.00	10.87
3.00	5.08	5.88	7.32	8.82	11.54	12.00	13.04
3.50	5.94	6.86	8.54	10.30	13.46	14.00	15.22
4.00	6.78	7.84	9.76	11.76	15.38	16.00	17.40
4.50	7.62	8.82	10.98	13.24	17.30	18.00	19.56
5.00	8.48	9.80	12.20	14.70	19.24	20.00	21.74

Table A.12. Seasonal Sales Expectancy—National Average

Month	Percentage of annual sales	Month	Percentage of annual sales
January	3.42	July	16.58
February	3.80	August	14.27
March	5.33	September	10.04
April	7.17	October	6.17
May	10.90	November	4.19
June	14.50	December	3.63

Table A.14.   City, County, or District Frozen Dessert Plant Inspection Form

Name...................................... Location...............
Sir: An inspection of your plant has this day been made, and you are notified of the defects marked below with a cross (x). Violation of the same item on two successive inspections calls for immediate degrading or suspension of permit.

(1) *Floors.*—Smooth finish, no pools ( ), wall joints and floor surface impervious ( ), trapped drains (cold storage rooms and counter freezer plants excepted), no sewage back-flow ( ), clean and free of litter ( )...........................( )

(2) *Walls and ceilings.*—Smooth, washable, light-colored finish (hardening and storage rooms excepted), good repair ( ), clean ( )..........................( )

(3) *Doors and windows.*—In fly season outer openings with effective screens and self-closing doors, or fly-repellent fans or flaps..................................( )

(4a) *Lighting.*—10 foot-candles 30 in. above floor (for natural light in new plants see Code)...( )

(4b) *Ventilation.*—No undue condensation and odors (cold storage rooms excepted)..( )

(5) *Miscellaneous protection from contamination.*—Tanks and vats covered, ports protected ( ), no woven-wire strainers, no straining pasteurized mix except through perforated metal ( ), no drip from mezzanine or overhead pipes ( ), flies under control ( ), processes partitioned (or approved enclosures in counter freezer plants) ( ), rooms of sufficient size ( ), ingredients not unloaded directly into processing rooms ( ), pasteurized product not in contact with equipment used for raw or lower grade products unless sterilized ( ), no plant operations in living quarters ( )....( )

(6) *Toilet facilities.*—Comply with plumbing code ( ), good repair ( ), clean ( ), outside ventilation ( ), no direct opening ( ), self-closing doors ( ), free of flies ( ), washing sign ( ), privies, if used, comply State standards ( )...............( )

(7) *Water supply.*—Sufficient outlets ( ), adequate ( ), safe, complies State standards ( )...( )

(8) *Hand-washing facilities.*—Adequate, convenient ( ), hot and cold water, soap, sanitary towels ( ), hands washed after toilet ( )...........................( )

(9) *Sanitary piping.*—Easily cleanable size, shape, and length ( ), smooth uncorroded surfaces ( ), sanitary fittings, interior surfaces accessible for inspection ( ) ....( )

(10) *Construction and repair of containers and equipment.*—Easily cleanable, smooth non-corrodible surfaces ( ), no open seams, good repair ( ), self-draining ( ), pressure-tight seats on submerged thermometers ( )..........................( )

(11) *Disposal of wastes.*—In public sewer or as approved by State board of Health ( ), no connection or back-siphonage into water supplies ( ), trash and garbage kept in covered containers ( )..( )

(12a) *Cleaning of containers and equipment.*—Multi-use containers thoroughly cleaned after each usage ( ), equipment each day ( )...............................( )

(12b) *Bactericidal treatment of containers and equipment.*—Containers treated after each cleaning in steam cabinet 170°F. for 15 min., or 200°F. for 5 min., or hot-air cabinet 180°F. for 20 min., or steam jet 1 min., or immersed in standard chlorine or 170°F. water for 2 min., or automatic washers (residual count not over 1 per cc of capacity, test 11), assembled equipment treated daily immediately before run, with flow of 200°F. steam or 170°F. water at outlets for 5 min. or standard chlorine flow for 2 min. (test 12); supplementary treatment for surfaces not thus reached ( )............( )

(13) *Storage of containers.*—In clean crates or racks above floor, protected from flies, splash, dust, inverted when practicable......................................( )

(14) *Handling of containers and equipment.*—No handling of surfaces to which ingredients or products are exposed ....( )

(15) *Storage and handling of single-service containers and utensils.*—Purchased in sanitary tubes or cartons ( ), kept therein in cabinet or other clean dry place ( ), sanitary handling ( )..( )

(16a) *Specifications for pasteurization thermometers.*—All Code specifications met by all new indicating and recording thermometers, by all replacements, and by recording thermometers under repair which require renewal of tube system ( ); existing thermometers meet at least accuracy and lag specifications (tests 1, 2, 3) ( ).........( )

(16b) *Maintenance of pasteurization time and temperature.*—Entire mix, excluding fruits, etc., pasteurized, no raw products bypass around pasteurizers ( ). Requirements for manual-discharge heated holders (for others see Code):
Temperature control.—Adequate agitation throughout holding period, agitator sufficiently submerged ( ); indicating and recording thermometers on each vat through-

Table A.14. City, County, or District Frozen Dessert Plant Inspection Form (Contd.)

out pasteurization ( ); recorder reads no higher than indicator (test 4) ( ); thermometer bulbs submerged ( )...( )

Time control.—Charts show 155°F. for 30 minutes, plus emptying time if cooling begun after outlet valve opened (also plus filling time when required) (test 6) ( ); no milk added after holding begun ( )...( )

Charts.—Used only 1 day, preserved 3 months ( ); must show date, location, daily check against indicating thermometer, amount and product represented, unusual occurrences, and operator's signature ( )...( )

(16c) *Inlet and outlet valves and connections.*—Any inlet and outlet valves used on single-vat installations must be leak-protector type, otherwise piping disconnected ( ), all multiple-vat installations have leak-protector inlets, also leak-protector outlets except where Code permits disconnecting outlet piping instead ( ), 30-minute tubular holders have leak-protector outlet or outlet piping disconnected until 30 minutes after filling begun ( ); leak-protector valves of approved design, effective in all closed positions, and installed in proper position (test 8) ( ); inlets and outlets below mix level have close-coupled valves ( ); plug-type valves have approved stops ( ); top inlets have air relief if submerged ( ). Valves kept fully closed except inlet while filling and outlet while emptying ( ); outlet valves sterilized automatically before opening if not leak protected or if mix accumulates in channel (test 9) ( ) ......( )

(16d) *Air heating.*—Air in vats and pockets heated to at least 5°F. above mix temperature during heating and kept at 160°F. or higher during holding, with approved device ( ), approved trap on steam line ( ), approved air thermometer (test 7), bulb at least 1 inch above mix ( ) ....( )

(16e) *Vat and pocket covers and cover ports.*—No drainage from top of cover into vat, open or closed ( ), ports surrounded by raised edges ( ), pipes, thermometers, etc., through cover have aprons unless joint watertight ( ); covers kept closed ( ) ....( )

(16f) *Preheating holders.*—Holders not used as heaters are preheated to pasteurization temperature just before run, also when empty after shutdown exceeding holding period, unless outlet has flow-diversion valve...( )

(17a) *Cooling.*—All fluid milk products cooled to 50°F. on receipt unless to be pasteurized within 2 hours ( ), pasteurizing mix cooled to 50°F. and held thereat until frozen ( ); header gap on surface coolers not less than $1/4$ inch or thickness of header at gap ( ), condensation and leakage from cooler supports and headers, unless completely enclosed in covers, directed away from tubes and milk trough ( ), recirculated water and refrigerant of required sanitary quality ( ), cooler covered or in separate room ( ), cooler shields tight fitting ( ), in regenerators, pasteurized-mix (or heat-transfer-medium) side automatically under greater pressure than raw mix at all times (see Code) ( )...( )

(17b) *Handling of mix.*—If not frozen where pasteurized, mix transported in sealed containers ( ), protected against contamination, no dipping, kept covered ( ) .....( )

(18) *Packaging.*—If not approved automatic equipment: no contact surfaces handled, packages adequately covered immediately after filling ( ); hands washed and disinfected before beginning moulding, wrapping, or packaging and after each interruption ( ), brick and fancy moulds handled in sanitary manner by trained persons ( )...( )

(19) *Overflow or spillage.*—Discarded...( )

(20) *Returns.*—No opened containers of mix or frozen desserts returned except for inspection...( )

(21) *Personnel, health.*—Required examinations and tests ( ), rejected persons not employed ( ), no person with infected wound or lesion ( )..........................( )

(22) *Personnel, cleanliness.*—Clean outer garment, washable for inside employees ( ), hands clean ( ) ....( )

(23) *Miscellaneous.*—*Vehicles:* Clean ( ), covered ( ), no contaminating substances transported ( ), distributor's name shown ( ). *Surroundings:* Kept neat and clean ( )...( )

(24) *Bacterial plate count of pasteurized mix or frozen desserts.*—Log average not over 50,000 ( ), 100,000 for grade B ( ) ....( )

(25) *Ingredients.*—Clean, fresh wholesome flavor, odor, and appearance ( ), stored above floor, kept covered, properly handled and refrigerated ( ); milk products meet bacterial standards ( ), also production standards, where locally required ( ); ingredients added after mix pasteurized are of approved quality ( ) ....( )

Table A.15. Federal Standards for Composition of Milk Products (as of January 1, 1980)

Product	Milkfat (%) Min.	Milkfat (%) Max.	Total milk solids (%) Min.	Total milk solids (%) Max.	Weight, min. (lb/gal)	Food solids, min. (lb/gal)
Plain ice cream	10.0	—	20.0[a]	—	4.5	1.6
Fruit, nut, or chocolate ice cream (bulky flavors)	8.0	—	16.0[b,c]	—	4.5	1.6
Frozen custard[d]	10.0	—	20.0[a]	—	4.5	1.6
Ice milk	2.0	7.0	11.0[e]	—	4.5	1.3
Fruit, nut or chocolate ice milk (bulky flavors)	2.0	7.0	11.0	—	4.5	1.3
Sherbet/water ice[f]	1.0	2.0	2.0	5.0	6.0	—
Mellorine	6.0[g]	—	2.7[h]	—	4.5	1.6

[a]MSNF not less than 6.0%.
[b]Must meet the standards for plain ice cream except for such reduction as is due to the addition of bulky flavoring ingredients, but in no case less than the minimum shown.
[c]To compensate for additional sweetening ingredients when bulky ingredients are used, the weight of chocolate or cocoa solids may be multiplied by 2.5; fruit or nuts by 1.4; partially or wholly dried fruits or juices by appropriate factors to obtain the original weights before drying and this multiplied by 1.4.
[d]Egg yolks, minimum 1.4%. When flavored, reduction to no less than 1.12% is permitted for addition of bulky ingredients.
[e]Caseinates may be added when the content of total milk solids is not less than 11.0%.
[f]When characterized by a fruit ingredient, shall have a titratable acidity of not less than 0.35%.
[g]Animal or vegetable fat; bulky flavors, 4.8%.
[h]Expressed as protein; bulky flavors, 2.2%.

Table A.16. Mix Proof Sheet for Checking Formula of 1000 liter Mix When the SI System Is Used[a]

$$\text{Density of mix} = \frac{100}{(10 \div 0.93) + (11 + 16 + 0.3 \div 1.58) + 62.7} = 1.10 \text{ kg/liter}$$

$$1000 \text{ liter} \times 1.10 = 1100 \text{ kg}$$

| | Mix formula | |
Ingredient	%	Weight (kg)
Fat	10.0	110.0
MSNF	11.0	121.0
Sugar	16.0	176.0
Stabilizer	0.3	3.3
TS	37.3	410.3

| | | | Proof sheet | | | |
Ingredient	Weight (kg)	Fat (kg)	MSNF (kg)	Sugar (kg)	Stabilizer (kg)	TS (kg)
Cream 40%	275.00	110.0	14.85	—	—	124.85
Skim milk powder	87.55	—	84.92	—	—	84.92
Dry whey	21.88	—	21.23	—	—	21.23
Sucrose	197.00	—	—	132.0	—	132.00
Glucose	55.70	—	—	44.0	—	44.00
Stabilizer	3.30	—	—	—	3.3	3.3
Water	459.57	—	—	—	—	—
Provided	1100.00	110.0	121.0	176.0	3.3	410.30
Desired	1100.00	110.0	121.0	176.0	3.30	410.3

[a]Ingredient densities are utilized extensively in determining the amount and the constituents supplied by each.

Table A.17. Mix Proof Sheet for Checking Formula of 1000 liter Mix Containing Vegetable Fat When the SI System Is Used

$$\text{Density of mix} = \frac{100}{(610 \div 0.93) + (32.55 \div 1.58) + 61.45} = \frac{100}{88.5} = 1.13 \text{ kg/liter}$$

$$1000 \text{ liter} \times 1.13 = 1130 \text{ kg}$$

| | Chocolate mix formula | |
Ingredient	%	Weight (kg)
Fat	6.0	67.8
MSNF	10.4	117.5
Sugar	19.0	214.7
Cocoa	2.8	31.6
Stabilizer	0.35	3.9
TS	38.55	435.5

| | | | | Proof sheet | | | |
Ingredients	Weight (kg)	Fat (kg)	MSNF (kg)	Sugar (kg)	Stabilizer (kg)	Cocoa (kg)	TS (kg)
Cocoa fat	68.48	67.8	—	—	—	—	67.80
NFDM	99.85	—	94.92	—	—	—	94.92
Whey	23.27	—	22.58	—	—	—	22.58
Cocoa	31.60	—	—	—	—	31.6	31.60
Sucrose	259.70	—	—	174.02	—	—	174.02
Glucose	51.49	—	—	40.68	—	—	40.68
Stabilizer	3.90	—	—	—	3.90	—	3.90
Water	593.71	—	—	—	—	—	—
Provided	1130.00	67.8	117.50	214.70	3.90	31.6	435.50
Desired	1130.00	67.8	117.50	214.70	3.90	31.6	435.5

Index

A

Absorption, description of, 46
Acacia gum, as ice cream stabilizer, 27, 34, 50, 85
Acid flavor in ice cream, source of, 315
Acidity
  of condensed milk, off flavors and, 65
  of ice cream mixes, 43
    effect on texture, 320, 321
  of ice cream and related products, 43
    federal requirements, 31 (*table*)
  of milk, 52
  of sherbets and ices, 290
  tests, for cream, ice cream mix, and milk, 361
Acids, as ice and sherbet ingredients, 51, 286, 288, 290
Acrylic polymers, as gums, 86
Advertising, of ice cream products, 380–381
Agar (agar-agar)
  as ice cream stabilizer, 27, 34, 50, 85, 89
  as ice stabilizer, 289, 294
  as sherbet stabilizer, 289
Aging of ice cream mix, 213–215
  changes occurring in, 214
Air, in ice cream, 36, 39
Air cell in ice cream, 234
  effects on body and texture, 316
  electron micrograph of, 235
  "fluffy" texture defect from, 318
  in low-temperature freezing, 245
Alcohol coagulation test for protein stability, 362
Aldolase, in milk, 57

Algebraic method, for milk and cream standardization, 122–125
Algin and alginates
  as ice cream stabilizers, 27, 34, 35, 85, 86, 87, 91
  advantages, 89
  for high-temperature processing, 205
  use, 91, 92
  as sherbet stabilizer, 288, 289
Alkalies, in ice cream, 27
All-vegetable frozen desserts, mix formulas for, 395
Allspice, in ice cream, 116
Almond toffee ice cream, mix formula for, 385
Almonds and almond flavor, in ice cream, 106, 115
Aluminum, in milk, 57
American Dairy Association, 447
American Dairy Science Association, 447
American Public Health Association, 369
Ammonia
  boiling point of related to gauge pressure, 347
  as refrigerant, 238, 247, 254
    advantages and disadvantages of, 344
  leak tests, 367–368
Amylase, in milk, 57
Animals, ice cream molds of, 301
Anisyl aldehyde, as synthetic vanilla flavor, 101
Annatto color, for ice cream, 117
Antibiotic residue tests, 369
Antioxidants, for ice cream, 91

453

W